Clinical Uses of Botulinum Toxins

Botulinum toxins now play a very significant role in the management of a wide variety of medical conditions; from headaches to hypersalivation, and from spasticity to sweating. In this book, a strong, international team of experts outline the basic neurochemistry of botulinum toxins and chart the progress of the drug from laboratory to clinic. Then individual chapters summarize their use for the main clinical indications in the context of other available treatments.

This book will be of interest to neuroscientists and practising clinicians working in a wide range of specialties, from neurology and dermatology to pediatrics, plastic surgery and rehabilitation medicine.

Anthony B. Ward is Director of the University Hospital of North Staffordshire Rehabilitation Centre in Stoke-on-Trent, and Senior Lecturer in Rehabilitation Medicine at the University of Keele. He is the President of the European Union of Medical Specialists (UEMS) Section of Physical and Rehabilitation Medicine.

Michael P. Barnes is Professor of Neurological Rehabilitation in the Academic Unit of Neurological Rehabilitation, University of Newcastle-upon-Tyne, and Consultant Neurologist and Consultant in Rehabilitation Medicine at Walkergate Park International Centre for Neurorehabilitation and Neuropsychiatry in Newcastle-upon-Tyne. He is President of the World Federation for Neurorehabilitation.

Clinical Uses of Botulinum Toxins

Edited by

Anthony B. Ward BSc, MB ChB, FRCP(Ed), FRCP
Consultant in Rehabilitation Medicine

and

Michael P. Barnes MD FRCP
Professor of Neurological Rehabilitation

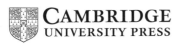
CAMBRIDGE
UNIVERSITY PRESS

CAMBRIDGE UNIVERSITY PRESS

Cambridge, New York, Melbourne, Madrid, Cape Town, Singapore, São Paulo

Cambridge University Press
The Edinburgh Building, Cambridge CB2 8RU, UK

Published in the United States of America by Cambridge University Press, New York

www.cambridge.org
Information on this title: www.cambridge.org/9780521833042

Printed in the United Kingdom at the University Press, Cambridge

A catalogue record for this publication is available from the British Library

Library of Congress Cataloguing in Publication data

Clinical uses of botulinum toxins/Anthony B. Ward & Michael P. Barnes.
  p. ; cm.
 Includes bibliographical references and index.
 ISBN-13: 978-0-521-83304-2 (hardback)
 ISBN-10: 0-521-83304-3 (hardback)
 1. Botulinum toxin. 2. Botulinum toxin – Therapeutic use. I. Ward,
Anthony B. II. Barnes, Michael P., 1952–
  [DNLM: 1. Botulinum Toxins – therapeutic use. QW 630.5.B2 C641 2007]

  QP632.B66C555 2007
  615′.329364 – dc22

                                                                2006025321
ISBN-13   978-0-521-83304-2   hardback
ISBN-10   0-521-83304-3   hardback

Contents

Colour plate section appears between pages 26 and 27

Contributors

Alberto Albanese
Istituto Nazionale Neurologico Carlo Besta
Università Cattolica del Sacro Cuore
Via G. Celoria, 11
20133 Milano
Italy

Khalid Anwar
Specialist Registrar in Rehabilitation
    Medicine
Hunters Moor Regional Neurological
    Rehabilitation Centre
Hunters Road
Newcastle upon Tyne, NE2 4NR
UK

Benjamin Anyanwu
New Jersey Neurosciences Institute
JFK Medical Center
Edison
New Jersey
USA

and

Seton Hall University School of Graduate
    Medical Education
South Orange
New Jersey
USA

Michael P. Barnes
Professor of Neurological Rehabilitation
Walkergate Park
International Centre for Neurorehabilitation
    and Neuropsychiatry
Berfrild Road
Newcastle upon Tyne, NE6 4QD
UK

Kenneth Beer
Director, Palm Bead Esthetic Centre
1500 North Dixie Highway, Suite 303
West Palm Beach, FL 33401
USA

Stephanie Benson
University of Colorado
School of Medicine
Denver
USA

Guiseppe Brisinda
Department of Surgery
Catholic School of Medicine
Catholic University Hospital Agostino
    Gemelli
Largo Agostino Gemelli 8
00168 Rome
Italy

Federica Cadeddu
Department of Surgery
Catholic School of Medicine
Catholic University Hospital Agostino
    Gemelli
Largo Agostino Gemelli 8
00168 Rome
Italy

Áine Carroll
Consultant in Rehabilitation Medicine
The National Rehabilitation Hospital
Rochestown Avenue
Dun Laoghaire
Co. Dublin
Ireland

Alastair Carruthers
Clinical Professor
Department of Dermatology
University of British Columbia
Vancouver BC
Canada

Joel L. Cohen
AboutSkin Dermatology and Derm Surgery
Englewood, CO
USA

Fiorella Contarino
Academic Medical Centre
Amsterdam
The Netherlands

David W. Dodick
Professor of Neurology
Mayo Clinic College of Medicine
13400 East Shea Boulevard
Scottsdale
Arizona 85259
USA

J. Oliver Dolly
International Centre for Neurotherapeutics
Dublin City University
Glasnevin
Dublin 9
Ireland

John Elston
Consultant Ophthalmic Surgeon
Oxford Eye Infirmary
Radcliffe Infirmary
Woodstock Road
Oxford OX2 6HE
UK

DeeAnna Glaser
Department of Dermatology
Saint Louis University School of Medicine
1402 S Grand Boulevard
St Louis, MO 63104
USA

Peter Hambleton
Health Protection Agency
Porton Down
Salisbury
Wilts SP4 0JJ

Philip A. Hanna
New Jersey Neurosciences Institute
JFK Medical Center
Edison
New Jersey
USA

and

Seton Hall University School of Graduate
    Medical Education
South Orange
New Jersey
USA

Maurice Hawthorne
Consultant in Ear, Nose and
    Throat Surgery
James Cook University Hospital
Middlesbrough TS1 5JE
UK

Joseph Jankovic
Professor of Neurology
Director, Parkinson's Disease Center and
    Movement Disorders Clinic
Department of Neurology
Baylor College of Medicine
6550 Fannin, Suite #1801
Houston, Texas 77030
USA

Gary Lawrence
International Centre for Neurotherapeutics
Dublin City University
Glasnevin
Dublin 9
Ireland

Giorgio Maria
Department of Surgery
Catholic School of Medicine
Catholic University Hospital Agostino
    Gemelli
Largo Agostino Gemelli 8
00168 Rome
Italy

Andrew M. Pickett
Ipsen Limited
190 Bath Road
Slough
Berkshire SL1 3XE
UK

Clifford C. Shone
Health Protection Agency
Porton Down
Salisbury SP4 0JG
UK

Anthony B. Ward
Consultant in Rehabilitation Medicine
North Staffordshire Rehabilitation Centre
The Haywood
Burslem
Stoke-on-Trent ST6 7AG
UK

1

Introduction

Michael P. Barnes[1] and Anthony B. Ward[2]

[1]Walkergate Park, International Centre for Neurorehabilitation and Neuropsychiatry, Newcastle upon Tyne, UK
[2]North Staffordshire Rehabilitation Centre, Stoke-on-Trent, UK

1.1 Introduction

This book has been written to highlight the remarkable progress in the application of botulinum toxin in medical practice. It is used across many specialties and has an increasing indication across a whole spectrum of diseases. As a result, its commercial sales have grown exponentially and its use in cosmesis has made 'BOTOX®' a household name. This is extraordinary after such a short time in this field and some other products have even gone so far as to add an '-ox' on the end of their brand name to attempt to capture some of the kudos (and market) of botulinum toxin. This is of course very different from when the drug was first marketed and when it was regarded as a highly dangerous product. The indications for botulinum toxin treatment are listed in Chapter 5. In many, there is still little or no evidence that it works, but in others, there is good evidence of its therapeutic benefit.

1.1.1 History of BoNT

Botulinum toxin was first identified as a poison in the nineteenth century. The toxin is a protein, which is produced by the Gram negative *Clostridium botulinum* bacterium. It is found in a variety of foods, but is most common in meat products. The name botulus means sausage and hence its terminology from its appearance in meat products. The features of botulism have been known since around the time of Christ and it was certainly described in the Middle Ages. However, it was not until 1817 that the German physician Justinus Kerner wrote on the role of an infective agent in food-borne poisoning[1]. He then published a monograph on poisoning in 1820 in which he described the features, made many original observations and commented on the possible causation, diagnosis and treatment[2]. He concluded that a toxin produced by an infective agent was responsible for the features of paralysis of skeletal and smooth muscles. He published

Clinical Uses of Botulinum Toxins, eds. Anthony B. Ward and Michael P. Barnes. Published by Cambridge University Press. © Cambridge University Press 2007.

a second monograph in 1822, in which he laid out his hypotheses on BoNT and described clinical evaluation of the problem through case histories of his patients and through post-mortem examination of patients with botulism[3]. He even ventured to infect himself and noted that while motor signals were always involved, sensation was always preserved. Most remarkably, he proposed that this toxin could be turned into a therapeutic agent for the control of chorea and other neurological diseases. It was left to the German physician, Muller, to coin the description, botulism, to connect the infection to meat products and, in particular, the sausage.

Pierre van Ermengem was Professor of Microbiology at the University of Ghent, Belgium, when he was asked to investigate an outbreak of botulism in the nearby village of Ellezelles. The illness appeared to follow a funeral ceremony and he was able to isolate the anaerobic bacterium *Bacillus botulinus* from the food and from the victims[4]. This was not the end of the story since there had been several outbreaks which confirmed the incriminating cause. Van Ermengem himself experimented on small animals and observed the typical features when they were fed with infected meat products. The isolated bacteria were the same anaerobic bacilli as before. Fortunately, efforts to control infection have been successful through better public health and meat hygiene standards. The bacterium was renamed in the twentieth century to *Clostridium botulinum*.

The potential for using the toxin in the military arena was also quickly realized and the USA led the way. The laboratory at the military camp, Fort Detrick, was used as a place to judge the effects of the toxin and much of our early knowledge of the agent comes from the studies carried out there. This followed work from Dr Hermann Sommer in the 1920s, which paved the way for identifying the toxin subtypes. He attempted to purify BoNT type A. Immunization against infection for workers at Fort Detrick was the first attempt to control the toxin. A toxoid was used as a vaccine.

1.1.2 History of BoNT as a therapeutic agent

The story starts in 1946 when Dr Carl Lammanna first crystallized BoNT type A. He described the toxin's components, but did not identify them as heavy and light chains. Fort Detrick produced purified toxin for other research groups, from which came a great deal of knowledge on the agent's structure, action and characteristics[5]. From this basic knowledge, came the crucial result of a British study group that botulinum toxin blocked the release of acetylcholine from synaptic vesicles at neuromuscular junctions[6]. It was thereafter a short step to deduce that the toxin may be able to block these junctions therapeutically in overactive muscles. The role of acetylcholine was described in neuromuscular control and in its responsibility for trophic activity in muscles[7]. Acetylcholine blockade by botulinum toxin resulted in muscle atrophy by paralysing the muscle[8]. Ophthalmological experiments started in the early 1970s, when Dr Alan Scott, an American ophthalmologist, experimented with several drugs in trying to find a suitable alternative to surgery for childhood strabismus. Botulinum toxin had immediate advantages through its relatively long action and he documented its promising role in 1973[9]. He also looked at other toxins during this period, but felt that BoNT had promise. Clinical studies in humans did not take place until 1977 when he injected a patient with strabismus. In his trial of 1982, he and his colleagues were able to observe that it was well tolerated and reversible and was also effective in nystagmus, blepharospasm, hemifacial spasm and even spasticity. Its activity will be described in Chapter 2 where reference will be made to early clinical studies[10,11].

The commercial preparations have received individual attention for registration purposes, as their characteristics are not identical. Both BOTOX® and Dysport® are licensed for the treatment of blepharospasm, hemifacial spasm and cervical dystonia and for the treatment of spastic lower leg problems in children with cerebral palsy over the age of two years. BOTOX® is now also licensed for upper limb post-stroke spasticity. Botulinum toxin type B (Myobloc (USA) or Neurobloc) entered the commercial arena in the late 1990s and received a licence for cervical dystonia in 2001 in the USA and many European countries. Recently, Merz, a German company, has released Xeomin which is a type A botulinum toxin free of complexing proteins (see Chapter 5).

Thereafter, its history has been well documented and has started to be used in patients with facial tics, blepharospasm, cervical dystonia and hemifacial spasm, and now many other indications — the subject of this book.

1.2 Why write this book?

Since this first usage there has been a steady increase in the number of clinical indications. There are now in excess of 100 reported uses of botulinum toxin in the world literature. Whilst many of these uses are still in the form of individual case reports and open studies there are nevertheless a significant number of indications that now have a robust and sound evidence base. Despite the dramatic increase in world literature on the clinical use of botulinum toxin there are surprisingly few textbooks that have tried to amalgamate the evidence into a single practical textbook — hence this volume.

We have several aims in writing this book. First we wanted leading clinicians in their field to write clear, practical chapters on their particular area of expertise.

The aim is for each author to provide a résumé and critique of the evidence base for the use of botulinum toxin in that particular clinical context. We have also asked each author to place the use of botulinum toxin in the context of other available treatment possibilities. In many conditions, such as spasticity, botulinum toxin is not a treatment in isolation but is simply part of the overall package of care for the individual patient. We also wanted each chapter to be clear and readable and offer a straightforward practical guide in the use of botulinum toxin. However, each chapter should not give the impression that there is a standard protocol for each individual use of botulinum toxin. This is certainly not the case. Each chapter should give a balanced review of the literature so that the individual clinicians can determine whether botulinum toxin is suitable and, if so, gain some idea of not only the usefulness of the technique but also the practicalities of the injection for each indication. Each patient is very different and thus each will need a personalized approach to the use of botulinum toxin for their particular problem.

1.3   Outline of the book

We have divided this book into two sections. The story of the clinical development of botulinum toxin is fascinating. This class of neurotoxin offers great future potential for the development of other therapeutic products. We feel that clinicians should have at least a basic understanding of the underlying chemistry and mode of action of the product, so one of the world's leading figures in the development of botulinum toxin – Professor Oliver Dolly – was asked to introduce the neurochemistry and mode of action of the toxin in Chapter 2. The commercial development of botulinum toxin is one of the success stories of recent years in terms of basic science being translated into practical clinical use in a relatively short period of time. Much of the early commercial development of botulinum toxin was at the Centre for Applied Microbiology and Research (CAMR) at Porton Down in the UK. CAMR developed a stable freeze-dried type A toxin formulation initially supplied to Moorfield's Eye Hospital in London. However, as the use of the toxin grew rapidly, CAMR developed the product commercially with Porton Products (now Ipsen Ltd) which eventually led to the approval by the Medicines Control Agency for licensed usage of strabismus, blepharospasm and hemifacial spasm in 1990. The product was also being developed commercially at the same time in the USA by Oculinum Inc. which was acquired in 1998 by Allergan. Ipsen now market the formulation, now called Dysport and Allergan market the formulation called BOTOX®. The story of the commercial development is outlined by Peter Hambleton, Andrew Pickett and

Clifford Shone in Chapter 3. This chapter also discusses the therapeutic potential of the botulinum neurotoxins as efficient neuronal delivery vectors as well as development of the neurotoxins as therapeutic analgesic agents.

The second section of the textbook brings together the evidence of the clinical efficacy of botulinum toxin for different indications. However, the principles of injection are generally similar and the practical issues of injection techniques are given by Tony Ward in Chapter 5. This chapter also outlines the side-effect profile as well as the practical differences between the different botulinum serotypes. The latter is a particularly important point as BOTOX® units are not the same as Dysport units. It is essential that clinicians understand that the two products do not have the same unit base. The situation is further complicated by the emergence of botulinum serotype B (Myobloc or Neurobloc – manufactured by Elan) and more recently Xeomin (manufactured by Merz) which is type A toxin free of complexing proteins. Clinicians new to the use of botulinum toxin should read this chapter prior to subsequent chapters on individual indications.

Although strabismus was the first clinical usage of botulinum toxin in man the product largely developed as a treatment of first choice for dystonia. Khalid Anwar maps the development of botulinum toxin for the management of cervical dystonia and discusses the various approaches to treatment of this disabling condition. Use of botulinum toxin for the management of focal dystonia has dramatically changed the lives of people with this condition. Prior to the advent of botulinum toxin there was very little that could be effectively done to manage dystonia but with success rates in excess of 90 per cent the condition can now usually be controlled and many individuals can go on to lead normal lives.

Although cervical dystonia is the commonest form of focal dystonia there are other rarer, but equally disabling types. Maurice Hawthorne and Khalid Anwar write about oromandibular and other laryngeal dystonias and dysphonias and they provide a good summary of the techniques behind these rare but important conditions (Chapter 7).

Although the management of dystonia has been revolutionized by botulinum toxin it is probably the use of botulinum toxin for the management of spasticity that has had most influence. There is a now a robust evidence base confirming the efficacy and safety of botulinum in the management of focal spasticity following stroke, traumatic brain injury, multiple sclerosis, cerebral palsy and a variety of other spastic conditions – in both adults and children. Tony Ward (Chapter 8) reviews the evidence and offers practical suggestions for the usage of botulinum toxin for these common problems. The chapter emphasizes that although botulinum has made a big impact it is not a treatment in its own right and needs to be combined with a range of other antispastic measures such as appropriate seating, physiotherapy, orthosis and the judicious use of oral medication. Botulinum toxin is an invaluable addition to our therapeutic armoury in the overall management of spasticity.

Although botulinum is mainly known for its muscle relaxation properties it also has profound and useful effects on the autonomic nervous system. It can have an extraordinary effect on hyperhidrosis (Chapter 9) as well as hypersalivation (Chapter 10). Such conditions can be extremely socially embarrassing and there are regrettably few practical alternative treatments. For example, many children with cerebral palsy have been socially isolated by constant dribbling. This is equally a source of embarrassment and isolation in the adult population with, for example, Parkinson's disease or motor neuron disease. Individuals with excessive sweating can also suffer major embarrassment and social and economic isolation as a result of their condition. Botulinum toxin can produce exceptional results for such people.

Botulinum toxin is also an analgesic agent and indeed Chapter 3 highlights the potential role of botulinum toxin in the management of chronic pain. The current usage in headaches (Chapter 11) and back and neck pain (Chapter 12) are discussed by David Dodick and Áine Carroll. The evidence of existing serotypes of botulinum toxin as an effective analgesic agent is not yet strong but nevertheless a number of good quality studies confirming the analgesic efficacy are now emerging. Botulinum is not likely to be a panacea for chronic pain but will clearly have a place, particularly for the various pain syndromes characterized by muscle spasm. Hopefully we will hear more in the future as botulinum toxin is further developed as an inhibitor of neurotransmission from pain conducting neurons.

One of the pioneers of the clinical use of botulinum toxin was John Elston when he was working in the early days of development at Moorfields Eye Hospital. He has written a wonderful chapter on the more established as well as the newer indications in clinical ophthalmology. Whilst botulinum still has a role to play in the management of strabismus it also has an important and thus a key role in the management of blepharospasm, hemifacial spasm and apraxia of eye opening as well as rarer indications such as post-facial palsy problems and the therapeutic induction of ptosis.

A fascinating and newer development has been the use of botulinum toxin for the management of bladder and bowel difficulties. This particularly includes the management of detrusor overactivity and the management of anal fissure. The practicalities and the place of botulinum in the management of these and other bladder and bowel problems are outlined in Chapter 14 by Giuseppe Brisinda.

Botulinum toxin continually features in the lay press. Such exposure is often useful as we have found in our clinics that after every press article there is a spate of new, and often appropriate, referrals for injection. However, the lay press have mainly focused on the use of botulinum toxin from the management of wrinkle lines and other cosmetic usages. There is little doubt that the practice of cosmetic surgery has been advanced by the safe and effective treatment of wrinkle lines with botulinum toxin. The techniques and results are demonstrated in Chapter 15.

Finally, there are a number of chronic neurological problems characterized by various degrees of muscle spasm. Many of these conditions are not particularly amenable to any intervention and botulinum toxin has been tried with some success in these conditions even though it is unlikely that such indications will ever be part of the therapeutic licence. These conditions include tics, myoclonus, stiff person syndrome, Parkinson's disease and tremor as well as the rarer forms of limb dystonia such as writer's cramp and other occupational cramps. These conditions are discussed by Mike Barnes in Chapter 16.

Overall, this book is not intended as a totally comprehensive review of all indications ever published for the use of botulinum neurotoxins. However, we hope that we have covered all the standard indications as well as reviewing the more important and the more promising indications that already provide further practical use of botulinum toxin and may do so increasingly in the future. The story of botulinum toxin has been a significant story of success and translation of basic neuroscience to practical reality. The story is not yet completed and there is every hope that botulinum neurotoxins will provide a platform for exciting clinical developments in the future. However, we hope that this textbook has provided the clinician, and the basic scientist, with a practical and readable guide to the development of this fascinating clinical entity.

REFERENCES

1. Kerner, J. (1817). Vergiftungdurch verdorbene Würste. *Ubinger Blätter Naturwissenschaften Arzneykunde*, **3**, 1−25.
2. Kerner, J. (1820). Neue Beobachtungen über die in Würtenburg so haufig vorfallenden todlichen Vergiftungen durch den Genuss geraucherter Würste. Tübingen: Osiander.
3. Kerner, J. (1822). Das Fettgift oder die Fettsäure und irhe Wirkungen afu der theirischen Organisnmus, ein Beytragzur Untersuchung des in verdobenen Würsten giftig wirkenden Stoffes. Stuttgart, Tübingen: Cotta.
4. Van Ermengem, E. P. (1897). Uber einen neuen aneroben Bacillus und sein Beziehung zum Botulismus. *Z. Hyg. Infektionskrankh*, **26**, 1−56.

5. Schantz, E. J. (1994). Historical perspective. In J. Jankovic and M. Hallett, eds., *Therapy with Botulinum Toxin*. New York: Marcel Dekker Inc, pp. xxiii–xxvi.

6. Burgen, A., Dickens, F. and Zatman, L. J. (1949). The action of botulinum toxin on the neuromuscular junction. *Journal of Physiology*, **109**, 10–24.

7. Drachman, D. (1964). Atrophy of skeletal muscles in chick embryos treated with botulinum toxin. *Science*, **145**, 719–21.

8. Drachman, D. B. and Houk, J. (1969). The effect of botulinum toxin on speed of muscle contraction. *American Journal of Physiology*, **216**, 1435–55.

9. Scott, A. B., Rosenbaum, A. and Collins, C. C. (1973). Pharmacological weakening of extra-ocular muscles. *Invest. Ophthalmol. Vis. Sci.*, **12**, 924–7.

10. Schiavo, G., Poulain, B., Rosetto, O., *et al.* (1992). Tetanus toxin is a zinc protein and its inhibition of neurotransmitter release and protease activity depend on zinc. *EMBO J.*, **11**, 3577–83.

11. Schiavo, G., Benefenati, E., Poulain, B., *et al.* (1992). Tetanus and botulinum B neurotoxins block neurotransmitter release by proteolytic cleavage of synaptobrevin. *Nature*, **359**, 832–4.

Mechanistic basis for the therapeutic effectiveness of botulinum toxin A on over-active cholinergic nerves

J. Oliver Dolly and Gary Lawrence

International Centre for Neurotherapeutics, Dublin City University, Dublin, Ireland

2.1 Introduction

Seven homologous variants (serotypes A–G) of botulinum neurotoxin (BoNT) are produced by different *Clostridium botulinum*, and closely-related toxins have been isolated from *C. butyricum* and *C. barati*[1]. All are proteins with $M_r \sim 150$ K which are activated by selective proteolytic cleavage to yield a heavy chain (HC) and a light chain (LC) linked by a disulphide bond and non-covalent interactions[2]. Each exhibits amazingly high specific neurotoxicities ($10^7 – 10^8$ mouse LD_{50} units/ mg) after separation from their naturally-occurring complexes with accessory proteins. The size and composition of such complexes differ for each serotype; for example, type A can be isolated as large assemblies (LL or L forms with $M_r \sim 900$ or 450 K) of the active moiety, BoNT, with non-toxic non-haemagglutinin and several haemagglutinin proteins[3].

Long before the recent spiralling interest worldwide in type A toxin as a therapeutic for weakening hyper-active muscles, BoNTs had been adopted as informative probes[4]. for delineating the fundamental process of quantal transmitter release[5]. This choice was based on their renowned abilities to induce neuromuscular paralysis by presynaptic inhibition of acetylcholine (ACh) release[6]. with exquisite specificity (i.e. without affecting any other measured parameters such as ion channels in the nerve terminal, ACh synthesis, etc.)[7]. Also, other toxins had been shown to be useful for the biochemical characterization of neurotransmitter receptors and cation channels[8,9]. Another attraction of using BoNTs was that motor nerves in frog paralysed with type D did not atrophy or undergo any detectable ultrastructural changes over ~ 50 days[10]; likewise, mammalian nerve endings treated with type A did not degenerate but, instead, underwent remodelling that culminated in full recovery of neuro-exocytosis after 90 days[11].

Clinical Uses of Botulinum Toxins, eds. Anthony B. Ward and Michael P. Barnes. Published by Cambridge University Press. © Cambridge University Press 2007.

2.2 Outline

In view of such unique potency and selective perturbation of a key step in synaptic transmission, which was very poorly understood in molecular terms despite Nobel prize winning contributions[12], it was prudent to expect that utilization of BoNTs as research tools would unveil a functionally important component. Nonetheless, some eminent scientists doubted the wisdom of working with such exotic and dangerous toxins. However, the commitment to this experimental approach yielded an even larger measure of success than needed to compensate for the difficulties in safely handling such potent neuroparalytic agents. Notable outcomes, to be reviewed herein in chronological order, include establishing molecular/mechanistic bases or evidence for the following:

(a) the targeting of BoNT/A and /B to cholinergic nerve endings in the periphery by binding to distinct ecto-acceptors located exclusively thereon, a step requiring the correct conformation of the HC;

(b) internalization of the toxic moiety by acceptor-mediated endocytosis and translocation to the cytosol, a process enhanced by neural stimulation;

(c) intracellular inactivation of ubiquitous target(s) essential for the release of all transmitters from small synaptic vesicles and large dense-core granules;

(d) light chain of type A inhibits ACh release at the neuromuscular junction, due to its reported Zn^{2+}-dependent endoprotease cleaving and disabling a SNARE protein, SNAP-25, which together with synaptobrevin and syntaxin — the substrates for BoNT/B/D/F/G and /C1 (reviewed in[13,14]) — were, thus, found to be responsible for Ca^{2+}-regulated exocytosis; and

(e) pinpointing factors contributing to the prolonged, but reversible, neuromuscular paralysis caused by BoNT/A including the persistence of its cleaved target, longevity of the protease activity and extended time course of the nerve sprouting/remodelling induced. Such an unique combination of remarkable multi-functional activities underpins the impressive success of type A toxin as a first-choice therapeutic for an ever-increasing number of conditions arising from over-activity of cholinergically-innervated muscles.

2.3 BoNT/A binds to 'productive' ecto-acceptors on motor and autonomic nerves: such targeting underlies its peripheral cholinergic specificity

Electrophysiological recordings in rodent phrenic nerve diaphragm[15] revealed that type A BoNT reduces the frequency of miniature end-plate potentials and blocks neurally-evoked end-plate potentials, without altering their

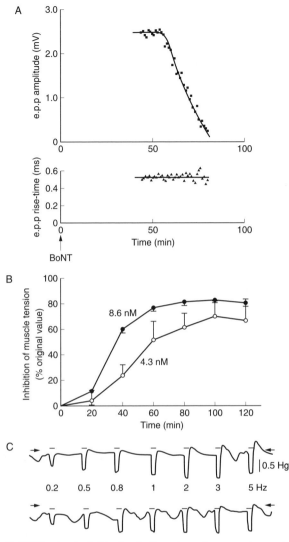

Figure 2.1   BoNT/A selectively blocks cholinergic motor neurotransmission. (A) Continuous monitoring of the amplitude (upper panel) and rise-time (lower panel) of post-synaptic end-plate potentials (e.p.p.s.) in a single fibre of mouse diaphragm, elicited by stimulation of the attached phrenic nerve. Plotted data represent the responses recorded following the addition of 10 nM BoNT/A (at 0 min). (B) Inhibition by BoNT/A (two concentrations) of smooth-muscle contractions upon transmural electrical stimulation of guinea-pig ileum. The force of contractions progressively declined following toxin addition. (C) Non-adrenergic inhibitory responses of guinea-pig taenia coli, elicited by 30 sec stimulation at the indicated frequencies in the presence of atropine and guanethidine (upper record), was unaffected by 2 hours exposure to 8.6 nM BoNT/A (lower trace).

rise-times (Figure 2.1A). These observations highlighted the pre-synaptic selectivity of this toxin and ability to reduce both spontaneous and evoked release of ACh. Cholinergic excitatory transmission in smooth muscle of guinea-pig ileum, elicited by transmural stimulation[16] can also be inhibited by BoNT/A (Figure 2.1B). Such susceptibility of neuronal ACh release in skeletal and smooth muscle preparations accords with the most pronounced and prevalent symptoms of human botulism[17] In contrast, non-adrenergic non-cholinergic inhibitory response of intestinal wall to field stimulation[16] is not affected by BoNT/A (Figure 2.1C). Similarly, the toxin was found to have minimal effect on nor-adrenergic excitatory response of rat anococcygeus muscle induced by field stimulation.

As a means of deciphering the basis of this preference for cholinergic nerves, BoNT/A and /B were radiolabelled to high specific radioactivities with ^{125}I whilst retaining their biological activities[18] and used to paralyse mouse diaphragm. Electron microscopic autoradiograms of this processed tissue showed very selective targeting of ^{125}I-BoNT type A (Figure 2.2A) and B[19] to motor nerve terminals. This involved saturable binding to ecto-acceptors on the unmyelinated presynaptic membrane because the labelling was diminished by the additional presence of an excess of non-radioactive toxin (Figure 2.2B). Moreover, type A and B toxins bound to distinct sites whose densities were determined to be 150 and 630 μm^{-2} of nerve terminal membrane[19,20]. Reduction of the disulphides in BoNT/A and alkylation of the thiols abolished its neurotoxicity, but abilities to bind to the ecto-acceptors and to inhibit transmitter release when applied intra-neuronally were retained[21]. In contrast, the separated HC of type A proved unable to prevent the 'productive' binding of BoNT/A to motor nerve terminals that led to muscle paralysis, being only capable of reducing 'non-productive' interaction[22]. Accordingly, the non-toxic derivative of the whole toxin, unlike the free HC, antagonized the neuromuscular paralytic activity of BoNT/A (Figure 2.3A) revealing that the conformation of HC required for 'productive' binding is maintained by its association with LC[22,23]. Importantly, the reduced alkylated BoNT/A failed to counteract the inhibition by serotypes B, F and E or the related tetanus toxin (Figure 2.3). This lack of cross-competition, together with the above-noted different acceptor densities for BoNT/A and /B, establish the existence of separate binding sites for the toxin serotypes examined. Notably, our conclusion is supported by the recent demonstrations that types B and G, but not A, bind to synaptotagmin I and II; such interaction of the former *only* requires ganglioside[24,25]. As these toxins just exploit the existence of multiple ecto-acceptors, an intriguing question arises as to the molecular nature and physiological roles of those for the other toxin serotypes that remain to be identified.

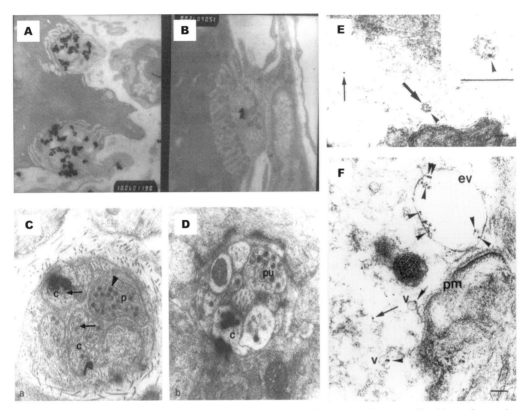

Figure 2.2   BoNT/A selectively binds at cholinergic motor end-plates and is internalized by endocytosis, followed by transfer to the pre-synaptic cytosol. Electron microscope autoradiograms of phrenic nerve muscle preparations (A, B) after exposure to 11 nM ^{125}I-labelled BoNT/A alone (A) or in the presence of 100-fold excess of the unlabelled toxin and (C, D) sections of mouse ileum after exposure to 20 nM ^{125}I-BoNT/A; note the deposition of silver grains on cholinergic endings but absence of labelling on peptidergic and purinergic varicosities. (E) Colloidal gold conjugated to BoNT/A revealed in 100 nm sections through mouse nerve-diaphragm. After silver enhancement, 10–20 nm grains were observed near the intra-lumenal membrane of intra-terminal endocytic structures such as coated vesicles [large arrow in (E) and (E, inset) at higher magnification], small smooth- and large-endocytotic vesicles [large arrowheads and ev, respectively, in (F)], and in the cytosol (small arrows).

It appears that binding is a prerequisite for the toxins' potent actions because fragments (e.g. LC-H$_N$, lacking the C-terminal half of HC) are unable to bind to motor nerve endings or antagonize the action of the intact toxin; also, these lack neuromuscular paralysing activity[26,27]. Accordingly, toxin-susceptible cholinergic nerves in ileum (cf. Figure 2.1B) could be labelled by ^{125}I-BoNT/A, unlike putative purinergic or peptidergic endings in the same sections[28], as seen in electron micrographs (Figure 2.2C, D).

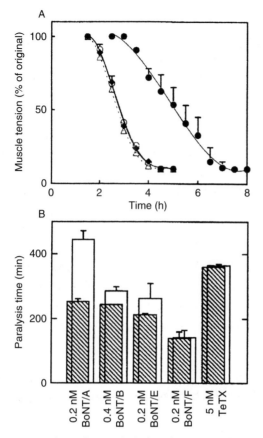

Figure 2.3   Antagonism of BoNT/A-induced neuroparalysis by an innocuous derivative shows that productive neuronal binding requires both associated HC and LC: the acceptor for BoNT/A is distinct from those for other serotypes and tetanus toxin. (A) Under conditions designed to be non-permissive for toxin internalization, 30 nM H_NLC fragment of BoNT/A ($\triangle$) or its HC ($\blacklozenge$) proved incapable of antagonizing the binding of 0.3 nM BoNT/A, as reflected by their inability to delay paralysis ($\bigcirc$) following the removal of toxin and nerve stimulation under permissive conditions. In contrast, 2.5 nM of a reduced and alkylated BoNT/A ($\bullet$) did impede BoNT/A-induction of paralysis. The derivative did not delay, or postponed only slightly, the onset of paralysis by other BoNT serotypes or tetanus toxin, indicating that BoNT/A binds to distinct functional acceptors.

2.4 ^{125}I-BoNT undergoes acceptor-mediated endocytosis in cholinergic nerves: enhancement by stimulation and acceleration of neuromuscular paralysis

Uptake of ^{125}I-labelled BoNT/A (Figure 2.2) and /B^{29} into motor nerve terminals occurs via a saturable process (i.e. blocked by excess of the respective unlabelled toxin) that is energy- and temperature-dependent, indicative of acceptor-mediated endocytosis. The relevance of this uptake process was high-lighted by its enhancement upon nerve stimulation[29] because the latter also shortens the toxin's paralysis time[30,31]. Furthermore, ammonium chloride and methylamine – lysosomotropic agents which interfere with the endocytotic pathway – attenuated toxin internalization[29] and, correspondingly, retarded the onset of BoNT-induced muscle paralysis[32]. Finally, efficient uptake of the neurotoxic moiety of type A toxin requires the presence of the inter-chain disulphide as well as the correct conformation of the HC which is, apparently, maintained by association with LC[21]. This observation underpins the need to use an innocuous mutant of intact BoNT to act as a cholinergic targeting vehicle for therapeutic adducts[33].

Involvement of endocytosis was reaffirmed by similar studies with BoNT/A conjugated to colloidal-gold[23] which unveiled gold particles associated with coated vesicles, small smooth- and large-endocytotic vesicles (Figure 2.2E, F). Some of the toxin molecules were seen close to the limiting membrane, pre-sumably awaiting translocation. Accordingly, gold particles could be detected in the cytoplasm, establishing that internalization occurred (Figure 2.2E).

2.5 Intra-neuronal inhibition by BoNT/A of the release of numerous transmitters from SSVs and LDCVs highlights an ubiquitous target essential for regulated exocytosis

The large size of neurons in *Aplysia* and ease of recording synaptic potentials were exploited for micro-injection of BoNT/A and monitoring of its effects; blockade of transmitter release was seen at both cholinergic (Figure 2.4A) and non-cholinergic synapses (Figure 2.4B) whereas only the former was susceptible to extracellularly-applied toxin[34]. Likewise, when BoNT/A gains access into cere-brocortical synaptosomes by use of relatively high concentrations[35], the Ca^{2+}-dependent evoked release of dopamine, GABA, noradrenaline, ACh (Figure 2.4C) or glutamate became inhibited[36]. Exocytosis from large dense-core granules of peptides (e.g. cGRP, substance P) and catecholamines is also inhibited by adequate exposure of neurons and endocrine cells to BoNT/A[37–39]. Clearly, this toxin inactivates an ubiquitous intracellular target that is essential for Ca^{2+}-regulated exocytosis and, thus, can block the release of a variety of messengers from neurons, endocrine (as discussed above) and exocrine cells[40] provided it can be delivered intracellularly by permeabilization or other methods. Its therapeutic applications (discussed below and elsewhere) are, therefore, only limited by the users' technical ingenuity. This is not a challenge in the case of peripheral cholinergic terminals because of their possession of 'productive' acceptors[22].

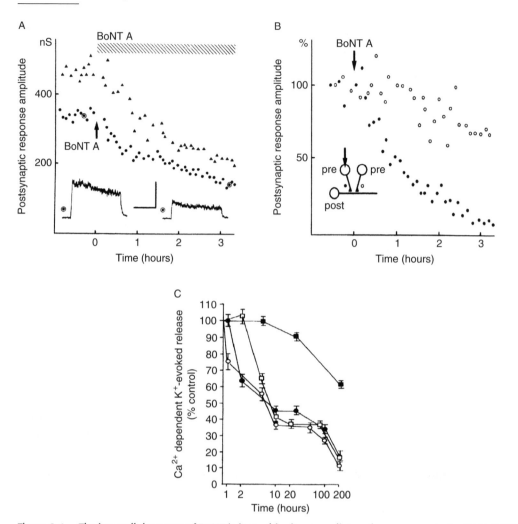

Figure 2.4   The intracellular target of BoNT/A is an ubiquitous mediator of neuro-exocytosis. (A) BoNT/A was bath-applied (hatched bar) at 7 nM (▲) or intracellularly injected to give a calculated intracellular concentration of 5 nM (●) in an identified cholinergic neuron (arrow) in the buccal ganglion of *Aplysia*. Neurally-evoked post-synaptic responses were monitored before and after administration of BoNT (Insets). Post-synaptic recordings at the point indicated in the control conditions (left) and during the decrease in ACh release (right) caused by intracellular administration of BoNT (◉). (B) Inhibition of post-synaptic potentials in the cerebral ganglia of *Aplysia* induced by intracellular injection of BoNT into a non-cholinergic pre-synaptic cell. Note that repetitive activation of this synapse reduces its activity over time; thus, responses to BoNT/A-injected neurons were compared directly with those to a non-injected pre-synaptic neuron afferent to the same cell. (C) Rat cerebrocortical synaptosomes were exposed for 30 min at 37°C to BoNT/A at the concentrations indicated and loaded with tritiated neurotransmitters acetylcholine (○), noradrenaline (●), dopamine (□) and γ-amino butyric acid (GABA; ■). Release of transmitter was elicited by 25 mM K^+ depolarization and the amounts released quantified.

2.6   LC of BoNT/A administered intracellularly blocks Ca²⁺-evoked exocytosis due to its proteolytic cleavage of SNAP-25

When LC isolated from BoNT/A was delivered into motor terminals[41], it abolished nerve-evoked muscle contraction (Figure 2.5A), as also observed when applied inside endocrine cells[38,42]. The discovery of clostridial neurotoxins being metallo-endoproteases[43] with BoNT/A cleaving off nine-residues from the C-terminus of SNAP-25[44,45], revolutionized this field and identified the final crucial step in the previously established multi-phasic mechanism outlined above. Cleavage of the SNARE protein by BoNT/A could be readily demonstrated in cerebellar granule neurons[46] and shown to correlate with the inhibition of glutamate release (Figure 2.5B). However, cleavage of only a minority of the total SNAP-25 by type A or E was observed in rat motor nerves (Figure 2.5C) despite neuromuscular transmission being abolished[47]. Apparently when minimal amounts of BoNT are used, proteolysis of a SNAP-25 subpopulation occurs that is critical for ACh release — probably at the active zone release sites, near its point of entry. In any case, SNAP-25 cleavage by BoNT/A definitely underlies blockade of exocytosis because synaptic transmission in leech is toxin-resistant due to a mutation at the scissile bond in SNAP-25[48]. Furthermore, exocytosis from chromaffin cells after inhibition by BoNT/A can be rescued by over-expression of a toxin-resistant SNAP-25 mutant (R198T), a feat not achievable with the wild-type SNARE (Figure 2.5D). The latter continued to be ineffective over 3 weeks after initial exposure to the toxin, indicating the persistence of its protease activity (Ref. 49; see later). Finally, it is noteworthy that BoNT/A and /E (which removes 26 C-terminal residues) have proved instrumental in establishing the role of SNAP-25 in exocytosis whilst the other serotypes have, likewise, been used to define the functional importance of the two SNAREs, syntaxin (/CI) and synaptobrevin (/B, /D, /F, /G)[14].

2.7   Prolonged neuromuscular paralysis and associated nerve sprouting induced by BoNT/A contrasts with the transient effect of type E: differences in the toxins' life-times and properties of /A- and /E-truncated SNAP-25

One of the many attractive features of type A BoNT for therapeutic applications is its prolonged duration (3—12 months in humans depending on the condition treated) of efficacy (detailed in other chapters). When injected into murine leg muscles, the induced weakness lasts for ∼30 days when measured crudely by the toe spread reflex assay (Figure 2.6A). In general agreement with this, /A-truncated SNAP-25 was shown to persist for 20—40 days in mouse motor nerve

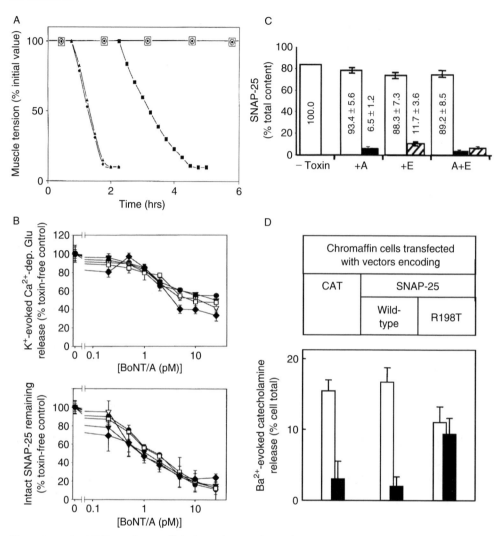

Figure 2.5   BoNT/A acts intra-cellularly to cleave selectively SNAP-25: delivery of the LC is adequate for inhibition. (A) Bath application to mouse nerve-diaphragms of liposomes encapsulating LC at a final concentration of 20 nM (**u**), 15 nM (**s**) and 9 nM (**■**) induced a progressive decrease in nerve-evoked muscle contractions, with higher doses having a more rapid effect. Empty liposomes (⊓) or those containing HC (**m**) had no effect. (B) Cultures of cerebellar granule neurons were exposed for 24 hours to the specified concentrations of BoNT/A and then returned to toxin free medium. After various times (● 0, **t** 7, ∇, □ 21 and **u** 31 days), the cells were loaded with [^{14}C]-labelled glutamine and Ca^{2+}-dependent K$^+$-depolarization evoked release of radiolabel was quantified (upper panel) before harvesting the cells and probing for full-length SNAP-25 by SDS-PAGE and Western blotting. Signal intensities were quantified from digitized images and normalized as a% of the toxin-free control (lower panel). (C) Mouse diaphragms were exposed to 2 nM BoNT/A, 0.5 nM BoNT/E or both toxins

endings (Figure 2.6C1), by using an antibody specific for the cleaved product in conjunction with fluorescent microscopy[47]. In vivo imaging of individual nerve terminals in mice, before and at various times after blockade with type A toxin[11], revealed that extensive nerve sprouting occurred up to 42 days. Although the original nerve ending remained devoid of endo-/exo-cytotic activity, vesicle recycling was visible in the new outgrowths and these formed functional extra-junctional synapses with the muscle which, apparently, mediated the observed return of the first phase of nerve-evoked muscle twitch[11]. By day 63, lengthening of the sprouts had ceased and vesicle recycling started to reappear in the parent terminal (Figure 2.6B2); after 93 days, the latter had fully recovered functionality and original shape with disappearance of all the sprouts (Figure 2.6B3).

In stark contrast, type E causes a much shorter transient effect (Figure 2.6A) consistent with the shorter lifetime of its cleaved product (Figure 2.6C2). Importantly, co-injection of type E with /A speeds up the functional recovery (Figure 2.6A), a striking phenomenon first observed with muscles in human volunteers[50]. In accord with these observations, BoNT/E was shown to hasten the removal of A-truncated SNAP-25[47]. BoNT/F, which cleaves a different target, synaptobrevin, and gives intermediate duration of action did not shorten the extended action of type A (Figure 2.6). This significant shift in time course not only suggests that BoNT/E further cleaves A-truncated SNAP-25 (as demonstrated clearly in vitro[46]) but, also, infers a lack of persistence of adequate activity of type A protease (when minimal doses are employed[46]) to resume its normal prolonged effect, after the transient action of /E[51]. On the other hand, BoNT/A activity has been reported to persist in chromaffin cells ($\gg$30 days; Figure 2.5D), cerebellar granule cells ($\gg$21 days; Figure 2.5B), cultured spinal cord neurons ($\sim$80 days) and rat muscle ($\gg$30 days)[51,52]. In this context, it is notable that LC of BoNT/A,

Caption for Figure 2.5 (*cont.*) simultaneously until nerve-evoked muscle contractions were completely blocked; control preparations were exposed to vehicle alone. The samples were then washed and end-plate regions dissected and solubilized with 2% CHAPS before immunoprecipitation of SNAP-25 using an antibody that binds full-length and C-terminally truncated SNAP-25 equally well. Precipitates were subjected to SDS-PAGE and probed for SNAP-25 by Western blotting. Signal intensities were quantified and normalized for full length- (open bars) and BoNT/A-truncated- (solid bars) and BoNT/E-truncated SNAP-25 (hatched bars). (D) Cultured bovine chromaffin cells were transiently exposed to BoNT/A, then maintained for a further 3 weeks before co-transfection with plasmids encoding human growth hormone (hGH, which localizes within secretory granules) and either chloramphenicol acetyl-transferase (CAT), wild-type SNAP-25 or a SNAP-25 with a mutation (R198 to T) that renders it insensitive to BoNT/A. Release of hGH from transfected cells was elicited with 2 mM Ba^{2+} and quantified by radio-immunoassay.

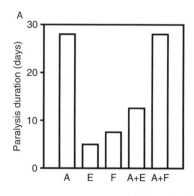

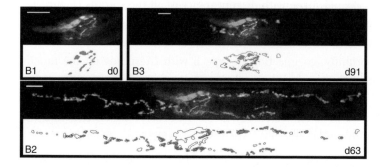

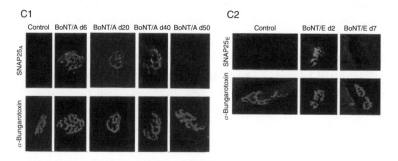

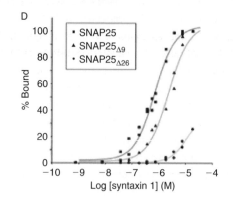

but not /E, displays ability to associate with the plasmalemma when expressed in PC-12 cells[53].

One possible interpretation[47] for these disparate findings is that A-truncated SNAP-25 squats at the release sites by associating with the other partnering SNAREs (syntaxin and synaptobrevin), as its ability to form a complex (albeit non-productive) persists[54]. By some such mechanism, the normal fast turnover of SNAP-25 is precluded. Interestingly, a recent study[55] lends some support to this notion; SNAP-25 truncated by BoNT/A retains considerable ability to bind syntaxin unlike the /E-truncated form (Figure 2.6D).

2.8 Therapeutic applications: present success and unique properties of BoNTs offer encouraging prospects for further advancement

This remarkable combination of unique properties established for BoNT/A (e.g. targeting to and internalization into cholinergic nerve endings, specificity in blocking ACh release, potency and long-lasting effects)[23,56]. underlies its unrivalled usefulness as the clinical treatment of an ever-increasing range of conditions arising from hyper-active motor nerves (detailed in other chapters).

Figure 2.6   Neuromuscular paralysis induced by BoNT/A is very prolonged compared to that produced by other serotypes, accords with the persistence of cleaved SNAP-25 and is accompanied by extensive and reversible remodelling of the end-plates. (A) Extent of paralysis was determined using the toe spread reflex (TSR) assay for mice injected (at day 0) in the hind leg with A, 5 pg BoNT/A; E, 50 pg BoNT/E; F, 4 ng BoNT/F; A+E, 2.5 pg BoNT/A + 25 pg BoNT/E and A+F, 2.5 pg BoNT/A + 2 ng BoNT/F, doses that had been predetermined to produce a maximum TSR score in the absence of any other symptoms of botulism. The plotted data indicate the time taken for the TSR score to return to baseline. (B) The lower panels represent localization of a nerve-terminal and its sprouts with the mitochondrial activity dye 4-di-2-ASP (outlined areas) and detection of vesicle-recycling with FM1-43 labelling (solid areas) in mouse sternamastoid muscle before the injection of 0.5 pg BoNT/A haemagglutinin complex (B1), the original terminal and extensive terminal sprouts at day 63 after injection (B2) and, at day 91, the original terminal with sprouts almost fully retracted (B3). The upper panels show composites of the images captured with each dye. (C) The products of SNAP-25 cleavage by BoNT/A (SNAP-25$_A$; C1) or BoNT/E (SNAP-25$_E$; C2) detected in mouse extensor digitorum longus muscles after injection of the requisite neurotoxin. Note that cleavage product can be detected up to 40 days after the injection of BoNT/A, but E-truncated SNAP-25 was removed within a week after administration of BoNT/E. (D) Increasing amounts of syntaxin 1 were incubated with resin-immobilized full-length SNAP-25 or truncated forms equivalent to the products of SNAP-25 cleavage by BoNT/A (SNAP-25$_{\Delta 9}$) or /E (SNAP-25$_{\Delta 25}$). Bound syntaxin was quantified by Western blotting. From Bajohrs et al. (2004). (For a colour version of this figure, please refer to the colour insert between pages 26 and 27.)

Likewise, the observed inhibitory effects of BoNT/A on different autonomic nerves[16] form a basis for its successful application as a therapy for over-active bladder[57], certain gastrointestinal disorders[58]. and hyperhidrosis, salivation or lacrimation[59]. However, there was a ~2 decade gap between the reported blockade by BoNT/A of smooth muscle and its later adoption in the clinic for that purpose. Thus, increased interaction/collaboration between basic and clinical scientists should further improve and extend BoNT therapies.

REFERENCES

1. Hatheway, C. L. (1990). Toxigenic clostridia. *Clin. Microbiol. Rev.*, **3**, 66–98.
2. DasGupta, B. R. (1989). In L. L. Simpson, ed., *Botulinum Neurotoxin and Tetanus Toxin.* New York: Academic Press, pp. 53–67.
3. Oguma, K., Fujinaga, Y. and Inoue, K. (1995). Structure and function of *Clostridium botulinum* toxins. *Microbiol. Immunol.*, **39**, 161–8.
4. Dolly, J. O., Halliwell, J. V., Black, J. D., Williams, R. S., Pelchen-Matthews, A., Breeze, A. L., Mehraban, F., Othman, I. B., and Black, A. R. (1984). Botulinum neurotoxin and dendrotoxin as probes for studies on transmitter release. *J. Physiol. (Paris)*, **79**, 280–303.
5. Simpson, L. L. (1981). The origin, structure and pharmacological activity of botulinum toxin. *Pharmacol. Rev.*, **33**, 155–88.
6. Burgen, A. S. V., Dickens, F. and Zatman, L. J. (1949). The action of botulinum toxin on the neuro-muscular junction. *J. Physiol. (Lond.)*, **109**, 10–24.
7. Gundersen, C. B. (1980). The effects of botulinum toxin on the synthesis, storage and release of acetylcholine. *Prog. Neurobiol.*, **14**, 99–119.
8. Dolly, J. O. and Barnard, E. A. (1984). Nicotinic acetylcholine receptors: an overview. *Biochem. Pharmacol.*, **33**, 841–58.
9. Catterall, W. A. (1988). Structure and function of voltage-sensitive ion channels. *Science*, **242**, 50–61.
10. Harris, A. J. and Miledi, R. (1971). The effect of type D botulinum toxin on frog neuromuscular junctions. *J. Physiol. (Lond.)*, **217**, 497–515.
11. de Paiva, A., Meunier, F. A., Molgó, J., Aoki, K. R. and Dolly, J. O. (1999). Functional repair of motor endplates after botulinum neurotoxin A poisoning: bi-phasic switch of synaptic activity between nerve sprouts and their parent terminals. *PNAS*, **96**, 3200–5.
12. Katz, B. (1972). In *Nobel Lectures, Physiology or Medicine 1963–1970*. Amsterdam: Elsevier.
13. Simpson, L. L. (2004). Identification of the major steps in botulinum toxin action. *Ann. Rev. Pharmacol. Toxicol.*, **44**, 167–93.
14. Schiavo, G., Matteoli, M. and Montecucco, C. (2000). Neurotoxins affecting neuro-exocytosis. *Physiol. Rev.*, **80**, 717–66.
15. Dolly, J. O., Lande, S. and Wray, D. (1987). The effects of *in vitro* application of purified botulinum neurotoxin at mouse motor nerve terminals. *J. Physiol. (Lond.)*, **386**, 475–84.

16. MacKenzie, I., Burnstock, G. and Dolly, J. O. (1982). The effects of purified botulinum neurotoxin type A on cholinergic, adrenergic and non-adrenergic, atropine-resistant autonomic neuromuscular transmission. *Neuroscience*, **7**, 997–1006.

17. Arnon, S. S. (2002). In M. F. Brin, J. Jankovic and M. Hallett, eds., *Scientific and Therapeutic Aspects of Botulinum Toxin*. Philadelphia: Lippincott Williams and Wilkins, pp. 145–50.

18. Williams, R. S., Tse, C.-K., Dolly, J. O., Hambleton, P. and Melling, J. (1983). Radio-iodination of botulinum neurotoxin type A with retention of biological activity and its binding to brain synaptosomes. *Eur. J. Biochem.*, **131**, 437–45.

19. Black, J. D. and Dolly, J. O. (1986). Interaction of ^{125}I-labelled botulinum neurotoxins with nerve terminals. I. Ultrastructural autoradiographic localization and quantitation of distinct membrane acceptors for types A and B on motor nerves. *J. Cell Biol.*, **103**, 521–34.

20. Dolly, J. O., Black, J., Williams, R. S. and Melling, J. (1984). Acceptors for botulinum neurotoxin reside on motor nerve terminals and mediate its internalization. *Nature*, **307**, 457–60.

21. de Paiva, A., Poulain, B., Lawrence, G. W., Shone, C. C., Tauc, L. and Dolly, J. O. (1993). A role for the interchain disulfide or its participating thiols in the internalization of botulinum neurotoxin-A revealed by a toxin derivative that binds to ecto-acceptors and inhibits transmitter release intracellularly. *J. Biol. Chem.*, **268**, 20838–44.

22. Daniels-Holgate, P. U. and Dolly, J. O. (1996). Productive and non-productive binding of botulinum neurotoxin A to motor nerve endings are distinguished by its heavy chain. *J. Neurosci. Res.*, **44**, 263–71.

23. Dolly, J. O., de Paiva, A., Foran, P., Lawrence, G., Daniels-Holgate, P. and Ashton, A. C. (1994). Probing the process of transmitter release with botulinum and tetanus neurotoxins. *Semin. Neurosci.*, **6**, 149–58.

24. Rummel, A., Karnath, T., Henke, T., Bigalke, H. and Binz, T. (2004). Synaptotagmins I and II act as nerve cell receptors for botulinum neurotoxin G. *J. Biol. Chem.*, **279**, 30865–70.

25. Dong, M., Richards, D. A., Goodnough, M. C., Tepp, W. H., Johnson, E. A. and Chapman, E. R. (2003). Synaptotagmins I and II mediate entry of botulinum neurotoxin B into cells. *J. Cell Biol.*, **162**, 1293–303.

26. Poulain, B., Wadsworth, J. D. F., Maisey, E. A., Shone, C. C., Melling, J., Tauc, L. and Dolly, J. O. (1989). Inhibition of transmitter release by botulinum neurotoxin A: contribution of various fragments to the intoxication process. *Eur. J. Biochem.*, **185**, 197–203.

27. Poulain, B., Wadsworth, J. D. F., Shone, C. C., Mochida, S., Lande, S., Melling, J., Dolly, J. O. and Tauc, L. (1989). Multiple domains of botulinum neurotoxin contribute to its inhibition of transmitter release in *Aplysia* neurons. *J. Biol. Chem.*, **264**, 21928–33.

28. Black, J. D. and Dolly, J. O. (1987). Selective location of acceptors for botulinum neurotoxin A on central and peripheral nerves. *Neuroscience*, **23**, 767–79.

29. Black, J. D. and Dolly, J. O. (1986). Interaction of ^{125}I-labeled botulinum neurotoxins with nerve terminals. II. Autoradiographic evidence for its uptake into motor nerves by acceptor-mediated endocytosis. *J. Cell Biol.*, **103**, 535–44.

30. Hughes, R. and Whaler, B. C. (1962). Influence of nerve-ending activity and of drugs on the rate of paralysis of rat diaphragm preparations by *Cl. botulinum* type A toxin. *J. Physiol. (Lond.)*, **160**, 221–33.

31. Simpson, L. L. (1980). Kinetic studies on the interaction between botulinum toxin type A and the cholinergic neuromuscular junction. *J. Pharmacol. Exp. Ther.*, **212**, 16–21.

32. Simpson, L. L. and DasGupta, B. R. (1983). Botulinum neurotoxin type E: studies on mechanism of action and on structure-activity relationships. *J. Pharmacol. Exp. Ther.*, **224**, 135–40.

33. Zhou, L. Q., de Paiva, A., Liu, D., Aoki, R. and Dolly, J. O. (1995). Expression and purification of the light chain of botulinum neurotoxin A: a single mutation abolishes its cleavage of SNAP-25 and neurotoxicity after reconstitution with the heavy chain. *Biochemistry*, **34**, 15175–81.

34. Poulain, B., Tauc, L., Maisey, E. A., Wadsworth, J. D. F. and Dolly, J. O. (1988). *Aplysia* as model for the study of the mechanism of inhibition of cholinergic transmission by botulinum neurotoxin.

35. Ashton, A. C. and Dolly, J. O. (1988). Characterization of the inhibitory action of botulinum neurotoxin type A on the release of several transmitters from rat cerebrocortical synaptosomes. *J. Neurochem.*, **50**, 1808–16.

36. McMahon, H. T., Foran, P., Dolly, J. O., Verhage, M., Wiegant, V. M. and Nicholls, D. G. (1992). Tetanus toxin and botulinum toxins type-A and type-B inhibit glutamate, γ-aminobutyric acid, aspartate, and met-enkephalin release from synaptosomes – clues to the locus of action. *J. Biol. Chem.*, **267**, 21338–43.

37. Lande, S., Pagel, C., Gibson, S. J., Kar, S., Dolly, J. O. and Polak, J. M. (1989). The immunocytochemical detection of motor end plates using antisera to protein gene product 95 (PGP 95). *Abstr. 9th Nat. Mtg. Bayliss & Starling Soc.*

38. Lawrence, G. W., Weller, U. and Dolly, J. O. (1994). Botulinum A and the light chain of tetanus toxins inhibit distinct stages of MgATP-dependent catecholamine exocytosis from permeabilised chromaffin cells. *Eur. J. Biochem.*, **222**, 325–33.

39. Welch, M. J., Purkiss, J. R. and Foster, K. A. (2000). Sensitivity of embryonic rat dorsal root ganglia neurons to *Clostridium botulinum* neurotoxins. *Toxicon*, **38**, 245–58.

40. Stecher, B., Ahnert-Hilger, G., Weller, U., Kemmer, T. P. and Gratzl, M. (1992). Amylase release from streptolysin O-permeabilized pancreatic acinar cells. Effects of Ca^{2+}, guanosine 5′-gamma-thio triphosphate, cyclic AMP, tetanus toxin and botulinum A toxin. *Biochem. J.*, **283**, 899–904.

41. de Paiva, A. and Dolly, J. O. (1990). Light chain of botulinum neurotoxin is active in mammalian motor nerve terminals when delivered via liposomes. *FEBS Lett.*, **277**, 171–4.

42. Penner, R., Neher, E. and Dreyer, F. (1986). Intracellularly injected tetanus toxin inhibits exocytosis in bovine adrenal chromaffin cells. *Nature*, **324**, 76–8.

43. Schiavo, G., Benfenati, F., Poulain, B., Rossetto, O., Delaureto, P. P., DasGupta, B. R. and Montecucco, C. (1992). Tetanus and botulinum-B neurotoxins block neurotransmitter release by proteolytic cleavage of synaptobrevin. *Nature*, **359**, 832–5.

44. Blasi, J., Chapman, E. R., Link, E., Binz, T., Yamasaki, S., De Camilli, P., Südhof, T. C., Niemann, H. and Jahn, R. (1993). Botulinum neurotoxin-A selectively cleaves the synaptic protein SNAP-25. *Nature*, **365**, 160–3.

45. Schiavo, G., Santucci, A., DasGupta, B. R., Mehta, P. P., Jontes, J., Benfenati, F., Wilson, M. C. and Montecucco, C. (1993). Botulinum neurotoxins serotypes A and E cleave SNAP-25 at distinct COOH-terminal peptide bonds. *FEBS Lett.*, **335**, 99–103.

46. Foran, P. G., Mohammed, N., Lisk, G. O., Nagwaney, S., Lawrence, G. W., Johnson, E., Smith, L., Aoki, K. R. and Dolly, J. O. (2003). Evaluation of the therapeutic usefulness of botulinum neurotoxin B, C1, E, and F compared with the long lasting type A. Basis for distinct durations of inhibition of exocytosis in central neurons. *J. Biol. Chem.*, **278**, 1363–71.

47. Meunier, F. A., Lisk, G., Sesardic, D. and Dolly, J. O. (2003). Dynamics of motor nerve terminal remodeling unveiled using SNARE-cleaving botulinum toxins: the extent and duration are dictated by the sites of SNAP-25 truncation. *Mol. Cell Neurosci.*, **22**, 454–66.

48. Bruns, D., Engers, S., Yang, C., Ossig, R., Jeromin, A. and Jahn, R. (1997). Inhibition of transmitter release correlates with the proteolytic activity of tetanus toxin and botulinus toxin A in individual cultured synapses of *Hirudo medicinalis*. *J. Neurosci.*, **17**, 1898–910.

49. O'Sullivan, G. A., Mohammed, N., Foran, P. G., Lawrence, G. W. and Dolly, J. O. (1999). Rescue of exocytosis in botulinum toxin A-poisoned chromaffin cells by expression of cleavage-resistant SNAP-25: identification of the minimal essential C-terminal residues. *J. Biol. Chem.*, **274**, 36897–904.

50. Eleopra, R., Tugnoli, V., Rossetto, O., De Grandis, D. and Montecucco, C. (1998). Different time courses of recovery after poisoning with botulinum neurotoxin serotypes A and E in humans. *Neurosci. Lett.*, **256**, 135–8.

51. Adler, M., Keller, J. E., Sheridan, R. E. and Deshpande, S. S. (2001). Persistence of botulinum neurotoxin A demonstrated by sequential administration of serotypes A and E in rat EDL muscle. *Toxicon*, **39**, 233–43.

52. Keller, J. E., Neale, E. A., Oyler, G. and Adler, M. (1999). Persistence of botulinum neurotoxin action in cultured spinal cord cells. *FEBS Lett.*, **456**, 137–42.

53. Fernandez-Salas, E., Steward, L. E., Ho, H., Garay, P. E., Sun, S. W., Gilmore, M. A., Ordas, J. V., Wang, J., Francis, J. and Aoki, K. R. (2004). Plasma membrane localization signals in the light chain of botulinum neurotoxin. *PNAS*, **101**, 3208–13.

54. Hayashi, T., McMahon, H., Yamasaki, S., Binz, T., Hata, Y., Südhof, T. C. and Niemann, H. (1994). Synaptic vesicle membrane fusion complex: action of *Clostridial* neurotoxins on assembly. *EMBO J.*, **13**, 5051–61.

55. Bajohrs, M., Rickman, C., Binz, T. and Davletov, B. (2004). A molecular basis underlying differences in the toxicity of botulinum serotypes A and E. *EMBO Rep.*, **5**, 1090–5.

56. Dolly, J. O. (1997). Therapeutic and research exploitation of botulinum neurotoxins. *Eur. J. Neurol.*, **4**, S5–10.

57. Smith, C. P. and Chancellor, M. B. (2004). Emerging role of botulinum toxin in the management of voiding dysfunction. *J. Urology*, **171**, 2128–37.

58. Brisinda, G., Bentivoglio, A. R., Maria, G. and Albanese, A. (2004). Treatment with botulinum neurotoxin of gastrointestinal smooth muscles and sphincters spasms. *Mov. Disord.*, **19** (Suppl. 8), S146–56.

59. Naumann, M. and Jost, W. (2004). Botulinum toxin treatment of secretory disorders. *Mov. Disord.*, **19** (Suppl. 8), S137–41.

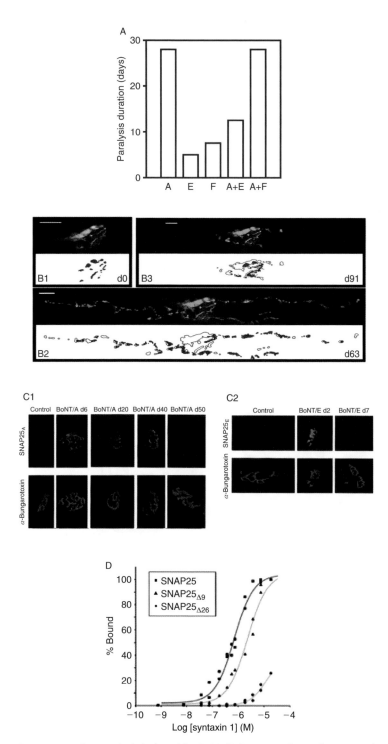

Figure 2.6   Neuromuscular paralysis induced by BoNT/A is very prolonged compared to that produced by other serotypes, accords with the persistence of cleaved SNAP-25 and is accompanied by extensive and reversible remodelling of the end-plates. (A) Extent of paralysis was determined using the toe spread reflex (TSR) assay for mice injected (at day 0) in the hind leg with A, 5 pg BoNT/A; E, 50 pg BoNT/E; F, 4 ng BoNT/F; A+E, 2.5 pg BoNT/A + 25 pg BoNT/E and A+F,

Caption for Figure 2.6 (*cont.*) 2.5 pg BoNT/A + 2 ng BoNT/F, doses that had been predetermined to produce a maximum TSR score in the absence of any other symptoms of botulism. The plotted data indicate the time taken for the TSR score to return to baseline. (B) The lower panels represent localization of a nerve-terminal and its sprouts with the mitochondrial activity dye 4-di-2-ASP (outlined areas) and detection of vesicle-recycling with FM1-43 labelling (solid areas) in mouse sternamastoid muscle before the injection of 0.5 pg BoNT/A haemagglutinin complex (B1), the original terminal and extensive terminal sprouts at day 63 after injection (B2) and, at day 91, the original terminal with sprouts almost fully retracted (B3). The upper panels show composites of the images captured with each dye. (C) The products of SNAP-25 cleavage by BoNT/A (SNAP-25$_A$; C1) or BoNT/E (SNAP-25$_E$; C2) detected in mouse extensor digitorum longus muscles after injection of the requisite neurotoxin. Note that cleavage product can be detected up to 40 days after the injection of BoNT/A, but E-truncated SNAP-25 was removed within a week after administration of BoNT/ E. (D) Increasing amounts of syntaxin 1 were incubated with resin-immobilized full-length SNAP-25 or truncated forms equivalent to the products of SNAP-25 cleavage by BoNT/A (SNAP-25$_{\Delta 9}$) or /E (SNAP-25$_{\Delta 25}$). Bound syntaxin was quantified by Western blotting. From Bajohrs *et al.* (2004).

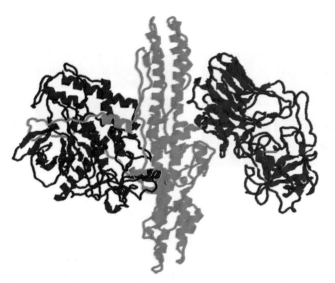

Figure 3.2   Structure and action of the botulinum neurotoxins. The figure shows a representation of the three-dimensional structure of a botulinum neurotoxin. The toxin exerts its neuroparalytic action via a four-step mechanism. Once in the blood stream, domains within the C-terminal portion of the toxin heavy chain (H$_C$ domain, shown in blue) bind to acceptors on the pre-synaptic nerve surface. After binding, the toxin is internalized into endosomes from where it is translocated across the membrane into the cytosol by the translocation domain (H$_N$ domain, shown in green). Once in the cytosol, the light chain (shown in red), which is a highly specific zinc-dependent protease, cleaves and inactivates an essential component of the neuroexocytosis apparatus.

Botulinum toxin: from menace to medicine

Peter Hambleton[1], Andrew M. Pickett[2] and Clifford C. Shone[1]

[1]Health Protection Agency, Porton Down, Salisbury, UK
[2]Ipsen Limited, 190 Bath Road, Slough, UK

3.1 Product development

The neurotoxins produced by the bacterium *Clostridium botulinum* that cause botulism are the most potent acute toxins known. There is no known cure for the flaccid muscular paralysis of botulism and for many people the disease evokes an emotive and fearful view of the toxins. Although rare, botulism is usually encountered as a food-borne disease that results from eating food contaminated with pre-formed toxin. Wound botulism and infant botulism are two other forms of the disease, although unlike food-borne botulism, these intoxications result from direct infection with the bacterium. The incidence of wound botulism has increased in recent years in drug users who inject heroin; infant botulism is now the most common form of the disease reported in the USA. Whilst these various forms of acquired botulism are frightening enough prospects, the toxins are now seen in the even more sinister context of use in weapons of biological warfare or bio-terrorism.

The perception of these potent microbial toxins is changing. Whilst the pharmaceutical industry annually spends many millions of pounds searching for or designing synthetic chemicals that have specific pharmacological activities, with the botulinum neurotoxins, nature has done all the work for us. Over aeons of time a family of molecules have evolved having a unique combination of biological activities that can be used to clinical benefit. Because of their high potency and exquisitely specific pharmacological activity, the botulinum toxins are increasingly being used to treat a range of clinical conditions involving uncontrolled muscle spasm, bringing relief of symptoms to many people for whom there was previously little in the way of effective treatment.

In the late 1960s Dr Alan Scott, an ophthalmologist at the Smith Kettlewell Institute in California was seeking less invasive alternatives to surgery as a means to correct strabismus. The possibility of using botulinum toxin to induce localized

Clinical Uses of Botulinum Toxins, eds. Anthony B. Ward and Michael P. Barnes. Published by Cambridge University Press. © Cambridge University Press 2007.

muscle weakness was raised in discussions with Dr Ed Schantz and in the 1970s Scott demonstrated, initially in non-human primates and in the early 1980s, clinically, the value of injecting small quantities of botulinum toxin into extraocular muscles as a means to treat strabismus[1,2]. The technique caught the imagination of ophthalmologists and neurologists around the world triggering an unusual drug development process. Largely through personal and published communications, the clinical efficacy of botulinum toxin was demonstrated and its use extended well beyond initial applications to include treatment of the symptoms of a range of relatively rare neurological disorders associated with involuntary muscle spasm, specifically focal dystonias[3-5]. Consequently, by the time the first marketing authorizations were granted the clinical therapeutic value of the toxin in treating the symptoms of a wide range of conditions had already become well established.

To meet the early demand for a therapeutic toxin formulation, Scott established Oculinum Inc. and the early formulation of type A toxin, Oculinum®, was granted Orphan Drug status by the US Food and Drug Administration (FDA) in 1978. In 1988, Allergan Inc. acquired the rights to distribute Oculinum® and responsibility for clinical trials to establish the effectiveness of the toxin for other indications. The following year the FDA granted approval for Oculinum® to be marketed in the USA as an orphan drug for the treatment of strabismus. Shortly afterwards, Allergan acquired Oculinum Inc. and successfully applied for FDA approval to change the product name to BOTOX®. In 2000 the indications for BOTOX® use were extended to include cervical dystonia and associated neck pain.

Ophthalmologists at the Moorfields Eye Hospital, London, were among the first clinicians in the UK to seek to apply Scott's new approach to correcting strabismus. Because of the, then, limited supply of Oculinum® they approached the Centre for Applied Microbiology and Research (CAMR) at Porton Down, a major centre of excellence for research on botulinum toxins. CAMR developed a stable freeze-dried type A toxin formulation that was initially supplied only to the Moorfields Eye Hospital but the use of toxin therapy grew rapidly and CAMR toxin was soon being used throughout the UK and in many European countries. CAMR's commercial partners Porton Products (now Ipsen Ltd.) successfully applied for marketing authorization in the UK and in 1990 the formulation Dysport® was approved by the Medicines Control Agency (MCA) for blepharospasm and hemi-facial spasm.

The type A toxin products now have approvals in many territories worldwide for a range of indications that include strabismus, blepharospasm, hemi-facial spasm, spasmodic torticollis, upper limb focal spasticity, treatment of dyskinesias (including cerebral palsy) in children, hyperhidrosis and cosmesis. The headline-grabbing use of toxin for the treatment of glabellar lines and facial hyperkinetic lines (facial wrinkles) has done much to raise awareness in the general public of the clinical value of botulinum toxins. Additionally, the toxins are in clinical studies to treat many, often rare, conditions involving uncontrolled focal muscle spasm. It is remarkable that well over 100 different potential clinical therapeutic applications for botulinum toxins have been described in the literature.

The success of these two products has stimulated the development of other products (Table 3.1). Neurobloc® (Myobloc® in the USA) is a serotype B toxin formulation, manufactured and distributed by Solstice Neurosciences, which is licensed for cervical dystonia. Locally developed type A toxin products are used in China and countries in the Far East. Toxins type C, E and F have also been used in the clinic.

The current product formulations are based on complexes of neurotoxin serotypes with other non-toxin proteins, some of which possess haemagglutination activity[13]. The manufacturing processes used differ for each product but at least one attempt to define the characteristics of therapeutic toxin preparations has been made[14]. It is known (P. Hambleton, unpublished) that purified neurotoxin preparations are effective. Formulations of neurotoxins are being developed and several clinical trials of purified neurotoxin have completed in Europe, sponsored by Merz with the now-licensed product in Germany, Xeomin®. The German company BioteCon have patent applications for the use of purified neurotoxin in treating Type A toxin non-responders (now assigned to Merz) and snoring[15,16]. It remains to be seen whether or not such products would offer clinical and

Table 3.1. *Therapeutic botulinum toxin products*

Toxin serotype	Product	Supplier	Approved indications
A	Dysport®	Ipsen	See text
	BOTOX®	Allergan	See text
	BoNT-A	Available in China	Strabismus, blepharospasm, hemifacial spasm
	Xeomin®	Merz	Focal dystomas
B	Neurobloc®	Solstice Neurosciences	Spasmodic torticollis
	Myobloc®		
C	No approved product	N/A	[a]See Refs 6 and 7
			[a]See Ref. 8
E	No approved product	Wako	
F	No approved product	N/A	[a]See Refs 9–12

[a]Non-approved use.

marketing advantages that would impact on the success of the current generation products. Whilst the relatively long duration of effect of toxin therapy is generally seen to be advantageous, neuromuscular blocking agents with both shorter and longer duration of action might have value; the development of botulinum toxin-based drugs with such properties may present significant scientific challenges.

3.2 Product assay

Product release tests that ensure product quality, safety and efficacy are defined for each approved toxin formulation. Examples of release tests for type A toxins are given in a Ph. Eur. Monograph[14], and a Chinese pharmacopoeial monograph[17]. Arguably, the most important test is that of potency, since this encompasses proof of both product efficacy and safety.

Therapeutic formulations of botulinum toxins are tested for potency using mouse lethality assays, with product activity being expressed in mouse LD_{50} units[18,19]. Such bioassays are inherently variable and although reproducibility can be achieved under stringent conditions, apparently minor differences in assay protocols can lead to significant variation in observed LD_{50}[19−23]. For example, the same number of mouse LD_{50} units of different formulations of type A toxin may not have equivalent biological (clinical) activities which has raised concerns with clinicians[24]. The assay diluent buffer used probably accounts for large differences in potency estimates[18,19] but other factors such as mouse strain, product formulation and assay design may also contribute to the observed differences[25]. Although alternative potency assays have been described (see examples in[21,25]) these may have subjective end points and have not, as yet, replaced the traditional mouse lethality assay. Whilst inter-laboratory variability may be resolved by expressing units of activity relative to that defined by a reference standard[27], it may be that no single bioassay can measure true clinical potency for all toxin formulations or therapeutic applications.

In recent years a number of in vitro assays have been developed to detect and quantify botulinum toxins. Immunoassays are capable of quantifying toxin[28,29] but suffer the disadvantage of not being able to distinguish between biologically active and inactive toxins, making them unsuitable as alternative potency, safety or stability tests[30]. Advances in understanding the molecular structure and mode of action of the botulinum toxins (see Section 3.7) have led to the development of sensitive in vitro quantitative assays of the enzymatic activity of the toxins that provide a basis for reducing the use of animals for potency testing[31]. Indeed, the in vitro enzymatic test for BoNT/A is now used to monitor the potency of clinical formulations[30]. Such progress is encouraging and suggests that it might soon be practicable to use a combination of in vitro assays to quantify the toxin mass and activity of clinical toxin formulations; if the performance of such test combinations could be validated they might replace the current potency bioassays. Bioassays do, however, demonstrate the full biological functionality of toxins (binding to receptors, internalization and enzymic activity) and may have a continuing role in the determination of in vivo activity

3.3   Production of botulinum toxins for clinical use

The manufacture of therapeutic-quality botulinum toxins for clinical use presents a number of challenging issues. The extreme toxicity of the proteins, the hazard categorization of the organism and the requirement to protect production staff from such hazards at all times, means that special measures must be taken to contain and perform production stages that would normally be straightforward to execute. The manufacturing processes themselves are straightforward and high yielding[32], therefore generally only carried out on a small scale. Although the volumes of material handled may be relatively low, the operation of laboratory-scale stages in containment conditions and in accordance with Good Manufacturing Practice (GMP), as required by licensing authorities, is not always straightforward. For example, even simple process steps such as centrifugation require careful risk assessments of exactly how materials are to be moved to and from the equipment, how primary and secondary containment of the processed materials and fractions is to be achieved; even the nature of the equipment to be used must be carefully specified. Detailed guidance is available and helpful[33], but is generally orientated towards the handling of toxin or organism in a clinical laboratory setting.

At all times, the manufacturing process must bring together and merge the GMP and the safety requirements. This is the case for both production of the toxin and for Quality Control testing. Manufacturing sites must meet all the requirements of the licensing authorities for each country where the product is to be marketed. Whilst there is commonality of such standards in Europe, other countries such as the United States and Japan have different emphases upon the common GMP theme. Successful manufacture through compliance with these differing requirements leads to global market access.

Generally, all toxin production equipment is contained within closed, negative pressure units (Figure 3.1) that serve to isolate the organism or the produced toxin from the facility environment and hence, by definition, from the operators. Such containment units have features similar to the equipment employed for the manufacture of cytotoxic drugs by chemical syntheses.

All production and laboratory equipment must go through full validation (from design through to procurement, acceptance, installation, operational and

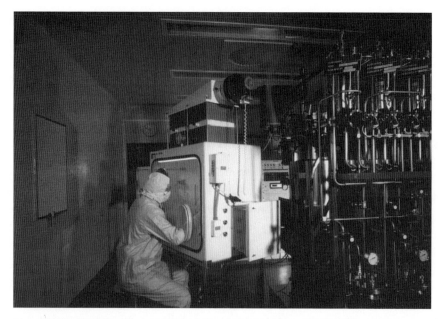

Figure 3.1   Class III microbiological safety cabinet. The safe manufacture of botulinum toxins requires containment of various unit processes in cabinets of this type that operate under negative pressure and provide a secure physical barrier between the product and the operator.

performance testing) to meet GMP. Fortunately, many of the tests performed at each stage are directly and highly applicable to containment and safety issues. Certain additional testing has to be carried out to meet the safety requirements but generally, this can be readily accommodated. Specific attention must be paid to the safe disposal of waste materials from such facilities; specialized equipment such as containment autoclaves and effluent treatment plants may be required, again dependent upon local requirements; exhaust gases from equipment and air from the facility must pass through appropriate sterilizing filters; production areas must be subject to validated rigorous disinfection and cleaning regimes.

The total manufacturing process is governed by a quality systems approach and by defined and inspected quality standards. This means that product made must not only be manufactured under defined and validated conditions that meet regulatory compliance but also must meet appropriate and defined standards of quality, safety, efficacy, purity and potency. Quality control testing is therefore carried out according to the same standards, examining each batch of final bulk toxin or finished dose form product for compliance with the required and approved specifications. Tests will examine potency and efficacy, generally by methods such as the mouse LD_{50} assay (see above); safety (including sterility of finished product) by pharmacopoeial methods; and purity by a series of tests as defined in the individual marketing authorizations. Other tests such as for product identity, examination for degradation products and presence/absence of impurities (such as compounds added during the purification process) may also be required. The monograph from the European Pharmacopoeia[14] specifies these requirements for a type A toxin clinical product.

3.4   Organisms used for clinical toxin manufacture

The strains of *Clostridium botulinum* used for the production of type A therapeutic toxin are likely to originate from those isolated and preserved by Ivan Hall in the early 1900s. Hall was Professor at both the University of California and, later, at the University of Colorado. His highly detailed publications, relating to the study and epidemiology of botulism food poisoning cases, are exceptional for the sheer numbers of organisms that he isolated and preserved. Type A strains he isolated were distributed to colleagues and universities throughout the world and deposited in various culture collections. Nevertheless, over the intervening years as a consequence of the inevitable numerous subcultures performed, any current 'Hall' type A strains may differ in various respects to the original isolates.

Recently, workers at Allergan have published the molecular characteristics of the type A Hall (Allergan) strain used for BOTOX® manufacture[34]. By molecular sequencing, they have demonstrated the gene cluster containing both the type A neurotoxin gene and related proteins which form their active toxin complex. This does not mean, of course, that these are the only components of the toxin complex used in the clinical formulation, as other clostridial proteins may become associated with the active core during production. In a comparison of the neurotoxin gene found in other type A Hall strains, a very high (but not absolute) level of identity and homology was shown, confirming that 'drift' in strains may have occurred.

The European Pharmacopoeia monograph for Type A toxin includes details of the type and degree of characterization of type A toxin-producing strains (seed lots) that is to be expected, including identity, microbial purity, phenotypic and genotypic characteristics. In particular, a requirement has been defined whereby each seed lot must not contain genes encoding other toxin serotypes. This requirement may not be met by certain type A toxin-producing strains as some are known to contain, for example, silent type B neurotoxin genes[35].

The only details available on the type B toxin producing strain employed by Elan for the manufacture of the active component of Myobloc®/Neurobloc® are contained in the prescribing information for the product: the strain is described as the Bean strain.

3.5 Formulation of therapeutic toxin products

The formulation of botulinum toxin into a therapeutic dosage form is a critical stage in the manufacture of a clinical product. The formulation procedure and final content of a therapeutic protein can significantly affect the stability, and even the potential immunogenicity, of the product. Protein formulation has been greatly studied over many years and using sophisticated technology, but in many cases the basic principles are the same. Therapeutic proteins often require the presence of a stabilizing agent, probably another protein and a bulking agent, often a sugar, in the final format. Various combinations of these excipients can be used to improve the storage conditions and extend the shelf life of the product. Products can be preserved frozen, refrigerated or at room temperature, as liquids or solids (possibly freeze dried). All four commercially available toxins are formulated and preserved with different components and in different formats, as shown in Table 3.2.

Generally, lower temperature storage permits a longer shelf life for protein therapeutics but this must be balanced commercially against the inconvenience for users of having to use freezers instead of normal refrigerators and the requirement

Table 3.2. Formulations of commercial botulinum toxins

Product	Toxin type	Dosage form	Unitage (LD_{50} per vial)	Excipients	Storage temperature	Shelf life (months)
DYSPORT®	A	Freeze dried	500	HSA Lactose	2–8°C	24
BOTOX®	A	Vacuum dried	100	HSA Sodium chloride	2–8°C	24
BoNT-A	A	Freeze dried	Variable[a]	Gelatin Dextran Sucrose	−5 to −20°C	36
NEUROBLOC®/ MYOBLOC®	B	Liquid	Variable[b]	HSA Sodium chloride Sodium succinate	2–8°C	36

HSA: human serum albumin.
[a]Different unit preparations are available (50 and 100 LD_{50} units per vial).
[b]Different unit preparations are available (2500 to 10 000 LD_{50} units per vial).

for complex cold-chain distribution systems. The inclusion of protein-rich excipients may also increase shelf life but the inclusion of animal-derived materials should be avoided. The acceptability of the gelatin-containing preparation from China (BoNT-A)[17] may therefore be questionable from this respect.

The use of different formulations and formats for the toxin products, including amino acids, poly-sugars and non-HSA containing formats has been investigated[36]. The use of recombinant HSA has also been examined and found to be an acceptable alternative to the human plasma-derived excipients currently included. Employment of cartridge and pen formats for administration is also a new field of work[36]. Different presentations for clinical use will assist administration, especially where multiple injections are required: typically, for use with treatment of glabellar lines or hyperhidrosis.

3.6 Therapeutic ratio of toxin products

With products of such toxicity, the therapeutic ratio (the ratio between the therapeutic dose and a toxic dose) is of concern. In particular, with toxin-containing products, data such as the LD_{50} for man are clearly not available! Therefore information must be obtained from animal studies and extrapolated to the human.

Gill[36], in his work covering bacterial toxins, indicated that the estimated lethal dose of botulinum toxin for man was approximately 1 ng per kilogram of body weight, equating to 70 ng for an adult of 70 kg body weight. With an estimated toxin content of about 5 ng per 100 LD_{50} units (per vial)[38] this approximates to about fourteen or more vials of BOTOX® product. This work was, however, some considerable time before the therapeutic use of the toxins. Later information published by the United States Food and Drug Administration[39] indicated a lethal i.m. dose in monkeys of 40 BOTOX® units per kilogram body weight, with a comment that 'the toxic dose for humans is estimated to be similar'. Based upon this estimate, again for a 70 kg adult, about 2800 BOTOX® LD_{50} units would be required for lethality in humans, or approximately 28 vials i.m.: clearly, this would not be an issue clinically.

Attempts to demonstrate that the therapeutic ratio for one toxin product may significantly differ from that of another and hence might be considered 'less safe' in clinical use[40–42] fail to take account of the fact that as described earlier, the measured units for one product cannot be extrapolated to another. In this case, the workers used the units labelled for each preparation at the time and did not translate the potency into a common unitage, so invalidating the study.

3.7   The future

3.7.1   Purified neurotoxins for clinical use

The presently available clinical formulations of botulinum toxins contain, in addition to the neurotoxin moiety, various other proteins which make up the toxin complex, the form in which it is secreted from the bacterium. These include the non-toxic, non-haemagglutinin protein (NTNH) and haemagglutinin (HA), the latter which comprises several heterologous subunits[43]. Together with the neurotoxin moiety, these accessory proteins form a large protein complex, which in the case of botulinum serotype A can be up to 900 000 Da. While the NTNH and HA play important roles in the protection and absorption of the neurotoxin from the mammalian gut[44], they are arguably superfluous within a preparation of botulinum toxin which is delivered by injection. Efficient protocols are available for the preparation of the various botulinum neurotoxin serotypes to over 95 per cent purity and hence the development of highly purified neurotoxin formulations for clinical use is a realistic objective.

Purified neurotoxins offer a number of potential advantages over products which contain NTNH and HA protein species. If, as seems likely, there is complete dissociation of the toxin protein complex within the blood, then the reduced size and protein load afforded by administration of purified neurotoxin may be clinically advantageous. The relative simplicity of the purified neurotoxin compared to its protein complex will certainly simplify product characterization and should also improve batch-to-batch reproducibility. In a study to compare the spread of the toxin from the site of injection, no significant difference between the spread of purified toxin compared to that of clinical formulations of the complex toxin was apparent[45]. As mentioned previously (see Section 3.1), clinical studies involving purified neurotoxin are currently have concluded in Europe.

3.7.2   Exploitation of engineered neurotoxin fragments

The neurotoxins of *C. botulinum* have evolved a powerful array of biological activities which are essential for their potent neuroparalytic actions (Figure 3.2). These include highly specific proteases, contained within the light chain of each neurotoxin, which are inhibitors of calcium-mediated secretion and heavy chain domains which bind nerve endings with high specificity and affinity. Modern protein engineering techniques allow these activities to be dissected out and expressed in discrete protein fragments. These fragments, which lack the toxicity of the parent molecule, provide a potential platform for a broad range of novel therapeutic agents.

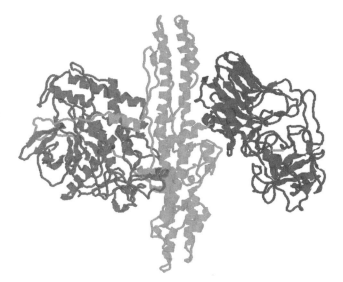

Figure 3.2   Structure and action of the botulinum neurotoxins. The figure shows a representation of the three-dimensional structure of a botulinum neurotoxin. The toxin exerts its neuroparalytic action via a four-step mechanism. Once in the blood stream, domains within the C-terminal portion of the toxin heavy chain (H_C domain, shown in blue) bind to acceptors on the pre-synaptic nerve surface. After binding, the toxin is internalized into endosomes from where it is translocated across the membrane into the cytosol by the translocation domain (H_N domain, shown in green). Once in the cytosol, the light chain (shown in red), which is a highly specific zinc-dependent protease, cleaves and inactivates an essential component of the neuroexocytosis apparatus. (For a colour version of this figure, please refer to the colour insert between pages 26 and 27.)

Exploitation of the light chain

Each of the botulinum neurotoxins contains within its light chain a highly specific zinc-dependent endopeptidase activity which acts on a small protein essential to the neuroexocytosis apparatus. Collectively, the botulinum neurotoxin family act on just three such proteins: vesicle-associated membrane protein (VAMP, also called synaptobrevin), synaptosomal protein of 25 kDa (SNAP-25) and syntaxin[46]. The various isoforms of these proteins form part of a large family of SNARE proteins (SNAP receptors) which act in cognate pairs to direct vesicular traffic within the cell. It is the damage to these proteins caused by the botulinum neurotoxins which results in the often long-lasting blockade of neurotransmitter release.

SNARE proteins are widely distributed and drive intracellular vesicular transport and secretion in both neuronal and non-neuronal cells. That several of the non-neuronal isoforms of VAMP\synaptobrevin and syntaxin are substrates for the botulinum neurotoxins opens up the possibility of extending their therapeutic range. It is the specific neuronal targeting properties of the C-terminal heavy chain region that defines the primarily neuroparalytic activity of the native botulinum toxins and modification of the targeting property of the native neurotoxins opens up the possibility of modulating secretion from selected cell populations. A variety of studies have demonstrated the susceptibility of non-neuronal secretory processes to the action of the clostridial neurotoxins including: the inhibition of insulin secretion from insulinoma cell lines[47], enzyme secretion from pancreatic acinar cells[48] and glucose uptake from adipocytes[49]. More recently, constructs have been designed to enable the targeted delivery of botulinum neurotoxin fragments to cells. In these constructs, the catalytically active light chain and translocation (N-terminal portion of the heavy chain) domains are retained while the C-terminal heavy chain receptor-binding domains are removed and substituted with alternative targeting ligands. Successful delivery of neurotoxin fragments and inhibition of secretion has been achieved using both nerve growth factor and wheat germ agglutinin as targeting ligands to block noradrenaline release from PC12 cells[50]. The wheat germ agglutinin construct was also effective in targeting HIT-T15 cells and blocking the stimulated release of insulin[51].

The above research paves the way for the development of a range of constructs designed to modulate secretion from a designated cell type. For the development of novel therapeutics to be successful, however, constructs must as far as possible mimic two key characteristics of the native neurotoxin: potency and longevity of action. The extremely high potency of the native botulinum neurotoxins allows very low therapeutic doses of only a few ng to be used and unwanted immune responses are relatively rare. If the potency of a novel toxin-derived therapeutic were to be significantly reduced compared to the native toxin, then immune responses may become problematic as a consequence of the increased doses required to obtain a therapeutic effect. Longevity of action is also highly desirable for a therapeutic which is likely to be delivered by injection and, as above, may reduce the likelihood of adverse immune responses. Provided these issues can be overcome, retargeted neurotoxin fragments may provide the means of treating a range of diseases where hyper-secretion is the underlying cause. Existing programmes of work to develop such therapeutics are described below.

Therapeutics for the treatment of chronic pain

Pain signals arise primarily from the activation of small diameter neurons known as A_δ and C-fibres and which have their cell bodies in the dorsal root ganglia that lie adjacent to the spinal cord. Signals transmitted from the periphery through synapses in the spinal cord to the brain lead to the sensation of pain. Severe chronic and neurogenic pain are poorly treated by existing drugs such as morphine, for which tolerance can quickly develop; there is an urgent need for novel and effective pain therapies.

While the native botulinum neurotoxins are potent inhibitors of neurotransmission from pain-conducting neurons[52], they are not selective for these neurons and block transmission from motor neurons even more efficiently[53]. The native neurotoxins, administered by intrathecal injection, are therefore likely to have poor safety profile as therapeutics for treatment of chronic pain. Recently, a programme of research has been undertaken to produce neurotoxin-derived drugs which are selective for the A_δ and C-fibres. In these studies, constructs were produced in which the native neurotoxin receptor-binding domain (Figure 3.2, shown in blue) was replaced with a lectin from *Erythrina cristagalli*[53]. The latter selectively binds A_δ and C-fibres compared to motor neurons and constructs were shown to block neurotransmitter release from cultures of dorsal root ganglia. Pain models, in which C-fibre function was assessed by in vivo electrophysiology, demonstrated these constructs to be effective analgesics[53]. Further studies are now required to enable the clinical development of these compounds.

Therapeutics for the treatment of allergy

IgE-induced secretion of various vasoactive amines, prostaglandins and leukotrienes from mast cells and basophils is the principle cause of acute allergy. Inhibition of secretion from these cells may therefore provide a mechanism for attenuating allergic responses. Early stage research to investigate the efficacy of IgE-targeted botulinum fragments to block secretion from mast cells and basophils is presently in progress[54].

3.7.3   Exploitation of the heavy chain

The heavy chain of botulinum neurotoxins (shown in green and blue in Figure 3.2) acts as an efficient neuronal delivery vector for the light chain warhead. Removal of the light chain renders the remaining fragment non-toxic leaving a potential neuronal delivery vehicle for drugs/macromolecules. Neuronal binding fragments derived from the clostridial neurotoxins possess a number of properties that make them attractive candidates from which to develop a range of novel delivery vectors: they bind their receptors with high affinity ($K_d < 10^{-9}$ M), they are specific for neuronal cells, and the targeted receptors are internalized into nerve endings. Also, since each neurotoxin serotype binds to a different pool of receptors, as a group they offer access to several distinct neuronal-specific markers. The isolated heavy chains of the clostridial neurotoxins also contain, in addition to the binding domain, a translocation domain which may aid the transport of drugs/macromolecules to the neuronal cytosol. Fragments derived from tetanus toxin also have an additional property in that they undergo efficient retrograde transport from the peripheral to the central nervous system and may have utility as vehicles to transport substances across the blood–brain barrier.

A number of studies have demonstrated the usefulness of the clostridial neurotoxins as neuronal delivery vectors and two strategies have evolved. The first is the use of the isolated heavy chain or C-terminal H_C fragments of the toxin as the targeting fragment. Studies using diphtheria toxin, in which the natural binding domain was replaced with tetanus toxin H_C fragment, showed the resulting hybrid to be a potent neuronal specific cytotoxic agent[55]. The H_C fragment of tetanus toxin has also been shown to be effective at targeting adenovirus[56] and condensed DNA[57] to neuronal cells albeit with relatively low efficiency. A construct consisting of a botulinum type A heavy chain coupled to a dextran has also been proposed as a potential drug delivery vehicle and shown to deliver fluorescent makers to neuronal cells[58].

A second strategy to exploit the clostridial neurotoxins as delivery vectors is to use whole toxin in which the light chain has been inactivated by mutagenesis. The payload is then fused to the inactive light chain portion of this vector. Neuronal delivery vector based on both botulinum toxin type A and tetanus toxin have been designed using this strategy[59,60]. Inactive botulinum neurotoxins have also been proposed as carriers for oral vaccines by virtue of their ability to cross gut and airway epithelial layers[61,62].

While the clostridial neurotoxins have significant potential for the delivery of therapeutics to the nervous system, a programme of work with a clear clinical target has yet to emerge.

REFERENCES

1. Scott, A. B., Rosenbaum, A. L. and Collins, C. C. (1973). Pharmaceutical weakening of extraocular muscles. *Invest. Ophthalmol.*, **12**, 924–7.
2. Scott, A. B. (1979). Botulinum toxin injection into extraocular muscles as an alternative to strabismus surgery. *Ophthalmol.*, **87**, 1044–9.
3. Marsden, C. D. and Quinn, N. P. (1990). The dystonias. Neurological disorders affecting 20,000 people in Britain. *Brit. Med. J.*, **300**, 139–44.
4. Jankovic, J. and Brin, M. F. (1991). Therapeutic uses of botulinum toxin. *New Engl. J. Med.*, **324**, 1186–94.
5. Jankovic, J. and Hallett, M. (eds.) (1994). *Therapy with Botulinum Toxin.* New York: Marcel Dekker Inc.
6. Eleopra, R., Tugnoli, V., Rossetto, O., Montecucco, C. and De Grandis, D. (1997). Botulinum neurotoxin serotype C: a novel effective botulinum toxin therapy in humans. *Neurosci. Lett.*, **224**, 91.

7. Eleopra, R., Tugnoli, V., Quatrale, R., Gastaldo, E., Rossetto, O., De Grandis, D. and Motecucco, C. (2002). *Clin. Neurophysiol.*, **113**, 1258−64.

8. Eleopra, R., Tugnoli, V., Rossetto, O., De Grandis, D. and Motecucco, C. (1998). Different time courses of recovery after poisoning with botulinum neurotoxin serotypes A and E in humans. *Neuroscience Lett.*, **256**, 135−8.

9. Chen, R., Karp, B. I. and Hallett, M. (1998). Botulinum toxin type F for treatment of dystonia: long term experience. *Neurology*, **51**, 1494−6.

10. Tugnoli, V., Marchese Ragona, R., Eleopra, R., De Grandis, D. and Montecucco, C. (2001). Treatment of Frey Syndrome with botulinum toxin type F. *Arch. Otolaryngol. Head Neck Surg.*, **127**, 339−40.

11. Sheean, G. L. and Lees, A. J. (1995). Botulinum toxin F in the treatment of torticillis clinically resistant to botulinum toxin A. *J. Neurol. Neurosurg. Psychiatry*, **59**, 601−7.

12. Greene, P. E. and Fahn, S. (1996). Response to botulinum toxin F in seronegative botulinum toxin A-resistant patients. *Movement Disorders*, **14**, 181−4.

13. Melling, J., Hambleton, P. and Shone, C. C. (1988). *Clostridium botulinum* toxins: nature and preparation for clinical use. *Eye*, **2**, 16−23.

14. Botulinum toxin type for injection. European Pharmacopoeia 5.8 (2007), 01/2005: 2113.

15. Bigalke, H. and Frevert, J. (1999). PCT patent application (PCT/DE00/0177) Therapeutic agent comprising a botulinum neurotoxin.

16. Bigalke, H. and Frevert, J. (1998). German patent application (DE19856897) Therapy for the control of snoring noises.

17. Requirements for Botulinum Toxin A for Therapeutic Use (2000). *Pharmacopoeia of the Peoples Republic of China*, 314−18.

18. McLellan, K., Gaines Das, R. E., Ekong, T. A. N. and Sesardic, D. (1996). Therapeutic botulinum type A toxin: factors affecting potency. *Toxicon*, **34**, 975−85.

19. Hambleton, P. and Pickett, A. M. (1994). Dose equivalence of botulinum toxin preparations (Letter). *J. R. Soc. Med.*, **87**, 719.

20. Pearce, L. B., Borodic, G. E., First, E. R. and McCallum, B. D. (1994). Measurement of botulinum toxin activity: evaluation of the lethality assay. *Toxic Appl. Pharmacol.*, **128**, 69−79.

21. Sesardic, D., McLellan, K., Ekong, T. A. N. and Gaines Das, R. E. (1996). Refinement and validation of an alternative bioassay for potency testing of therapeutic botulinum type A toxin. *Pharmac. Toxic.*, **78**, 283−8.

22. Sawtell, J. A. and Ream, A. J. (1995). Observations on the effect of the diluent used for diluting challenge toxin the clostridium botulinum potency assay. *Biologicals*, **23**, 249−51.

23. Schantz, E. J. and Kautter, D. A. (1978). Microbiological methods: standardization assay for *Clostridium botulinum* toxins. *J. Ass. Analyt. Chem.*, **61**, 96−9.

24. Brin, M. F. and Blitzer, A. (1993). Botulinum toxin: dangerous terminology errors (Letter). *J. R. Soc. Med.*, **86**, 493−4.

25. Sesardic, D. (2002). Alternatives in testing of bacterial toxins and antitoxins. In F. Brown, C. Hendrikson, D. Sesardic and K. Cussler, eds., Advancing science and elimination of the use of laboratory animals for development and control of vaccines and hormones. *Dev. Biol. Stand.*, **111**, 101−8.

26. Peng, K., Merlino, G., Addeo, J., Foster, S., Spanoyannis, A. and Aoki, K. R. (1998). Botox® is six-fold more potent than Dysport® in the Mouse Digit Abduction Scoring Assay Movement Disorder Society 50th International Congress of Parkinson's Disease and Movement Disorders P2.102.

27. Sesardic, D., Gaines Das, R. E. and Corbel, M. J. C. (1997). Botulinum toxin. *J. R. Soc. Med.*, **87**, 307.

28. Shone, C. C., Appleton, N., Wilton-Smith, P., Hambleton, P., Modi, N., Gatley, S. and Melling, J. (1986). *In vitro* assays for botulinum toxins and antitoxins. In I. Davidson and W. Hennessen, eds., Reduction of animal usage in the development and control of biological products. *Dev. Biol. Stand.* Basel: Karger, **64**, 141−5.

29. Ekong, T. A. N., McLellan, K. and Sesardic, D. (1995). Immunological detection of *Clostridium botulinum* toxin type A in therapeutic preparations. *J. Immun. Methods*, **180**, 181−91.

30. Sesardic, D. (2002). Alternatives in testing of bacterial toxins and antitoxins. In F. Brown, C. Hendrikson, D. Sesardic and K. Cussler, eds., Advancing science and elimination of the use of laboratory animals for development and control of vaccines and hormones. Basel: Karger, **111**, 101−8.

31. Hallis, B., James, B. A. F. and Shone, C. C. (1996). Development of novel assays for botulinum type A and B neurotoxins based on their endopeptidase activities. *J. Clin. Microbiol.*, **34**, 1934−8.

32. Schantz, E. J. and Johnson, E. A. (1992). Properties and use of botulinum toxin and other microbial neurotoxins in medicine. *Microbiological Reviews*, **56**(1), 80−99.

33. The Management, Design and Operation of Microbiological Containment Laboratories HSE Books, 2001, ISBN 0717620344.

34. Li Zhang, Wei-Jen Lin, Shengwen Li and Roger Aoki, K. (2003). Complete DNA sequences of the botulinum neurotoxin complex of *Clostridium botulinum* type A-Hall (Allergan) strain. *Gene*, **315**, 21−32.

35. Bradshaw, M., Dineen, S. S. and Johnson, E. A. (2001). Regulation of Botulinum Neurotoxin Expression reviewed in Annual Report of the University of Wisconsin Food Research Institute, **2001**, 13−15.

36. Hunt, T. J. (2000). PCT patent application (PCT/US01/03641) Botulinum Toxin Pharmaceutical Compositions.

37. Gill, D. M. (1982). Bacterial toxins: a table of lethal amounts. *Microbiological Reviews*, **46**(1), 86−94.

38. Prescribing information for BOTOX® (Botulinum Toxin Type A) Purified Neurotoxin Complex, July 2002.

39. Food and Drug Administration Medical Officer's review of BOTOX® submission for treatment of glabellar facial lines, November 9, 2001 and March 4, 2002, page 10 (as published by FDA).

40. Aoki, K. R. (1999). Preclinical update on Botox (botulinum toxin type A)-purified neurotoxin complex relative to other botulinum toxin preparations. *European Journal of Neurology*, **6**(Suppl. 4), S3–S10.

41. Aoki, K. R. and Wheeler, L. (2000). A comparison of the efficacy and safety of Botox® and Dysport® in mice. *Movement Disorders*, **15**(Suppl. 3), 35.

42. Aoki, K. R. and Guyer, B. (2001). Botulinum toxin type A and other botulinum toxin serotypes: a comparative review of biochemical and pharmacological actions. *European Journal of Neurology*, **8**(Suppl. 5), 21–9.

43. Inoue, K., Fujinaga, Y., Watanabe, T., Ohyama, T., Takeshi, K., Moriishi, K., Nakajima, H., Inoue, K. and Oguma, K. (1996). Molecular composition of *Clostridium botulinum* type A progenitor toxins. *Infect. Immun.*, **64**, 1589–94.

44. Ohishi, I., Sugii, S. and Sakaguchi, G. (1977). Oral toxicities of *Clostridium botulinum* in reponse to molecular size. *Infect. Immun.*, **16**, 107–9.

45. Dodd, S. L., Rowell, B. A., Vrabas, I. S., Arrowsmith, R. J. and Weatherill, P. J. (1998). A comparison of the spread of three formulations of neurotoxin A as determined by effects on muscle function. *Eur. J. Neurol.*, **5**, 181–6.

46. Schiavo, G., Matteoli, M. and Montecucco, C. (2000). Neurotoxins affecting neuro-exocytosis. *Physiol. Rev.*, **80**, 717–66.

47. Boyd, R. S., Duggan, M. J., Shone, C. C. and Foster, K. A. (1995). The effect of botulinum neurotoxins on the release of insulin from insulinoma cell lines HIT-15 and RINm5F. *J. Biol. Chem. (Commun.)*, **270**, 18216–18.

48. Gaisano, H. Y., Sheu, L., Foskett, J. K. and Trimble, W. S. (1994). Tetanus toxin light chain cleaves a vesicle-associated membrane protein (VAMP) isoform-2 in rat pancreatic zymogen granules and inhibits secretion. *J. Biol. Chem.*, **269**, 17062–6.

49. Chen, F., Foran, P., Shone, C. C., Foster, K., Melling, J. and Dolly, O. (1997). Botulinum type B inhibits insulin-stimulated glucose uptake into adipocytes and cleaves cellubrevin unlike type A toxin which failed to proteolyze the SNAP-23 present. *Biochemistry*, **36**, 5719–28.

50. Chaddock, J. A., Purkiss, J. R., Duggan, M. J., Quinn, C. P., Shone, C. C. and Foster, K. A. (2000a). A conjugate composed of nerve growth factor and a non-toxic derivative of botulinum neurotoxin type A can inhibit neurotransmitter release *in vitro*. *Growth Factors*, **18**, 147–55.

51. Chaddock, K., Purkiss, J., Friss, L., Broadbridge, J., Duggan, M., Shone, C., Quinn, C. and Foster, K. (2000b). Inhibition of neurotoxin release by a retargeted endopeptidase derivative of *C. botulinum* type A. *Infect. Immun.*, **68**, 2587–93.

52. Welch, M. J., Purkiss, J. R. and Foster, K. A. (2000). Sensitivity of embryonic rat dorsal root ganglia neurons to *Clostridium botulinum* neurotoxins. *Toxicon*, **38**, 245–58.

53. Duggan, M. J., Quinn, C. P., Chaddock, J., Purkiss, J. R., Alexander, F., Doward, S., Fooks, S. J., Friis, L., Hall, Y., Kirby, E., Leeds, N., Moulsdale, H. J., Dickenson, A., Green, M., Rahman, W., Suzuki, R., Shone, C. C. and Foster, K. A. (2002). Inhibition of release of neurotransmitters from rat dorsal root ganglia by a novel conjugate of a *Clostridium botulinum* toxin A endopeptidase fragment and *Erythrina cristagalli* lectin. *J. Biol. Chem.*, **277**, 34846–52.

54. Bigalke, H. and Frevant, J. (2003). US patent application (US2003059912): Hybrid *protein* for inhibiting the degranulation of mastocytes and the use thereof.

55. Francis, J. W., Brown, R. H., Figueiredo, D., Remington, M. P., Castillo, O., Schwarzschild, M. A., Fishman, P. S., Murphy, J. R. and vanderSpec, J. C. (2000). Enhancement of diphtheria toxin potency by replacement of the receptor binding domain with tetanus toxin C-fragment: a potent vector for delivering heterologous proteins to neurons. *J. Neurochem.*, **74**, 2528–36.

56. Schneider, H., Groves, M., Muhle, C., Reynolds, P. N., Knight, A., Themis, M., Carvajal, J., Scaravilli, F., Curiel, D. T., Fairweather, N. F. and Coutelle, C. (2000). Retargeting of adenoviral vectors to neurons using the Hc fragment of tetanus toxin. *Gene Ther.*, **18**, 1584–92.

57. Knight, A., Carvajal, J., Schneider, H., Coutelle, C., Chamberlain, S. and Fairweather, N. (1999). Non-viral neuronal gene delivery mediated by the Hc fragment of tetanus toxin. *Eur. J. Biochem.*, **259**, 762–9.

58. Goodnough, M. C., Oyler, G., Fishman, P. S., Johnson, E. A., Neale, E. A., Keller, J. E., Tepp, W. H., Clark, M., Hartz, S. and Adler, M (2002). Development of a neuronal delivery vector for the intracellular transport of botulinum neurotoxin agonists. *FEBS Lett.*, **513**, 163–8.

59. Li, Y., Foran, P., Lawrence, G., Mohammed, N., Chan-Kwo-Chion, C. K., Lis, G., Aoki, R. and Dolly, J. O. (2001). Recombinant forms of tetanus toxin engineered for examining and exploiting neuronal trafficking pathways. *J. Biol. Chem.*, **276**, 31394–401.

60. Dolly, J. O., Wheeler, L. A., Aoki, R. K. and Garst, M. A. (2001). US Patent application (US62003794): Modification of clostridial toxins for use as transporter proteins.

61. Simpson, L. L., Maksymowych, A. B. and Kiyatkin, N. (1999). Botulinum toxin as a carrier for oral vaccines. *Cell. Mol. Life Sci.*, **56**, 47–61.

62. Park, J. B. and Simpson, L. L. (2003). Inhalation poisoning by botulinum toxin and inhalation vaccine with its heavy chain component. *Infect. Immun.*, **71**, 1147–54.

Botulinum toxin: primary and secondary resistance

Benjamin Anyanwu[1], Philip A. Hanna[1] and Joseph Jankovic[2]

[1]New Jersey Neuroscience Institute, JFK Medical Center, Edison, NJ, USA; Seton Hall University School of Graduate Medical Education, South Orange, NJ, USA
[2]Parkinson's Disease Center and Movement Disorders Clinic, Baylor College of Medicine, Houston, Texas, USA

4.1 Introduction

Botulinum toxin (BoNT), the most potent biologic toxin, is a highly effective therapeutic tool in a variety of neurologic and other disorders. In minute doses it has the ability to block Ach release and, therefore, has been exploited to relieve disease symptoms associated with muscle hyperactivity. Intramuscular injection of BoNT produces a chemodenervertion at the neuromuscular junction that results in reversible partial paralysis. While used primarily for conditions characterized by abnormal, excessive, or inappropriate muscle contractions[1,2], BoNT is also increasingly used in the management of a variety of ophthalmologic, urologic, gastrointestinal, orthopedic, cosmetic and dermatologic disorders[2-4].

As the use of BoNT continues to increase, the antigenicity of BoNT and development of immunoresistance secondary to blocking antibodies has continued to be a pressing concern. A certain percentage of patients receiving repeated injections develop blocking antibodies (immunoresistance) against BoNT (BoNT-Abs) causing them to be completely resistant to the effects of subsequent BoNT injections[5-12]. This is termed secondary resistance. Primary resistance refers to lack of response to initial BoNT treatment, which is extremely rare, and may be due to pre-existing BoNT-Abs, possibly as a result of prior immunization against botulism. The frequency of neutralizing or blocking antibodies (immunoresistance) against BoNT is not known. This lack of information is partly due to a paucity of well-designed epidemiological studies utilizing appropriate assays to determine the frequency of blocking antibodies in a prospectively followed population of BoNT-treated patients. Furthermore, nearly all published data on secondary resistance to BoNT-A (BOTOX®) is based on studies of the original

Clinical Uses of Botulinum Toxins, eds. Anthony B. Ward and Michael P. Barnes. Published by Cambridge University Press. © Cambridge University Press 2007.

preparation of BOTOX®, used until 1998 rather than the currently used preparation (see below)[12]. These studies reported the frequency of antibodies to be as low as 4.3 per cent[6] and as high as 10 per cent[13]. Still unpublished data, reported only in the labeling information, showed that 33 of 192 (17%) patients previously treated with the original BOTOX® for cervical dystonia had BoNT-Abs[14]. In another study involving 446 patients treated with BoNT-B (MYOBLOC™) 18 per cent developed BoNT-Abs after 18 months of treatment[15].

Some of the more common causes of clinical failure include such factors as patient selection. For example, although it is estimated that at least 80 per cent of patients with primary cervical dystonia have a moderate or marked improvement after BoNT treatment, post traumatic cervical dystonia manifested chiefly by neck spasms and shoulder elevation without dystonic tremor probably represent a distinct disorder that is relatively resistant to BoNT injections[16]. In addition, inappropriate selection of injection sites, inadequate dose, and decreased potency due to drug handling and denaturing of the protein can also result in clinical failure. Furthermore, some patients may have overactivity of muscles that are very difficult to inject because of inaccessible anatomic location. Also, contractures and skeletal abnormalities may also limit the efficacy of BoNT. Finally, patients may have unrealistic expectations, including the anticipation of complete resolution of the abnormal movements or symptoms after the first injection. For the purposes of this chapter, we will focus on therapy failure due to immunoresistance.

4.2 Primary resistance

Pre-existing immunoresistance has been postulated as a possible cause of primary response failure, but this is very unlikely and BoNT-Abs are rare even in patients surviving botulism. Also, there has been debate as to whether chronic exposure to BoNT in childhood botulism can produce stable BoNT antibody titers. Cross-reactivity with other antibodies such as tetanus toxin antibodies have also been postulated, but could not be detected in control series[17]. Historically, neutralizing antibodies have been used for the treatment and prevention of botulism. While we are not aware of specific instances where primary resistance was clearly linked to prior immunization to botulism, there may be a subset of patients in which prior immunization may lead to subsequent resistance to the therapeutic use of botulinum toxin.

Botulinum toxin type B (BoNT-B) therapy failure due to formation of BoNT type B antibodies (BoNT-B-Abs) had only been reported in patients with botulinum toxin type A antibodies (BoNT-A-Abs). However, two patients with no apparent previous exposure to BoNT have been found to have evidence of BoNT-B-Abs[18]. In the first patient, complete therapy failure occurred after a single exposure to 14 400 mouse units (MU) BoNT-B (NeuroBlock®). The mouse diaphragm assay (MDA) revealed a BoNT-B-AB titer in excess of $10\,mU\,ml^{-1}$. No effect was elicited with doubling the BoNT-B dose. In the second patient, a single exposure to 7200 MU BoNT-B led to a complete therapy failure. MDA testing revealed a BoNT-B-AB tite in excess of $10\,mU\,ml^{-1}$. Again, doubling the BoNT-B dose did not elicit any effects. However, application of 180 MU BoNT-A (BOTOX®) produced the original response on three consecutive occasions. Although BoNT-AB formation can occur after a single exposure to BoNT, this is highly unusual. Dressler and colleagues[19] concluded that since therapy failure occurred after the first-ever BoNT exposure, short intervals between injections as well as use of booster injections can be excluded as causes for BoNT-B-AB formation in both patients and therefore a more likely cause may be the substantially higher amount of antigenic protein administered with the BoNT-B therapy[19].

4.3 Secondary resistance

Secondary resistance, although now quite rare, is still the most likely cause of treatment failure. By definition, patients who develop secondary resistance have shown prior clinical response to BoNT, but subsequently lose the benefit. Although the mechanisms of secondary resistance are now well understood, we review here the relevant data about the immunology of BoNT.

Clinically used BoNT consists of neurotoxin, the protein responsible for BoNT toxic or therapeutic effect in combination with a large number of non-toxic proteins[20]. All of those proteins are antigens capable of inducing antibody production. The clinically relevant BoNT-Abs are those that reduce the therapeutic action of BoNT by interfering with its binding to the presynaptic membrane receptor, hence the term 'blocking' or 'neutralizing' antibodies.

4.4 Developing resistance

There are many factors that determine antigenicity of BoNT, including the amount of complex protein. In contrast to the original BOTOX® (lot 79–11), which contained 25 ng of neurotoxin complex protein per 100 units, the current BOTOX® preparation (2024), approved by the FDA in 1997, and utilized in clinical practice since 1998, contains only 5 ng of the complex protein per 100 units[21]. The two preparations seem to have similar efficacy and adverse effect profile[12,22–24]. The current BOTOX® has been shown to have less antigenicity than the original preparation when tested in rabbits[21]. In one multicenter, retrospective analysis of 191 randomly selected patients with cervical dystonia who had received at least two consecutive treatments with original BOTOX®, followed by at least three consecutive treatments with current BOTOX®, the mean doses of original and current BOTOX® were comparable (245 and 250 units, respectively). Using the current BOTOX®, patients were exposed to less neurotoxin complex protein (~12 ng/250 units) than with the original (~61 ng/245 units) formulation. Response rate per period averaged 90 per cent for both original and current BOTOX®. Adverse events of any type were reported by an average of 14.4 per cent of patients per period receiving original BOTOX® compared to an average of 19.4 per cent of patients per period receiving current BOTOX®. The conclusion of the study was that the efficacy and safety of current US BOTOX® were comparable to original BOTOX® in the treatment of cervical dystonia and that the treatment with current BOTOX® results in lower exposure to neurotoxin complex protein and may therefore result in reduced antigenicity compared to treatment with original BOTOX®[12].

There is compelling evidence that the lower risk of BoNT-Abs formation with the current BoNT type A compared to the original BoNT type A (used before 1998) may be attributed to the lower protein load in the current BoNT type A. In a study comparing the efficacy and immunogenicity of the original and the current BoNT type A in the treatment of cervical dystonia, 4 of 42 (9.5%) patients treated with the original BoNT type A developed detectable blocking antibodies, as against none of the 119 patients treated with the current BoNT type A exclusively[12].

The appearance of BoNT-Abs responses is closely linked to duration of treatment and frequency. Greene et al.[6] found that BoNT resistant patients had a shorter interval between injections, more 'boosters,' as well as a higher dose at the 'non-booster' injection as compared to non-resistant patients treated during the same period. Thus clinicians are warned against using booster injections and are encouraged to extend the interval between treatments as long as possible, certainly at least 2 months, and to use the smallest possible doses. We and others have observed that typically if immunoresistance does develop, it tends to occur within the first 1–4 years of treatment, and BoNT-AB formation seems less likely after this treatment period.

In addition to the quantity of antigens, the quality of antigens can affect the immunogenic properties of a protein. Important determinants of these properties include:

(1) the presence of foreign proteins, whose role is to enhance the immune response or act as adjuvants, without affecting its efficacy;

(2) such intrinsic properties, as size, shape or subunits of the proteins;

(3) the presence of denatured antigen, given that denaturation of proteins causes various degrees of conformational changes and may change the regions that are recognized by the immune system;

(4) the presence of polymerized antigens as these may enhance the immuno-genicity of small proteins; and

(5) changes of the covalent structure which often can drastically alter the antigenic properties of proteins, as in cleavage of disulfide bonds, in certain proteins[25].

Unnicked or 'nonactivated,' single chain, neurotoxin may also contribute to the overall neurotoxin protein load without contributing to the therapeutic efficacy of the BoNT. In this regard, it is notable that BoNT-A (and BoNT-F) are released in the nicked form whereas the nicking in BoNT-B is more variable depending on the strain and preparation.

Besides overall protein load, another factor that may contribute to the development of antibodies is serum cross-reactivity between different BoNT serotypes. Although traditionally considered immunologically distinct, the different BoNT serotypes share a remarkable homology in the various epitopes[26]. Epitopes are small (6–8 amino acid residues) components of the protein that have distinct boundaries, occupy surface locations and are limited in number. The antibody response to each epitope is under separate genetic control and therefore varies with the host. T-cells, under H-2 gene control (explain H-2, etc.), also recognize the epitopes recognized by antibodies, but may in addition recognize other sites to which antibodies have not been mounted. Because of the marked homology (in some cases involving up to 13 residues), there is a strong possibility that BoNT-Abs directed against one type of BoNT can also cross-react and cross-neutralize other BoNT serotypes.

Previous studies have shown that in a set of homologous proteins, the regions of immune recognition occur at structurally equivalent locations[27]. For instance the tetanus toxin and BoNT-Abs show extensive homology[26] and, therefore, it is expected that these proteins would show significant immunological cross-reactivity. Certain serotypes of BoNT, such as A, B, C1, and E, can cross react with tetanus toxin[28]. While there is no evidence that immunization against tetanus increases the risk of BoNT-Abs, cross-reactivity with tetanus has been offered as a possible explanation for the detection of BoNT-B antibodies in rare individuals even without exposure to BoNT-B[29,30]. Mice treated with BoNT-A fragments develop antibodies that cross-reacted with other serotypes[31]. In one study, patients with spasticity who received BoNT-A produced measurable titers of antibodies against several other serotypes[29]. Further studies are needed to determine whether immunoresistance to one type of BoNT increases the risk of developing blocking antibodies to another type of BoNT, but the practice of alternating between two different BoNT serotypes suggested by some may increase the risk of immunoresistance to both. Finally, it should be noted that there are many other factors, besides protein antigenicity and protein load, such as the patient's immunologic status, that play a role in determining whether a patient develops blocking antibodies or not.

4.5 Detecting antibodies

Several in-vitro as well as in-vivo techniques have been developed to detect BoNT antibodies, but the in vivo mouse protection assay (MPA) is considered the 'gold standard' for detecting neutralizing (blocking) antibodies[32]. This assay evaluates the ability of increasing dilutions of a patient's serum to protect experimental mice from lethal test doses of BoNT. Four Swiss Webster mice are injected intraperitoneally with a mixture of lethal dose of BoNT and patient's test serum. If at least three of the four mice die, this indicates absence of blocking antibodies. The presence of antibodies in the test serum is indicated if there are no deaths or only one mouse dies, suggesting that the mice were protected by blocking antibodies in the patient's serum. Using the MPA assay, we compared 22 randomly selected BoNT antibody negative patients with 20 patients who were immunoresistant and found that the resistant patients had an earlier age at onset (mean age: 31.8 ± 16.7 vs. 43.4 ± 10.5; $P < 0.05$), higher mean dose per visit (249.2 ± 32.5 vs. 180.8 ± 68.7, $P < 0.0005$), and higher total cumulative dose (mean dose: 1709 ± 638 vs. 1066 ± 938; $P < 0.01$).

Another assay for BoNT-AB is the mouse protection assay of the diaphragm (MPDA), also referred to as the mouse diaphragm assay (MDA)[33]. In the MDA assay, the left phrenic nerve and the left hemi diaphragm are excised from a mouse and placed in an organ bath[33]. The phrenic nerve is then stimulated and isometric contractions are recorded with a force transducer. The time required for reduction of the twitch amplitude by 50 per cent is called 'paralysis time'. If the paralysis time is outside of 2 standard deviations of the mean paralysis time of the control population the test result is considered positive. The MDA has a potential advantage over the MPA in that it requires only one mouse per sample tested, and the results can be available within hours. The concordance between the MPA and the MDA, however, is only 63 per cent and further studies are needed to determine the relative sensitivity and specificity of the MDA assay.

The clinical utility of in-vitro assays such as the western blot assay (WBA) and patient-based clinical tests such as the frontalis-type A test (F-TAT) or unilateral brow injection (UBI) in the detection of BoNT-AB has been studied extensively. Some of these assays apart from utilizing in vitro rather than in vivo techniques may have an advantage over the MPA as they appear to be more sensitive. We compared the MPA assay to the Western blot assay (WBA) in detecting antibodies (Ab) against BoNT-B and correlated the assay results with clinical responses to BoNT-A injections[10]. MPA and WBA were compared in 51 patients

(34 non-responders and 17 responders) who received BoNT-A injections, mainly for cervical dystonia. A subset of patients received a test injection into either the right brow (14) or right frontalis, the frontalis-type A test (F-TAT) (12). In this test 15 U of BoNT-A is administered as two doses of 7.5 U each into the right frontalis muscle. The patient is considered to be type A resistant if they were able to wrinkle both right and left frontalis muscles symmetrically (type-A responsive patient cannot wrinkle the injected right frontalis muscle). Patients who are resistant to BoNT and are injected into the right brow frown symmetrically, whereas responsive patients frown asymmetrically by contracting only the left corrugator/procerus muscle. We prefer injecting the right brow (unilateral brow injection or 'UBI') rather than the frontalis muscle (F-TAT) since some patients have difficulty voluntarily raising their brows and thus their response to a frontalis injection is difficult to determine. Furthermore, the brow injections are more cosmetically acceptable in that the asymmetric responses are present only during voluntary contractions whereas unilateral disappearance of frontal wrinkles may not be desirable. In the UBI test, 20 units of BOTOX® or 1000 units of MYOBLOC™ is injected, by convention, into the right eyebrow. One or two weeks later the patient is instructed to look in the mirror and frown. If the medial eyebrows contract symmetrically this would indicate that the right medial eyebrow muscles (procerus and corrugator) were not paralyzed, thus suggesting immunoresistance. On the other hand, asymmetrical frown indicates unilateral medial brow paralysis, hence no blocking antibodies (Figure 4.1).

The specificity of the MPA was 100 per cent on all three parameters (clinical, eyebrow and frontalis injections) while the WBA specificity was only 71 per cent for clinical response but 100 per cent for both eyebrow and frontalis responses. Sensitivities for both assays were low (33–53%). Of the 16 patients previously antibody positive by MPA, seven became negative on retesting after a mean interval of 33 months (range, 6–93 months). We concluded that UBI and F-TAT correlated well with MPA results and with clinical responses and may have a utility in the evaluation of BoNT non-responders.

Other methods of antibody detection such as the immunoprecipitation assay (IPA), which quantitatively assesses the degree of immunoresistance[34] has been shown to be more sensitive than MPA and may have a predictive value in determining impending or future unresponsiveness[11]. In a study comparing the IPA and MPA for the detection of BoNT-Abs, we found that both assays had high specificity although the sensitivity of IPA was higher than MPA (the sensitivity for the MPA was low; 50 per cent for clinical, 38 per cent for eyebrow and 30 per cent for frontalis responses while the IPA sensitivity was much higher at 84 per cent for clinical ($P < 0.001$), 77 per cent for eyebrow ($P = 0.111$, NS) and 90 per cent for frontalis responses ($P < 0.02$). Additionally, IPA seems to

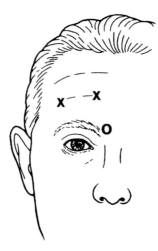

O = 20 Units of BOTOX® or 1,000 Units of MYOBLOC™ (UBI)
X = 10 Units of BOTOX® or 500 Units of MYOBLOC™ (F-TAT)

Figure 4.1   Clinical test for BoNT responsiveness unilateral brow injection (UBI) or frontalis type A toxin or (F-TAT) injection.

display positivity earlier than the MPA and could prognosticate future non-responsiveness. Eyebrow and frontalis 'test' injections also correlated well with clinical and immunological results and are therefore useful in the assessment of BoNT non-responders[11].

In addition to such patient based testing such as the F-TAT and UBI, the extensor digitorum brevis test (EDB test) as well as the sternocleidomastoid test (SCM test) has also been utilized for BoNT-AB detection. In the SCM test, measurement of isometric activation before and after BoNT application is made[35]. Dressler *et al.* found that a reduction of maximal voluntary contraction as measured by EMG of the sternocleidomastoid muscle more than 2 standard deviations below non-disease control values correlated well with BoNT-AB status as measured by the MDA assay. The EDB test employs similar monitoring of motor functioning[36]. The compound muscle action potentials (CMAPS) elicited by electric stimulation of the peroneal nerve before, and a few weeks after, injection of the EDB muscle with BoNT are compared. In patients who are serologically antibody negative, a marked decrease (usually about 50 per cent) in CMAP can be detected in the injected EDB. The test therefore provides a simple quantitative method of detecting resistance to BoNT, with a sensitivity approaching 80 per cent and specificity of nearly 94 per cent.

Another way to test for BoNT immunoresistance is by taking advantage of the observation that BoNT inhibits sweating. Using iodine starch staining and quantified used capacitance hygrometry, this sudometric technique shows that sweating persists in BoNT non-responders after subcutaneous injection of 12.5 U of BoNT-A, whereas this dose quite reliably inhibits sweating in control responders[37]. Unfortunately standardization of this test has been difficult.

Besides WBA and IPA, there are other in-vitro assays, including the SLIDA[38], enzyme-linked immunosorbent assay (ELISA)[39], and a monoclonal antibody-based immunoassay[40], that have been reported to detect BoNT-Abs. However, the presence or absence of antibodies measured by these assays do not correlate well with the observed clinical response.

Dot blot is another in-vitro assay that evaluates patient serum sample for its ability to bind to non-denatured BoNT immobilized on a nitrocellulose membrane in a 96-well format[21]. Strips of nitrocellulose membrane containing duplicate 'dots' of BoNT and appropriate controls are incubated overnight with the diluted sera at 4°C. Standard immunochemical methods are used to visualize captured human immunoglobulins on the nitrocellulose membrane. Positive samples (color development) are then tested with serial dilutions beginning from 1/300 to estimate an antibody titer.

Recently, studies with such primary cell cultures as rat embryonic spinal cord cells have proven to substantially increase the sensitivity of assaying for BoNT-Abs and are capable of detecting as low titers as $2-10\,\mathrm{mU\,ml^{-1}}$. These tests utilize the ability of antisera capable of neutralizing endopeptidase, as well as translocating and cell binding of the toxin, with sensitivity better than the MPA[41].

4.6   Overcoming resistance

A subset of patients who develop BoNT-Abs later become BoNT-AB negative after an average of 30 months (range: $10-78$)[42]. When these BoNT-AB negative patients are re-injected with BoNT-A they usually benefit with a response comparable to their earlier experience. Most, however, lose their clinical response to subsequent injections and when re-tested are found to be antibody positive again. In another study using MDA, Dressler et al.[33] estimated the onset of decrease in antibody titer to occur about $2-5$ years after the last injection, with the average estimated latency to non-detectable levels of 2000 days (5.6 years). This is substantially longer than the estimated duration found in the study by Sankhla et al.[42] and the one-year latency estimated from immunization experiments with pentavalent botulinum toxoid[43]. The difference could be possibly due to the higher doses of BoNT per session (546 U) used by Dressler, and high sensitivity of the MDA.

BoNT-A resistant patients usually benefit from injections with other serotypes of BoNT, such as BoNT-B, BoNT-C or BoNT-F[44-52]. A combination of BoNT-A and BoNT-F used in a double-blind controlled trial of blepharospasm produced no prolongation of the beneficial effect[53]. A recent study[46] demonstrated a high antigenicity of BoNT-B using novel mouse protection assay.

Besides using a different serotype, some investigators have suggested that plasma exchange and immunoabsorption on a protein A column provides an alternative therapy for these secondary non-responders[54]. Furthermore, intravenous immunoglobulin and other methods have been used, largely unsuccessfully, to deplete the BoNT-A antibodies[55]. Finally, mycophenolate, an immunosuppressant commonly used to prevent transplant organ rejection, at 750 mg twice a day starting 48 hours before BoNT treatment and continuing for 10 days, has been reported anecdotally to possibly prevent BoNT antibody formation[56].

Prevention of immunoresistance, by using preparations of BoNT with the lowest possible antigenicity and by keeping the dose per treatment session as low as possible and the inter-dose interval as long as possible (particularly in young women), is of paramount importance in maintaining the beneficial response to this most effective treatment.

REFERENCES

1. Comella, C. L., Jankovic, J. and Brin, M. F. (2000). Use of botulinum toxin type A in the treatment of cervical dystonia. *Neurology*, **55**(Suppl. 5), S15–S21.

2. Jankovic, J. (2004). Botulinum toxin in clinical practice. *J. Neurol. Neurosurg. Psychiatry*, **75**, 951–7.

3. Gracies, J.-M. and Simpson, D. M. (2000). Botulinum toxin therapy. *Neurologist*, **6**, 98–115.

4. Brin, M. F., Hallett, M. and Jankovic, J. (2002). *Scientific and Therapeutic Aspects of Botulinum Toxin*. Philadelphia, PA: Lippincott Williams & Wilkins.

5. Zuber, M., Sebald, M., Bathien, N. *et al.* (1993). Botulinum antibodies in dystonic patients treated with type A botulinum toxin: frequency and significance. *Neurology*, **43**, 1715–18.

6. Greene, P., Fahn, S. and Diamond, B. (1994). Development of resistance to botulinum toxin type A in patients with torticollis. *Mov. Disord.*, **9**, 213–17.

7. Jankovic, J. and Schwartz, K. (1995). Response and immunoresistance to botulinum toxin injections. *Neurology*, **45**, 1743–6.

8. Borodic, G., Johnson, E., Goodenough, M. and Schantz, E. (1996). Botulinum toxin therapy, immunologic resistance, and problems with available materials. *Neurology*, **46**, 26–9.

9. Göschel, H., Wolhfart, K., Frevert, J. *et al.* (1997). Botulinum A toxin therapy: neutralizing and non-neutralizing antibodies – therapeutic consequences. *Experimental Neurology*, **147**, 96–102.

10. Hanna, P. A. and Jankovic, J. (1998). Mouse bioassay versus Western blot assay for botulinum toxin antibodies: correlation with clinical response. *Neurology*, **50**, 1624–9.

11. Hanna, P. A., Jankovic, J. and Vincent, A. (1999). Comparison of mouse bioassay and immunoprecipitation assay for botulinum toxin antibodies. *J. Neurol. Neurosurg. Psychiatry*, **66**, 612–16.

12. Jankovic, J., Vuong, K. D. and Ahsan, J. (2003). Comparison of efficacy and immuno-genicity of original versus current botulinum toxin in cervical dystonia. *Neurology*, **60**, 1186–8.

13. Kessler, K. R., Skutta, M. and Benecke, R. (1999). Long-term treatment of cervical dystonia with botulinum toxin A: efficacy, safety, and antibody frequency. German Dystonia Study Group. *J. Neurol.*, **246**(4), 265–74.

14. BOTOX® (Botulinum Toxin Type A) (2000). Purified Neurotoxin Complex, Product Information, http://www.botox.com/prescribing_info.html.

15. MYOBLOC™ http://www.myobloc.com/product_information/full_prescribing_info.pdf

16. Truong, D. D., Dubinsky, R., Hermanowicz, N. *et al.* (1991). Posttraumatic torticollis. *Arch. Neurol.*, **48**, 221–3.

17. Dolimbek, B. Z., Jankovic, J. and Atassi, M. Z. (2002). Cross reaction of tetanus and botulinum neurotoxins A and B and the boosting effect of botulinum neurotoxins A and B on a primary anti-tetanus antibody response. *Immunol. Invest.*, **31**, 247–62.

18. Dressler, D. (2004). Clinical presentation and management of antibody-induced failure of botulinum toxin therapy. *Mov. Disord.*, **19**(Suppl. 8), S92–S100.

19. Dressler, D. and Bigalke, H. (2004). Antibody-induced failure of botulinum toxin type B therapy in de novo patients. *Eur. Neurol.*, **52**, 132–5.

20. DasGupta, B. R. (1994). Structures of botulinum neurotoxin, its functional domains and perspectives on crystalline type A toxin. In J. Jankovic and M. Hallett, eds., *Therapy with Botulinum Toxin*. New York: Marcel Dekker, pp. 15–40.

21. Aoki, K. R., Merlino, G., Spanoyannis, A. F. and Wheeler, L. A. (1999). BOTOX® (Botulinum Toxin Type A) Purified Neurotoxin Complex prepared from the new bulk toxin retains the same preclinical efficacy as the original but with reduced antigenicity. *Neurology*, **52**(Suppl. 2), A521–2.

22. Benabou, R., Brin, M. F. and Doucette, J. T. (1999). Cervical dystonia: a retrospective study on safety and efficacy of BOTOX lots 79–11 and 2024. *Neurology*, **52**(Suppl. 2), A117–18.

23. Racette, B. A., McGee-Minnich, L. and Perlmutter, J. S. (1999). Efficacy and safety of a new bulk toxin of botulinum toxin in cervical dystonia: a blinded evaluation. *Clin. Neuropharmacol.*, **22**, 337–9.

24. Jankovic, J., Davis, T., Wooten-Watts, M. and the BOTOX Cervical Dystonia Retrospective Study Group. (2005). The safety of BOTOX® (Botulinum Toxin Type A) prepared from new US bulk toxin is comparable to the original in cervical dystonia treatment: a retrospective analysis. *Mov. Disord.*, **15**(Suppl. 2), 31.

25. Atassi, M. Z. (2004). Basic immunological aspects of botulinum toxin therapy. *Mov. Disord.* **19**(Suppl. 8), S68–84.

26. Atassi, M. Z. and Oshima, M. (1999). Structure, activity, and immune (T and B cell) recognition of botulinum neurotoxins. *Critical Reviews Immunol.*, **19**, 219−60.

27. Kazim, A. L. and Atassi, M. Z. (1980). A novel and comprehensive synthetic approach for the elucidation of protein antigenic structures. Determination of the full antigenic profile of the alpha-chain of human haemoglobin. *Biochem. J.*, **191**(1), 261−4.

28. Halpern, J. L., Smith, L. A., Seamon, K. B. *et al.* (1989). Sequence homology between tetanus and botulinum toxins detected by an antipeptide antibody. *Infect. Immun.*, **57**, 13−22.

29. Doellgast, G. J., Brown, J. E., Koufman, J. A. *et al.* (1997). Sensitive assay for measurement of antibodies to *Clostridium botulinum* toxins A, B, and E: use of hapten-labeled-antibody elution to isolate specific complexes. *J. Clin. Microbiol.*, **35**, 578−83.

30. Aoki, K. R. (1999). Preclinical update on BOTOX (botulinum toxin-A)-purified neurotoxin complex relative to other botulinum toxin preparations. *Eur. J. Neurol.*, **6**(Suppl. 4), S3−S10.

31. Dertzbaugh, M. T. and West, M. W. (1996). Mapping of protective and cross-reactive domains of the type A neurotoxin of *Clostridium botulinum*. *Vaccine*, **14**, 1538−44.

32. Hatheway, C. L. and Dang, C. (1994). Immunogenicity of the neurotoxins of *Clostridium botulinum*. In J. Jankovic and M. Hallett, eds., *Therapy with Botulinum Toxin*. New York, NY: Marcel Dekker, Inc., 93−108.

33. Dressler, D., Lange, M., Bigalke, H. (2005). Mouse diaphragm assay for detection of antibodies against botulinum toxin type B. Mov. Disord., **12**, 1617−9.

34. Palace, J., Nairne, A., Hyman, N. *et al.* (1998). A radioimmunoprecipitation asssay for antibodies to botulinum A. *Neurology*, **50**, 1463−6.

35. Dressler, D., Bigalke, H. and Rothwell, J. C. (2000). The sternocleidomastoid test: an in vivo assay to investigate botulinum toxin antibody formation in humans. *J. Neurol.*, **247**, 630−2.

36. Kessler, K. R. and Benecke, R. (1997). The EBD test − a clinical test for the detection of antibodies to botulinum toxin type A. *Mov. Disord.*, **12**(1), 95−9.

37. Birklein, F. and Erbguth, F. (2000). Sudomotor testing discriminates between subjects with and without antibodies against botulinum toxin A − A preliminary observation. *Mov. Disord.*, **15**, 146−9.

38. Siatkowski, R. M., Tyutyunikov, A., Biglan, A. W. *et al.* (1993). Serum antibody production to botulinum A toxin. *Ophthalmology*, **100**, 1861−6.

39. Notermans, S. and Nagel, J. (1989). Assays for botulinum and tetanus toxins. In L. L. Simpson, eds., *Botulinum Neurotoxin and Tetanus Toxin*. San Diego: Academic Press, pp. 319−31.

40. Shone, C., Wilton-Smith, P., Appleton, N. *et al.* (1985). Monoclonal antibody-based immunoassay for type A *Clostridium botulinum* toxin is comparable to the mouse bioassay. *Appl. Environ. Microbiol.*, **50**, 63−7.

41. Hall, Y. H., Chaddock, J. A., Moulsdale, H. J. *et al.* (2004). Novel application of an in vitro technique to the detection and quantification of botulinum neurotoxin antibodies. *J. Immunol. Methods*, **288**, 55−60.

42. Sankhla, C., Jankovic, J. and Duane, D. (1998). Variability of the immunologic and clinical response in dystonic patients immunoresistant to botulinum toxin injections. *Mov. Disord.*, **13**, 150–4.

43. Siegel, L. S. (1988). Human immune response to botulinum pentavalent (ABCDE) toxoid determined by a neutralizing test and by an enzyme-linked immunoabsorbent assay. *J. Clin. Microbiol.*, **26**, 2351–6.

44. Eleopra, R., Tugnoli, V., Quatrale, R. *et al.* (2006). Clinical use of non-A botulinum toxins: botulinum toxin type C and botulinum toxin type F. Neurotox Res., **9**, 127–31.

45. Greene, P. E. and Fahn, S. (1996). Response to botulinum toxin F in seronegative botulinum toxin A-resistant patients. *Mov. Disord.*, **11**, 181–4.

46. Jankovic, J., Hunter, C., Dolimbek, B. Z. *et al.* Clinico-Immunologic Aspects of botulinum toxin type B treatment of cervical dystonia. Neurology (in press).

47. Eleopra, R., Tugnoli, V., Rossetto, O. *et al.* (1997). Botulinum neurotoxin serotype C: a novel effective botulinum toxin therapy in human. *Neurosci. Lett.*, **224**, 91–4.

48. Lew, M. F., Adomato, B. T., Duane, D. D. *et al.* (1997). Botulinum toxin type B (BotB): A double-blind, placebo-controlled, safety and efficacy study in cervical dystonia. *Neurology*, **49**, 701–7.

49. Houser, M. K., Sheean, G. L. and Lees, A. J. (1998). Further studies using higher doses of botulinum toxin type F for torticollis resistant to botulinum toxin type A. *J. Neurol. Neurosurg. Psychiatry*, **64**, 577–80.

50. Chen, R., Karp, B. I. and Hallett, M. (1998). Botulinum toxin type F for treatment of dystonia: long-term experience. *Neurology*, **51**, 1494–6.

51. Brashear, A., Lew, M. F., Dykstra, D. D. *et al.* (1999). Safety and efficacy of Neurobloc (botulinum toxin type B) in type A-responsive cervical dystonia. *Neurology*, **53**, 1439–46.

52. Brin, M. F., Lew, M. F., Adler, C. H. *et al.* (1999). Safety and efficacy of NeuroBloc (botulinum toxin type B) in type A-resistant cervical dystonia. *Neurology*, **53**, 1431–8.

53. Mezaki, T., Kaji, R., Brin, M. F. *et al.* (1999). Combined use of type A and F botulinum toxins for blepharospasm: a double-blind controlled trial. *Mov. Disord.*, **14**, 1017–20.

54. Naumann, M., Toyka, K. V., Taleghani, M. *et al.* (1998). Depletion of neutralizing antibodies resensitizes a secondary nonresponder to botulinum A neurotoxin. *J. Neurol. Neurosurg. Psychiatry*, **65**, 924–7.

55. Dressler, D., Zettl, U., Bigalke, H. and Benecke, R. (2000). Can intravenous immunoglobulin improve antibody mediated botulinum toxin therapy failure? *Mov. Disord.*, **15**, 1279–81.

56. Duane, D., Monroe, J. and Morris, R. E. (2000). Mycophenolate in the prevention of recurrent neutralizing botulinum toxin A antibodies in cervical dystonia. *Mov. Disord.*, **15**, 365–6.

5

Introduction to botulinum toxin in clinical practice

Anthony B. Ward

North Staffordshire Rehabilitation Centre, Stoke-on-Trent, UK

5.1 Introduction

This section introduces the use of botulinum toxin (BoNT) in clinical practice. It will address aspects that are common to the drug's application in all the conditions described later in the book and will cover the following.

- Botulinum Toxin Serotypes
  - practical differences
  - dosage differences
- Commercial Production
- Indications and Licensing
- Storage Issues
- Injection Techniques
  - patient preparation
  - dilution
  - target organ location
    - electromyography
    - nerve/muscle stimulation
    - ultrasound
    - other imaging
  - disposal
  - repeated injections
- Side effects
- Safety and Adverse Events
- Helpful Hints
- Training Issues

Clinical Uses of Botulinum Toxins, eds. Anthony B. Ward and Michael P. Barnes. Published by Cambridge University Press. © Cambridge University Press 2007.

5.2   Botulinum toxin serotypes

Chapter 2 has given details of botulinum toxin subtypes. Research continues to identify further subtypes and to determine the possibility of new commercially available products, but commercial production is limited to three drugs of type A and one of type B. BoNT-A is marketed as BOTOX®, which is produced in the USA and Ireland by Allergan, a global company based in California, USA and as Dysport®, which is produced in the United Kingdom by Ipsen Ltd, an Anglo-French company based in England. Recently, Merz in Germany have marketed a type A toxin free of complexing proteins, called Xeomin (see end of chapter). There is a Chinese-produced BoNT-A, of which little is known of its characteristics, production or of its safety record. BoNT-B is produced in the USA by Elan, again of California and is marketed as Myobloc™ in the USA and as Neurobloc in Europe. Differences in their applications exist and the different nature of their production accounts for this[1].

Table 5.1, shows how the different preparations behave differently and this is best seen in their diffusion characteristics. Most is known about the diffusion of BoNT through muscles. It spreads through tissue planes and can cross about 4–5 sarcomeres to reach the neuromuscular junctions. While BOTOX® and Dysport® both utilize pre-synaptic nerve terminal cytoplasmic SNAP25 to be transported to the synaptic vesicle membranes, their uptake is different and the amount of neurotoxin protein and the optimal working pH are thought to be important[2]. In addition, the spread to distant sites may also be different, but this has still to be determined accurately[3].

There is quite a difference in patients' response to doses of BoNT and more than one injection may be required to find the optimal dose for that person.

Table 5.1. Characteristics of commercially-produced toxins

	BOTOX®	Dysport®	Myobloc™/ Neurobloc™
Serotype	A	A	B
Complex molecular weight[a]	900 kDa	~900 kDa	700 kDa
Package (units)	100	500	2500, 5000, 10 000
Neurotoxin protein per vial (ng)	~5	12.5	25, 50, 100
Form	Vacuum-dried	Lypholized	Solution
pH	~7	~7	5.6
Manufacturer	Allergan (US)	Ipsen (UK)	Elan (US)
Year of approval	1989	1991	2000

[a]The largest complex for type B is 500 kDa, whereas that for type A is 900 kDa.

Table 5.2. Characteristic dosages of BoNTs

	BOTOX®	Dysport®	Myobloc™ /Neurobloc™
Maximal dose per visit	400–600 U	1200–1500 U	25 000
Maximal dose per injection site	50 U	150 U	4000
Typical doses			
Cervical dystonia	100–200	350–700	7500–12 000
Spasticity	180–400	500–1200	10 000–25 000

The responsiveness to BoNT can be grossly predicted by an injection of a small amount of succinylcholine into a muscle[4]. This produces weakness for a few hours; however, it does not predict the optimal dose and it is probably easier and more informative just to give the BoNT.

Bioassay methods have resulted in different units, as can be seen from Table 5.2 and these are based on the lethality of intra-peritoneal injections of the toxin into a population of Swiss-Webster mice[2]. One unit or mouse-unit is sufficient to kill 50 per cent of these mice (LD_{50}). The companies have not been able to find consistent results between their products and, as a result, attempts have been made to find a standardized dose. This too has not been successful to date. The bioassay differences may also reflect the activity of the different species used in the production of BoNT-A.

Several attempts have been made to find a conversion ratio between the products and this too has caused considerable controversy. There is no concrete data to support a conversion ratio and fairly wild variations have been proposed. Magar's study[5] has plenty of inaccuracies, but has shown some subjective relationship between BOTOX® and Dysport®. He and his colleagues took 29 patients with cervical dystonia and blepharospasm, who had been stabilized on Dysport® for a minimum of 2 years. They then switched them to BOTOX® and carried out a further 456 injections. This retrospective study then looked at the dose given to gain an equivalent clinical effect. Although this was open labelled and did not produce data for objective equivalence, the investigators were experienced enough in the expected response from BoNT treatment to have a fairly good idea of what constituted an equivalent effect from injections. Certainly, there were no significant differences between treatment frequencies, which would be expected. Their conclusion was that:

- There is a wide range of dose ratios between BOTOX® and Dysport®
- More than 80 per cent of patients utilized a ratio of 4 : 1 or more
- There is no fixed dose ratio between BOTOX® and Dysport® and that differences even occur within different muscles within the same patient.
  Figures 5.1 to 5.4 show this effect more clearly.

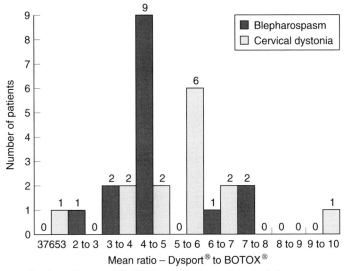

Figure 5.1   Distribution of mean ratio blepharospasm and cervical dystonia.

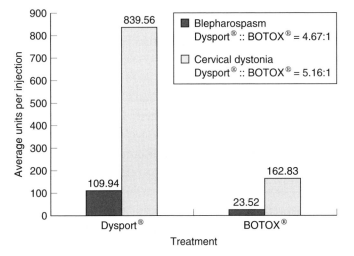

Figure 5.2   Mean dose per injection blepharospasm and cervical dystonia.

It is important to state that there is no fixed dose ratio between the two BoNT-As, as this will prevent a lot of potential confusion. It is much better to learn the expected effect of one particular preparation in a patient and base treatment on proper experiences. There is also potential confusion for inexperienced doctors, when switching from one product to another. First, it is important to recognize that the products have different doses and then upon what ratio should the dose be calculated? Most people work on the basis of about 4–5 Dysport® to 1 BOTOX® and to 50 Myo/Neurobloc. The report approved by the Royal College of Physicians

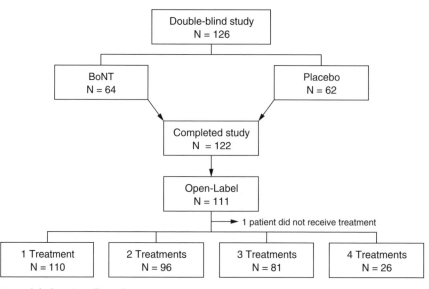

Figure 5.3   Open label patient flow chart.

of London Clinical Effectiveness and Evaluation Unit on 'The Management of Adults with Spasticity – Guidelines for the Use of Botulinum Toxin Type A' has an appendix giving the doses of BOTOX® and Dysport® and used a comparator of about 4:1, but this is for adults with spasticity. Little is known about the dosage requirements and differences between preparations for non-neurological indications. All the companies have posted data on their recommended dosages. Those of BOTOX® and Neurobloc™ have been posted on the webpage of the American organization for people with movement disorders, WeMove[6]. For the sake of convenience, however, Odergren's ratio of 3–5 Dysport® units to 1 of BOTOX® (calculated usually at 4:1) and 50:1 for Myobloc™/Neurobloc™ BOTOX®[7].

Standard dosage ranges are also well-documented and examples are given in Chapter 8 for spasticity.

5.3 Commercial production

This has already been addressed, but the companies have perhaps to a greater degree than those for other drugs been very supportive in the training of medical staff and physiotherapists. The botulinum toxin that comes for clinical practice is very different from the naturally found product. It is highly purified and produced to stringent biological standards. BoNT is not cheap, but its effect lasts for several months and the cost can equate to about £1 ($1.40) per day. Put like that, it is not so expensive, as many drugs are of this order of cost. Because it is not cheap, it should only be used when there is clear benefit, but it has no rival

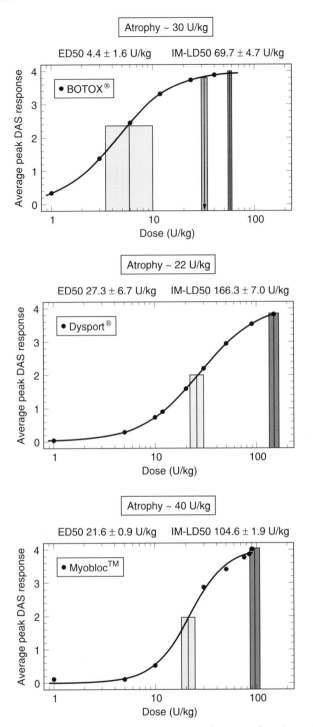

Figure 5.4   Safety and diffusion margins for BOTOX®, Dysport® and Myo/Neurobloc.

Table 5.3. Study of selected use in > 100 conditions

Indication for use		Class of evidence for use			
		A	B	C	D
Focal dystonia	Blepharospasm[a,b]		Y		
	Cervical dystonia[a,b,c]	Y		Y	
	Foot dystonia			Y	
	Meig's Syndrome				Y
	Occupational m. dystonia[a]			Y	
	Oromandibular dystonia		Y		
	Spasmodic dysphonia			Y	
	Writer's cramp				
Hemifacial spasm[a,b]			Y		
Tremor	Essential tremor				Y
	Palatal tremor		Y		
Spasticity	Cerebral palsy[a]	Y			
Upper limb[a]	Multiple sclerosis	Y			
Lower limb[a]	Stroke[a]	Y			
	Spinal cord injury	Y			
	Traumatic brain injury	Y			
Autonomic disorders	Focal hyperhidrosis[a]		Y		
(secretory)	Gustatory sweating		Y		
	Sialorrhoea				Y
	Excess lacrimation				Y
Urological	Bladder hyper-reflexia		Y		
	DSD		Y		
	Vaginismus			Y	
	Urethral Syndrome				Y
Cranial nerve disorders incl.	Strabismus[a,b]			Y	
ophthalmic indications	Sixth N (Abducens) palsy			Y	
	Facial nerve disorders				Y
	Nystagmus and oscillopsia				Y
Pain	Migraine			Y	
	Tension headache			Y	
	Spinal pain (neck and back)				Y
	Muscle spasm		Y		
	Myofascial Pain Syndrome			Y	
	Fibromyalgia				Y
Gastrointestinal disorders	Achalasia				Y
	Oesophageal reflux				Y
	Sphincter of Oddi spasm				Y
	Anal fissure		Y		

Table 5.3. (*Cont.*)

Indication for use		A	B	C	D
		\multicolumn{4}{c}{Class of evidence for use}			
	Constipation				Y
	Anismus				Y
Cosmetic	Wrinkles − glabellar lines[b]			Y	
	Brow furrow				Y
	Focal hyperhidrosis[a]		Y		
	Myokymia				Y
Other	Bruxism and other TMJ disorders				Y
	Rigidity				Y
	Tics − Gilles de la Tourette Syndrome				Y
	Stiff Person Syndrome				Y

[a]Indicates a licence within a European Union member state.
[b]Indicates approval for BOTOX® by the US Federal Drug and Food Administration.
[c]Indicates approval for Myobloc™ by the US Federal Drug and Food Administration.

Table 5.4. Characteristics of the commercial preparations of BoNT

	BOTOX®	Dysport®	Neurobloc™
Serotype	A	A	B
Complex MW	900 kDa	∼9000 kDa	700 kDa
Package(units)	100	500	2500/5000/10 000
Neurotoxin protein per vial (ng)	∼5	12.5	25/50/100
Form	Vacuum dried	Lypholized	Solution
pH	∼7	∼7	5.6
First year of approval	1989	1991	2000

as treatment for certain conditions. For this reason, it has been well-regarded in many clinical conditions and the range is described later in the book. Rather than looking solely at its cost, it should be remembered that the alternative treatments may also have a significant economic and human cost. For instance, the cost of 300 U BoNT (plus syringes, etc.) given for adductor spasticity may come to about £450 ($720). In contrast, a bilateral obturator nerve block with 6 per cent phenol in aqueous solution may achieve a similar result at a fraction of the price for the drug. The treatment may, however, take over an hour of specialist time to do and this and the higher incidence of adverse effects starts to equate the costs quite well. When phenol is injected into nerves with a sensory component, there is a real chance of inducing a painful dysaesthesia, which would require at least six weeks of gabapentin treatment to reduce symptoms. The cost of gabapentin would certainly equate to a very great cost of the order of magnitude of the BoNT itself.

There is now a well-established line of toxin production and the clinical experience is of a consistent patient response to the drug. Access to the drug depends very much on the health care system differences between countries. Reimbursement is established in most developed countries, but depends on the indication. Similarly, state health systems have funded the drug, but there are concerns that its wider availability for other indications will result in a further pressure on drug budgets. There is thus a sentiment that health services will fund the drug, where clear functional benefits are seen and where there is well-audited use of the drug by services. Cost-effectiveness therefore becomes an important issue for BoNT in contrast to other drugs used in medical practice.

5.4 Indications and licensing

BoNT has a wide number of indications, which are listed below. The history of the product has already been described, but it is a truly remarkable drug. Wherever acetylcholine exists, there is an opportunity for its function to be blocked by BoNT. As a result, there are many potential indications, but the task now is to identify where its use can be justified on clinical and pharmaco-economic grounds. There is no doubt, for instance, that it relieves acute muscle spasm in back pain, but can one justify its use for a transient self-limiting episode, when cheaper, well-proven and easier to administer alternatives exist, such as simple analgesics? On the other hand, its use in chronic conditions may be more straightforward, particularly if the cost and tolerance/safety profile of the alternatives are significant. Therefore, this book will look at the role of BoNT in the pharmacological armamentarium of these conditions.

Similarly, BoNT has a number of licences under its commercial preparations. Europe is perhaps a little in advance of the USA in this respect, which may reflect a different approach to the collection of evidence and justification for general use. Nevertheless, BoNT is widely used in clinical practice for licensed and non-licensed indications and there is a sufficiently wide experience of the drug, that physicians and surgeons could claim protection by the body of professional opinion in its efficacy. It should be noted, however, that practice should follow any guidelines that may exist[8].

5.5 Storage issues

The presentation of BoNT is now very straightforward and gone are the days when clinicians would have to don gowns, gloves, masks and goggles to dilute the pure toxin to therapeutic concentrations. The three purified commercial preparations are now presented as standardized dose vials and their storage is given on the datasheets.

These are:

BOTOX®	Comes as a freeze-dried 100 U/vial
	Storage between 4−5°C in refrigerator
	Use preparation within 6 hours of dilution
Dysport®	Comes as a powder for dilution with 2.5 ml normal saline.
	500 mU/vial.
	Storage between 4−5°C in refrigerator
	Use preparation within 4 hours of dilution
Myobloc™	Neurobloc™/Myobloc™ comes as a a ready-to-use liquid formulation, that does not require reconstitution and is available in three convenient vial configurations of 2500 Units in 0.5 mL, 5000 Units in 1.0 mL; and 10 000 Units in 2.0 mL 2500 U/vial.
Neurobloc™	Storage at room temperature

The storage differences exist because the preparations are not the same. Different strains of *C. botulinum* are used in manufacture and different methodologies are undertaken to purify and formulate the drugs. It is also noted that the immunogenic load of BOTOX® is significantly less than the other types, but its clinical significance is unclear.

Once diluted, the preparations should be used within the above time frames, but all are remarkably resilient drugs. Their re-use has been shown to be still potent 24 hours after dilution[9].

5.6   Injection techniques

This section is a practical approach to injecting BoNT.

5.6.1   Drawing up

(1) BOTOX® and Dysport® come in standard vials of 100 U and 500 mU respectively and require dilution with normal saline. The section below discusses dilution characteristics more fully. There is a negative vacuum which draws in the diluent. Neurobloc™/Myobloc™ presents already diluted and simply requires drawing up. Always add a slightly larger volume of saline than intended (e.g. add 1.1 ml for a 1 ml, 2.2 for 2 ml or 5.3 ml for a 5 ml dilution), as the BoNT has a tendency to stick to the glass vial. This may create a situation where there may be less volume than expected and would be important, for instance, where the volume obtained in the syringe for a 2 ml dilution was only 1.85 ml. If one wished to inject 40 U BOTOX® (0.8 ml) into the flexor

digitorum profundus muscle, 40 U (0.8 ml) into the flexor digitorum superficialis muscle and 20 U (0.4 ml) into the flexor pollicis longus muscle,
one may find that there would only be 0.25 ml available for the latter muscle.
Therefore, injecting slightly more saline than required would allow a full 2 ml
of BoNT and all the target organs would receive the correct volume and any
errors would thus be 'diluted'.

(2) Do not shake the BOTOX® and Dysport® vials, as vigorous shaking has the
potential to denature the neurotoxin protein. Simply roll the vial between your
fingers and the toxin dissolves easily.

(3) The easiest way to draw up the contents is to separate the needle from the
syringe after inserting it into the vial and this will equalize the pressures. Then
carefully draw up the full contents of the vial.

(4) Always be tidy and well-organized to avoid the risk of discarding a full or half-
full vial. Clinicians use multiple vials and may not use their complete contents.
Vials can be used for more than one patient and there is a potential for
inefficient use of resources. I have seen on two occasions when full vials were
thrown away by accident.

5.6.2 Dilution

The effects of dilution have been thought to be important for some time,
but Gracies et al. have highlighted this[8]. They set out to verify the effects of
dilution and endplate targeting in a controlled study in patients with spasticity,
utilizing previously histologically mapped endplates in human biceps brachii[10].

As optimal dilutions were unknown and injection techniques varied in the
treatment of spasticity, this was the first paper to produce some hard data.
Previous studies in animal and in small human muscles in healthy volunteers had
shown a correlation between the degree of muscle paralysis after BoNT injection
and injected volume[11,12]. Animal studies had also shown a greater block by BoNT
when the drug was injected near the motor endplates[9,11,13].

This is the first double-blind evidence that:

• injecting biceps brachii muscle with BoNT type A in spasticity with a high-
volume/low potency dilution (20 U/ml, i.e. 5 ml per vial of BoNT-A) provides
significantly greater neuromuscular block and spasticity reduction than with
a low-volume/high-potency dilution (100 U/ml, i.e. 1 ml per vial);

• an endplate targeting technique achieves greater blocking effects than random
injection.

It was postulated that differential changes in elbow extensor co-contraction
during isometric flexor efforts might contribute to this discrepancy, but the
conclusion is that a high dilution (e.g. 20 U/ml) is used for injecting larger
muscles (such as those in the lower limb or in upper limb muscles above

the elbow), we recommend using high dilution, particularly when the primary goal is to improve passive function.

5.6.3   Patient preparation

BoNT is safe and patient information literature should make this clear. Intramuscular injections are a common way of delivering this treatment and most will be carried out by physicians as an outpatient or ambulatory procedure. Most patients will not need any special preparation, but those requiring sedation or anaesthesia (such as for gastrointestinal procedures, those unable to tolerate injections, etc.) will need to be prepared as for any other minor procedure.

The subject of obtaining a signed patient consent form is contentious, for it could be argued that the very appearance of the patient at the clinic for a simple outpatient procedure without sedation implies consent. It is probably wise, however, to obtain written consent, as this will allow the clinician to go through the benefits and risks of the procedure. Good medical practice would do this anyway, but a signed consent form only partially protects a doctor in any event. Explaining the possibility of, albeit infrequent, side effects, such as dysphagia, or mild transient weakness and myalgia will maintain patient confidence.

Patients should take an active part in deciding the goals of their treatment. They should therefore know the expected outcome of treatment and that BoNT only treats the neurogenic problem and not the biomechanical one. It is an adjunct to other treatments, such as physical treatment in spasticity. It takes about 1–4 days to see any change after the injection and that recurrent injections may unusually result in non-response (see below). Patients with spasticity should therefore be set up in a rehabilitation programme in conjunction with the injection, so that they can gain most benefit. Patients should also be told that the treatment itself lasts for some 3 to 4 months, but that its effects are completely reversible. In some conditions, this may be longer and the secretory disorders anecdotally seem to demonstrate this.

The procedure requires accurate placement of the injection into the target organ and it is therefore important for both the patient and the injector to be comfortable. Patients should be warned that injections of some less accessible muscles may take some time and that injecting some muscles may be more painful than others. Since the skin of the hand and feet is more sensitive, the small intrinsic muscles should be injected first, when the EMG needle is sharpest. The injector will require assistance to draw up the BoNT and to position the patient, as many will be significantly disabled.

Some practices are set up to inject patients on a different occasion from the assessment process. This has the major disadvantage that the patient has to attend twice for treatment and that more medical and nursing time will be used. To offset this, the amount of BoNT consumed will be lessened, as an injection session can match patients' requirements, so that little or no BoNT is wasted unused. For instance, a patient requiring 220 U BOTOX® can be matched with another patient requiring 180 U and 400 U can be ordered. Patient discussion takes place in the clinic and the injection sessions focus purely on the procedure itself, thus making for a smooth process. In this way also, the nurses can assist heavily dependent patients in getting on and off the bed, preparing for the injection, etc., while the injector can be getting on with injecting patients.

5.6.4   Target organ location

It is right that clinicians should learn how to achieve accurate placement of the injection. If an accurate diagnosis has been made and the patient has been prepared for a specific treatment, then he or she needs to know that the technical aspects of the injection have been correctly addressed. A number of techniques exist and Table 5.5 gives some of the advantages and disadvantages. Whichever is used depends on the expertise and training of the injector, on the facilities available and on the patient throughput.

There is no evidence for one technique over another and there has been one report of no advantage over an EMG technique over a blind approach[14]. However, it is probably difficult to defend a purely blind approach to injecting small muscles in the hope that BoNT diffusion will give a therapeutic effect. There has to date also been no hard evidence that accurate placement of the needle allows a decrease in the dose amount of BoNT given, but Gracies *et al.* supports the common sense view, which suggests that the closer the injection to the motor point, the better the uptake and the better the blocking[8]. A trial of different treatment doses would therefore be the next logical step.

The difficulty is that injecting small muscles with high volume low potency dilutions may give rise to nociceptive feedback and will be painful. My own personal recommendation is to restrict these larger volumes to upper arm muscles (pectoralis major, deltoid, triceps, biceps brachii and brachialis muscles), hip and thigh muscles (hip and knee flexors and extensors) and gastrocnemius and soleus muscles. For the others a 2 ml dilution is recommended. When injecting the bladder or oesophageal muscle, a 1 ml dilution is suggested and a 0.5 ml per 100 U BOTOX® allows for any dilution by salivary or exocrine glands. These are purely personal preferences and are not based on hard evidence.

Table 5.5. Techniques for muscle location

Technique	Advantages	Disadvantages
Electromyography	• Allows good assessment of muscle activity in neurological disorders • Reasonably accurate needle placement when organ function persist • Simple cheap EMG amplifiers available	• Does not greatly help needle placement when there is no residual organ function, although there are a number of techniques to assist accuracy. • Sometimes painful • Difficult if muscle greatly wasted
Nerve/muscle stimulation	• Accurate method to locate muscle and to ascertain muscle function, particularly in the presence of absent volitional activity • Simple cheap nerve/muscle stimulators available	• Need to locate motor points to achieve good stimulation. • May be painful, if stimulus increased. • Difficult if muscle greatly wasted
Ultrasound	• Accurate method to locate muscle • Non-invasive	• Need ultrasonographer/ radiologist expertise at examination, which increases technical logistics and procedure cost • Cost of ultrasound machine • No information on muscle activity
Other imaging	• CT gives accurate needle placement	• Cannot justify CT radiation level • MR not recommended for needle placement
None	• Cheap and easy, if injector knows relative anatomy and surface anatomy • Justified in *large*, easily identified upper arm and leg muscles	• Not accurate for locating small muscles, even in skilled hands • Potential waste/misuse of BoNT

Ultrasonography has considerable advantages in that it is non-invasive and highly accurate once the technique has been learnt. However, most clinicians use imaging personnel to assist them and thus the procedure becomes expensive and requires a formal approach, lest it becomes difficult to organize. To acquire good accurate images requires adequate equipment, which further increases the cost[15].

5.6.5 Disposal

Disposal of BoNT is the same as for all other biologic products. It is a safe product and contamination by a used vial is most unlikely to cause a public health problem. Nonetheless, disposal through the hospital contamination and 'sharps' system is advised.

5.7 Repeated injections

Chapter 2 has dealt with this topic to a large extent, but clinicians need to appreciate the reversibility of BoNT. The drug has such a variety of uses that its combined clinical characteristics cannot be described adequately. Its use in cervical dystonia is to relax muscles for the period of its activity and further injections are required. It has similar characteristics in secretory disorders, such as focal hyperhidrosis, where the condition starts to return after 3 to 4 months of the drug action. Its use in spasticity and in other neuromuscular conditions (e.g. gastrointestinal and urological) demonstrates an ability to change the impairment and possibly the functioning of the patient and here the drug is an adjunct to other more definitive treatments, such as physical management in spasticity, where the patient may experience motor learning changes[16]. As a result, the need for repeated injections differs from condition to condition.

For instance, in glabellar lines it can maintain the effect of laser surgery to give a more polished and refined result[17].

The longer term effects are now becoming well known and Jitpimolmard *et al.* reported on the long term efficacy and side effects of the treatment of hemifacial spasm with Dysport® over 12 treatments[18]. The median number of treatments was four and produced a response rate of 97 per cent. The overall mean duration of improvement was 3.4 months, but this varied between 2.60 to 3.71 months from the first to the twelfth treatment. The response rate persisted in the range 70.00 to 78.10 per cent with duration of improvement lasting for 2.65 to 4.31 months. Similar findings were found using BOTOX® and showed a consistent efficacy and reliability, which too was similar to that of BOTOX®[19].

Brashear *et al.* have also shown good responses in the repeated treatments for post-stroke upper limb spasticity[20]. Patients were followed up for 42 weeks in an open label study following a 12 week randomized control trial of BOTOX® versus placebo. They were treated according to local standard practice and given up to four further treatments over the 54 week period.

The primary measures were the Principal Therapeutic Intervention Target on a Disability Assessment Scale and the Ashworth Scale and significant changes were a one-point gain on the PTIT Disability Assessment or more or a one-point drop or more in wrist flexor muscle tone on the Ashworth Scale. The duration of benefit was also assessed. Significant improvements from baseline were seen at 6 weeks for each treatment cycle across all efficacy measures. The average number of treatment cycles per patient was 2.72 out of a potential four treatment cycles and 7.4 per cent of patients demonstrated improvement for at least 24 weeks. In summary, BoNT improved tone and function over the 54-week period and 200−240 U of BOTOX® appeared to be an effective long-term therapy in producing sustained improvement in functional disability.

Many patients only ever need one or two treatments with BoNT, but people with chronic spasticity, such as those with multiple sclerosis and spinal cord injury may need it more regularly. There are no hard and fast rules, but the recommendation is for no more than three monthly injections and use of the smallest dose necessary to gain a clinical effect. The former appears to be the more important criterion and the latest formulation of BOTOX® has a smaller quantity of neurotoxin protein and is hence less likely to generate resistance and non-response. On the other hand, however, the bigger the dose, the longer the clinical effects are likely to last[21].

5.8 Side effects

5.8.1 General

Clinically relevant side effects are few when one considers the potential of this drug as a neurotoxin. One must also separate unwanted effects from side effects, as many of the recognized features, such as dysphagia, are in fact simply the spread of the desired pharmacological effects of the drug. However, some, such as dysphagia, are potentially dangerous and measures should actively be employed to prevent them. If they do occur, patients should have the knowledge to recognize them and seek appropriate medical advice. It is perhaps simple therefore to divide up these effects as:

• Unwanted therapeutic effects
• Unwanted effects worth tolerating for the overall benefit of the treatment
• Side effects

They are more common after certain treatments than for others. For instance, limb spasticity, particularly when large muscles are treated, is very unlikely to give rise to unwanted effects, whereas cervical and facial injections are more frequently associated. They are common to all BoNT types, but differences exist in their incidence between the toxin types and commercial preparations. The critical factor appears to relate to the characteristics of and differences of the toxin types' retention within injected muscle and its diffusion[22]. The term *Safety Margin* is the therapeutic window and is a measure of diffusion from the injection site to systemic circulation. The *Diffusion Margin* is the index of undesirable escape (i.e. local toxicity) in the absence of systemic effects. Aoki *et al.* looked at a population of mice and showed a log-scale relationship between the local effect (in this scale digit abduction function, measured on a digit abduction score – DAS) and a local muscle effect, which corresponded with the ED_{50} dose[23,24]. There was a relatively constant for mean peak DAS response and the toxin dose, at which the maximum local effect gave rise to systemic effects and thus to the ED_{50}.

The findings may thus help explain the different side-effect profiles of all three preparations and, in particular, the differences between the two type A products[25,26].

The whole question of immune resistance is addressed in Chapter 4, but clinicians treating chronic spasticity, as a general rule, give the smallest dose necessary and leave an interval of at least 3 months between injections to minimize the risk of secondary non-response. They would also avoid giving booster injections, except that some patients after an acute disabling condition may only ever need one or two treatments and it is thus safe to give those whenever they are clinically indicated.

5.9   Safety and adverse events

There are a few well-known contraindications to BoNT, which are not dose-dependent. The paralytic effects of the toxin are antagonized by certain aminoquinoline antimalarial compounds, such as chloroquine through interaction with a selective, stereo-specific site, that is not well correlated with anti-malarial activity. Although BoNT does not influence the spinal cord anterior horn cell, its systemic effect has the potential to worsen anterior horn cell disorders, such as myasthenia gravis, the Lambert–Eaton Syndrome, poliomyelitis and progressive muscular atrophy[27,28]. 3,4-Aminopyridine has been used to treat the Lambert–Eaton Syndrome and inhibits BoNT effectively in animal studies in the early stages of its effect and in reducing the paralysis. However, this is not confirmed in in-vitro analysis[28,29]. All peripheral nerve dysfunction is liable to give rise to problems, but invariably does not[30]. Care should be taken with the dose[31,32].

Interaction with aminoglycoside antibiotics, such as gentamicin, is also recognized and the BoNT should be withheld until the antibiotic is no longer required[33].

5.10 Helpful hints

(1) The uptake of BoNT is increased in active muscles and programmes have been devised to stimulate activity either physically, or, where voluntary activity is not possible, electrically. The evidence for this is not convincing, but the hypothesis makes sense and many clinicians do it.

(2) The cost-pressure on the spasticity budget in the UK (and possibly also in other social health care systems) is built around the cost of the drugs and costs can be controlled by injecting patients at a separate session to the assessment session. In this way, the amount of BOTOX® used can be predicted and best use made of it. There are other advantages, as, for instance, a heavily dependent patient can be helped on to a couch by care staff, while another more mobile patient is injected. This speeds up the clinic time and makes best use of medical time.

(3) Always inject areas of greatest sensitivity first, as needles are sharpest the first time they are inserted. This applies particularly to the palm of the hand and to the soles of the feet.

5.11 Training issues

- Specific training is required for clinicians involved in a specialized spasticity service. This applies to doctors, therapists and nurses and should cover all aspects of spasticity management and not just BoNT. Training should be geared towards those referring patients and those injecting. Guidelines have been produced in both the USA and in Europe and have been focused towards adult spasticity[34], cerebral palsy[35], dystonia[36] and focal hyperhidrosis[37].

- What goes into acquiring expertise in this area of medicine? Certainly, acquiring knowledge and natural history of the underlying disorder; knowing when to intervene is usually clear, but knowing when not to is perhaps even more important. As BoNT has so many applications, clinicians will have to develop expertise in certain fields and a thorough knowledge of that field is required, so that the place of BoNT in treatment can be appreciated. The development of BoNT clinics or services is therefore undesirable, whereas specialized services for spasticity, hyperhidrosis, etc. can deliver high quality care.

- The content of training is subject to the needs and development of that area of treatment. The demonstration of competency is important and this treatment should be a part of the formal specialist training programme in the field. General practitioners and nurse/therapist require specific training and mentoring by the specialized service to develop confidence. Guidelines are being produced for the former in the UK, which are designed to help the quality of referral rather than produce GP specialists in the field. Very few will be able to devote the time to take this on, but many will review patients following stroke and will need to know the indications for spasticity treatment. Most of the conditions amenable to BoNT treatment are relatively uncommon and acquired spasticity is one of the more common.

Additional information regarding xeomin

After preparation of this book, Xeomin was licensed in Germany. This is a type A toxin free of complexing proteins[38]. Experience is currently limited but early reports indicate that it is of similar efficacy to the other type A toxins with a similar side-effect profile[39,40]. It is yet to be determined whether the absence of proteins will result in a lower risk of antibody development.

REFERENCES

1. McLellan, K., Das, R. E., Ekong, T. A. and Sesardic, D. (1996). Therapeutic botulinum toxin type A toxin: factors affecting potency. *Toxicon*, **34**, 975–85.
2. Aoki, K. R. (2001). A comparison of the safety margins of botulinum toxin serotypes. *Journal of Neurology*, **248**(Suppl. 1), 3–10.
3. Jankovic, J. and Orman, J. (1987). Botulinum A toxin for cranial-cervical dystonia: a double-blind placebo-controlled study. *Neurology*, **37**, 616–23.
4. Walker, F. O., Scott, G. E. and Butterworth, J. (1993). Sustained focal effects of low dose intramuscular succinylcholine. *Muscle & Nerve*, **16**, 181–7.
5. Ahmed, F., Magar, R., Marchetti, A. and Ferguson, I. (2003). *European Journal of Neurology*, **10**(Suppl. 1), 162.
6. WeMove – Website. http://www.wemove.org
7. Odergren, T., Hjaltason, H., Kaakkola, S., Solders, G., Hanko, J., Fehling, C., Marttila, R. J., Lundh, H., Gedin, S., Westergren, I., Richardson, A., Dott, C. and Cohen, H. (1998). A double blind, randomised, parallel group study to investigate the dose equivalence of Dysport and Botox in the treatment of cervical dystonia. *Journal of Neurology, Neurosurgery and Psychiatry*, **64**(1), 6–12.

8. Turner-Stokes, L. and Ward, A. B. (2002). The management of adults with spasticity using botulinum toxin. *Clinical Medicine*, **2**(2), 128–30.

9. Gracies, J.-M., Weisz, D. J., Yang, B. Y., Flanagan, S. and Simpson, D. (2002). *Effects of Botulinum Toxin Type A Dilution and Endplate Targeting Technique in Upper Limb Spasticity.* Presented to American Neurological Association Meeting.

10. Sanders, I., Mu, L., Amirali, A. *et al.* (1998). Motor endplate mapping of the human biceps brachii muscle. Abstract. *Ann. Neurol.*, **44**, 501.

11. Shaari, C. M. and Sanders, I. (1993). Quantifying how location and dose of botulinum toxin injections affect muscle paralysis. *Muscle Nerve*, **16**, 964–9.

12. Bigalke, H., Wohlfarth, K., Irmer, A. and Dengler, R. (2001). Botulinum A toxin: Dysport improvement of biological availability. *Exp Neurol.*, **168**(1), 162–70.

13. Childers, M. K., Kornegay, J. N., Aoki, R., Otaviani, L., Bogan, D. J. and Petroski, G. (1998). Evaluating motor end-plate-targeted injections of botulinum toxin type A in a canine model. *Muscle Nerve*, **21**(5), 653–5.

14. Koko, C. and Ward, A. B. (1997). Management of spasticity. *British Journal of Hospital Medicine*, **58**(8), 400–5.

15. Berweck, S., Feldkamp, A., Francke, A., Nehles, J., Schwerin, A. and Heinen, F. (2002). Sonography-guided injection of botulinum toxin A in children with cerebral palsy. *Neuropediatrics*, **33**(4), 221–3.

16. Richardson, D. (2002). Physical therapy in spasticity. *European Journal of Neurology*, **9**(Suppl. 1), 17–22.

17. Carruthers, J. and Carruthers, A. (1998). The adjunctive usage of botulinum toxin. *Dermatologic Surgery*, **24**(11), 1244–7.

18. Jitpimolmard, S., Tiamkao, S. and Laopaiboon, M. (1998). Long term results of botulinum toxin type A (Dysport) in the treatment of hemifacial spasm: a report of 175 cases. *Journal of Neurology, Neurosurgery and Psychiatry*, **64**(6), 751–7.

19. Dodel, R. C., Kirchner, A., Koehne-Volland, R., Kunig, G., Ceballos-Baumann, A., Naumann, M., Brashear, A., Richter, H. P., Szucs, T. D. and Oertel, W. H. (1997). Costs of treating dystonias and hemifacial spasm with botulinum toxin A. *Pharmacoeconomics*, **12**(6), 695–706.

20. Brashear, A., Zafonte, R., Corocran, M., Galvez-Jimenez, N., Gracies, J.-M., Gordon, M. F., Mcafee, A., Ruffing, K., Thompson, B., Williams, M., Lee, C.-H. and Turkel, C. (2002). Inter- and intra-rater reliability of the Ashworth Scale and the Disability Assessment Scale in patients with upper limb post-stroke spasticity. *Archives of Physical Medicine & Rehabilitation*, **83**(10), 1349–54.

21. Sampaio, C., Ferreira, J. J., Simoes, F., Rosas, M. J., Magalhaes, M., Correia, A. P., Bastos-Lima, A., Martins, R. and Castro-Caldas, A. (1997). DYSBORT: a single-blind, randomized parallel study to determine whether any differences can be detected in the efficacy and tolerability of two formulations of botulinum toxin type A – Dysport and Botox – assuming a ratio of 4 : 1. *Movement Disorders*, **12**(6), 1013–18.

22. Aoki, K. R. and Guyer, B. (2001). Botulinum toxin type A and other botulinum toxin serotypes: a comparative review of biochemical and pharmacological actions. *European Journal of Neurology*, **8**(Suppl. 5), 21–9.

23. Aoki, K. R. (2001). A comparison of the safety margins of botulinum neurotoxin serotypes A, B, and F in mice. *Toxicon*, **39**, 1815−20.

24. Aoki, K. R. (2002). Botulinum neurotoxin serotypes A and B preparations have different safety margins in preclinical models of muscle weakening efficacy and systemic safety. *Toxicon*, **40**, 81−6.

25. Nussgens, Z. and Roggenkamper, P. (1997). Comparison of two botulinum-toxin preparations in the treatment of essential blepharospasm. *Graefes Archive for Clinical and Experimental Ophthalmology*, **235**(4), 197−9.

26. Ranoux, D., Gury, C., Fondarai, J., Mas, J. L. and Zuber, M. (2002). Respective potencies of Botox and Dysport: a double blind, randomised, crossover study in cervical dystonia. *Journal of Neurology, Neurosurgery and Psychiatry*, **72**(4), 459−62.

27. Erbguth, F., Claus, D., Engelhardt, A. and Dressler, D. (1993). Systemic effect of local botulinum toxin injections unmasks subclinical Lambert−Eaton myasthenic syndrome. *Journal of Neurology, Neurosurgery and Psychiatry*, **56**(11), 1235−6.

28. Bachmeyer, C., Benz, R., Barth, H., Aktories, K., Gilbert, M. and Popoff, M.R. (2001). Interaction of *Clostridium botulinum* C2 toxin with lipid bilayer membranes and Vero cells: inhibition of channel function by chloroquine and related compounds in vitro and intoxification in vivo. *FASEB Journal*, **15**(9), 1658−60.

29. Davis, L. E., Johnson, J. K., Bicknell, J. M., Levy, H. and McEvoy, K. M. (1992). Human type A botulism and treatment with 3,4-aminopyridine. *Electromyography and Clinical Neurophysiology*, **32**, 379−83.

30. Mezaki, T., Kaji, R., Kohara, N. and Kimura, J. (1996). Development of general weakness in a patient with amyotrophic lateral sclerosis after focal botulinum toxin injection. *Neurology*, **46**(3), 845−6.

31. Glanzman, R. L., Gelb, D. J., Drury, I., Bromberg, M. B. and Truong, D. D. (1990). Brachial plexopathy after botulinum toxin injections. *Neurology*, **40**(7), 1143.

32. Klein, A. W. (2002). Complications and adverse reactions with the use of botulinum toxin. *Disease-A-Month*, **48**(5), 336−56.

33. Wang, Y. C., Burr, D. H., Korthals, G. J. and Sugiyama, H. (1984). Acute toxicity of aminoglycoside antibiotics as an aid in detecting botulism. *Appl. Environ. Microbiology*, **48**, 951−5.

34. Turner Stokes, L. and Ward, A. B. (2001). *The Management of Adults with Spasticity − Guidelines for the Use of Botulinum Toxin Type A*. Byfleet: Hourds.

35. Graham, H. K., Aoki, K. R., Autti-Rämo, I., Boyd, R. N., Delgado, M. R., Gaebler-Spira, D. J., Gormley, M. E., Guyer, B. M., Heinen, F., Holton, A. F., Matthews, M., Molenaers, G., Motta, F., García-Ruiz, P. J. and Wissel, J. (2000). Recommendations for the use of botulinum type A in the management of cerebral palsy. *Gait and Posture*, **11**, 67−9.

36. Berardelli, A., Abbruzzese, G., Bertolasi, L., Cantarella, G., Carella, F., Curra, A., De Grandis, D., DeFazio, G., Galardi, G., Girlanda, P., Livrea, P., Modugno, N., Priori, A., Ruoppolo, G., Vacca, L. and Manfredi, M. (1997). Guidelines for the therapeutic use of botulinum toxin in movement disorders. Italian Study Group for Movement Disorders, Italian Society of Neurology. *Italian Journal of Neurological Sciences*, **18**(5), 261−9.

37. Lowe, N. J., Sandeep, C., Halford, J., Jones, H., Payne, S. and Poyner, T. (2003). Guidelines for the primary care treatment and referral of focal hyperhidrosis. *Guidelines*, 381–91.

38. Jost, W. H., Kohl, A., Brinkmann, S. and Comes, G. (2005). Efficacy and tolerability of a botulinum toxin type A free of complexing proteins (NT 201) compared with commercially available botulinum toxin type A (BOTOX) in healthy volunteers. *J. Neural. Transm.*, **112**, 905–13.

39. Roggenkamper, P., Jost, W. H., Biharia, K., Comes, G. and Grafe, S. (2006). Efficacy and safety of a new Botulinum Toxin Type A free of complexing proteins in the treatment of blepharospasm. *J. Neural. Transm.* **113**, 303–12.

40. Benecke, R., Jost, W. H., Kanovsky, P., Ruzicka, E., Comes, G. and Grafe, S. (2005). A new botulinum toxin type A free of complexing proteins for treatment of cervical dystonia. *Neurology*, **64**, 1949–51.

6

Cervical dystonia

Khalid Anwar

Hunters Moor Regional Neurological Rehabilitation Centre, Newcastle upon Tyne, UK

6.1 Introduction

The term dystonia is defined as a sustained, involuntary contraction of muscle that produces an abnormal posture and frequently causes twisting and turning[1]. Cervical dystonia is the most common form of adult-onset focal dystonia[2]. It is defined as involuntary twisting and turning of the neck caused by abnormal involuntary muscle contractions[1]. This abnormal posture may be associated with spasms, jerks or tremors or a combination of these features. Cervical dystonia also has been referred to as spasmodic torticollis but this term does not reflect the dystonic nature of the problem. It implies that spasms are an essential feature of the disease although these can be absent in 25—30 per cent of the patients with cervical dystonia[3]. Torticollis on the other hand is the physical sign of the twisted neck and may result from many non-dystonic causes.

It is well known that due to variable presentation of this disease cervical dystonia is frequently misdiagnosed and accurate diagnosis is often delayed[4]. The aetiology and pathogenesis of cervical dystonia remains unclear. However it is generally agreed that genetic factors, trauma, altered sensory input, primary vestibular abnormality and impaired basal ganglia function may all have some role in the development of this disease. Adult-onset cervical dystonia usually does not become generalized although there may be segmental spread with involvement of arms jaws or trunk[5]. A small percentage of patients can have a spontaneous remission but it is usually short lived and incomplete[6-8]. In terms of treatment, botulinum toxin therapy remains the most effective symptomatic treatment of cervical dystonia since its introduction in late 1980s. The development of neutralizing antibodies occurs in 5—10 per cent of cases and seems to be dependent on dosage and interval between the treatments. Other treatments, which are available although not as effective as botulinum toxin therapy, include anti-cholinergics, benzodiazepines and baclofen. These are usually used if the response to botulinum toxin therapy is not adequate. Surgical treatment is available for the treatment of cervical dystonia but is reserved for refractory cases and includes intrathecal baclofen and high frequency bilateral stimulation of globus pallidus internus.

This chapter concentrates on the use of botulinum toxin therapy in the treatment of cervical dystonia in the context of other treatment options. Greater emphasis is put on the practical aspects of botulinum toxin therapy.

6.2 Epidemiology

The true prevalence of cervical dystonia is difficult to estimate. It has been estimated at nine cases per 100 000 population in Rochester, Minnesota, USA[9] that is based on a retrospective chart review. Cervical dystonia is the most common adult-onset focal dystonia[10]. The incidence seems to be sex and age related. Women are affected 1.5—1.9 times more than men[11,12]. The maximum incidence of cervical dystonia is in its fifth decade of life and does not differ between men and women with 70—90 per cent of cases presenting between the fourth and sixth decade[11].

6.3 Natural history

The cervical dystonia typically begins insidiously with patients complaining of a 'pulling' or 'drawing' in the neck or an involuntary twisting or jerking of the head[10]. Initial non-specific symptoms often result in an incorrect diagnosis and thus often a delay in correct diagnosis occurs[13]. There is a great heterogeneity in the speed of progression of symptoms from onset to maximal severity[4]. Symptoms tend to worsen on average 3—5 years, with a range of one month to 18 years[14]. The disease then tends to stabilize even slightly improving before stabilizing[10]. In most cases cervical dystonia remains confined to the neck but can spread beyond the neck to the adjacent areas in about one third of them[15]. It is very rare for cervical dystonia to spread beyond adjacent areas and to progress to generalized dystonia. Spontaneous remissions of cervical dystonia occur in up to 20 per cent of patients but are usually short lived and incomplete[6-8]. Remissions usually occur in the initial period of the disease but may occur late in the disease as well. Remission is usually followed by relapse in almost all the cases within 5 years and a cycle of remission and relapse may occur[10].

6.4 Clinical features

Symptoms depend upon the severity of the disease, duration of the disease, the muscles involved and the different neck and head positions and postures assumed.

Patients seek treatment due to a variety of reasons that include pain, abnormal neck position, head tremor and social embarrassment and depression. All these factors can have an impact on the quality of life of the patient and can result in some degree of disability. Questioning patients about disability and clarifying the contributing factors is crucial for optimum care of patients with cervical dystonia[10].

6.4.1 Pain

There is a high incidence of pain in this disease, which distinguishes this from other focal dystonias[17]. Pain is present in almost 75 per cent of patients at sometime during their illness and contributes to disability[12,14–16]. It usually affects the neck and the shoulders with some radiation and is described as an aching sensation. Pain is increased by constant head turning, greater degree of head turning and the presence of spasms[16]. The pain can be intermittent or continuous and typically is diffuse and widespread[18].

6.4.2 Motor symptoms

Cervical dystonia manifests itself as involuntary muscle contractions that cause twisting or turning of the neck. A wide variety of abnormal head postures may be assumed, and deviations may produce head turning (torticollis), leaning (laterocollis), or pulling forward (anterocollis), backward (retrocollis), or a combination of these postures[4]. In the majority of patients the abnormal posture is present most of the time, but it may change during the course of the illness[3]. Cervical dystonia may be associated with dystonia in another body part, or with postural limb tremor in as many as one third of the patients[3,10,12,15].

6.4.3 Head tremor

Two types of tremors affect the head. The tremor is termed 'dystonic' if there is a directional preponderance and it increases in amplitude when the head is deviated away from the direction of the involuntary movement. If the tremor is rhythmical, symmetrical and does not change considerably with head movement, it is 'essential'[4]. One report of 300 patients found dystonic tremor in 37 per cent of the patients and essential tremor in another 30 per cent[12]. It is unclear whether essential tremor in the head or in the hand is an additional manifestation of a primarily dystonic disorder or a separate associated movement disorder similar or identical to essential tremor[10].

6.4.4 Social embarrassment

Cervical dystonia can result in social withdrawal and isolation. Patients often become very anxious and self-conscious. They often curtail social engagements and try to avoid interaction with other people. Thus cervical dystonia can affect their social, private and professional life[19].

6.4.5 Depression

Previously disagreement existed about whether cervical dystonia was a psychiatric illness, but now it is well recognized as a neurological illness[10]. At the same time it is well known that depression is associated with this disease in almost a quarter of the patients[20].

6.5 Disability and quality of life

Disability and functional impairment is common in cervical dystonia. It can have an impact on all the different aspects of life including work, leisure activities and activities of daily life. In one series some degree of disability was found in 99 per cent of 220 patients with cervical dystonia[21]. Disability is caused by combination of physical discomfort, functional impairment, social embarrassment, isolation and depression. Disability is also caused by task specific limitations such as inability to drive and inability to participate in leisure activities. Questioning patients about disability and exploring the contributing factors is crucial for the optimal care of the patients with cervical dystonia. The impact of cervical dystonia on quality of life is significant and is comparable to patients with Parkinson's disease, mild to moderate multiple sclerosis and moderate epilepsy[22].

6.6 Provocative and palliative factors

Several provocative and palliative factors are characteristic of idiopathic dystonia[10]. Most important is the so-called 'sensory trick' or *geste antagoniste* to relieve the cervical dystonia[23]. This involves touching the chin, face or head. Other effective tricks include pulling the hair, sucking on a pen, pulling an earlobe, leaning against a high-backed chair or placing something in the mouth. These tricks are more effective early on in the disease and are not helpful in all patients. How these tricks work is not entirely clear but these do suggest that dystonia may have a sensory element to it[24−32]. Other less common palliative factors include alcohol, relaxation and rest. Anxiety, stress, fatigue, walking and self-consciousness usually aggravate cervical dystonia[33]. These palliative and provocative factors can vary between patients as well. Lying supine, relaxation and sleep helped 40 per cent of 72 patients but made it worse in 16−25 per cent in one study[34].

6.7 Classification of cervical dystonia

Cervical dystonia can be classified in various ways.

1. **On the basis of aetiology**
   - Idiopathic (primary) cervical dystonia.
   - Secondary cervical dystonia: Table 6.1[4].

2. **On the basis of dominant head position**
   - Torticollis: this is the most common type, present in about 50 per cent of patients[35–37].
   - Laterocollis: lateral tilt present in 10–15 per cent of patients.
   - Retrocollis: backward head tilt present in 10–15 per cent of patients.
   - Anterocollis: forward flexion of the neck is rare.
   - Propulsion: forward shift of the head on the trunk.
   - Lateropulsion: sideway shift of the head on the trunk.
   - Complex cervical dystonia: variable head position with different combinations and is a feature in 10–15 per cent of patients.

6.8 Pathogenesis

Although pathogenesis of cervical dystonia remains unclear, there has been great progress in understanding the different factors that might be involved in the development of this disease. This is especially true of the genetic factors as there is growing evidence that some adult-onset focal dystonias are genetically based[38–42]. Trauma has long been implicated in the pathogenesis of cervical dystonia[11,12,43] and physiological studies have also implicated the sensory system, particularly in view of the effectiveness of sensory tricks[44–47]. Theories of vestibular impairment producing impaired postural feedback have lost favour[10,48] but evidence is increasing to support a role for impaired basal ganglia functioning in the development of this disease[49–53].

6.9 Diagnosis

The diagnosis of cervical dystonia is a clinical diagnosis. The diagnosis is often delayed, due to the variable presentation of the disease and poor recognition of the spectrum of its clinical manifestations[43]. Two issues must be settled to arrive at the diagnosis of idiopathic cervical dystonia[10]. First, it must be confirmed that we are dealing with dystonia and not with many non-dystonic causes of an abnormal neck posture[54]. It must be borne in mind that torticollis is a physical sign and not a disease. Second, all the secondary causes of dystonia should be excluded by history, physical examination and laboratory investigations. In practice most of these are easily distinguished clinically from the true idiopathic

Table 6.1. Secondary causes of cervical dystonia[4]

Metabolic causes
- Wilson disease
- Kernicterus
- Amino acid disorders
  - Glutamic acidemia
  - Methylmalonic acidemia
  - Homocystinuria
  - Hartnup's disease
  - Tyrosinosis
- Lipid disorders
  - Metachromatic leukodystrophy
  - Ceroid lipofuscinosis
  - Dystonic lipidosis
  - Gangliosidoses
  - Hexosaminidase A and B deficiency
- Mitochondrial encephalopathies
  (e.g. Leigh disease, Leber disease)
- Vitamin E deficiency
- Biopterin deficiency
- Triosephosphate isomerase deficiency
- Lesch Nyhan syndrome

Vascular causes
- Cerebrovascular, or ischemic injury
- Arteriovenous malformation
- Perinatal cerebral injury

Infections
- Viral encephalitis
- Subacute sclerosing panencephalitis
- AIDS
- Creutzfeldt–Jakob disease

Tumour
- Brain tumour

Toxins
- Carbon monoxide
- Manganese
- Carbon disulphide
- Methanol
- Disulfiram
- Wasp sting

Table 6.1. (*Cont.*) Secondary causes of cervical dystonia

Drugs
- Levodopa
- Dopamine agonist
- Antipsychotics
- Metoclopramide
- Fenfluramine
- Flecainide
- Ergot agents
- Anticonvulsants
- Certain calcium channel blockers

Neurodegenerative disorders
- Progressive supranuclear palsy
- Multiple systems atrophy
- Corticobasal–ganglionic degeneration
- Hallervorden–Spatz disease
- Hypobetalipoproteinaemia, acanthocytosis, retinitis pigmentosa, pallidal degeneration (HARP syndrome)
- Neuroacanthocytosis
- Spinocerebeller ataxia, types 1, 2, 3
- Ataxia telangiectasia
- Huntington's disease

Demyelinating disorders
- Multiple sclerosis

cervical dystonia and no further investigation is needed[55]. Magnetic resonance imaging (MRI) and/or computed tomography (CT) scans in a group of 149 patients with clinically idiopathic cervical dystonia found no abnormalities that altered management[56]. Some of the common non-dystonic causes of abnormal neck posture are shown in Table 6.2[4].

6.10   Treatment of cervical dystonia

With the introduction of botulinum toxin therapy, treatment of cervical dystonia has improved substantially[57]. It is the treatment of choice for cervical dystonia[58]. Unfortunately it still remains symptomatic treatment and is not a cure. Oral pharmacological therapy continues to play an important part in alleviating symptoms of cervical dystonia either alone or in increasing numbers in combination with botulinum toxin therapy. The role of surgery is confined to a small number of patients with significant disability despite maximal medical therapy, or who have become resistant to botulinum toxin therapy[57].

Table 6.2. Non-dystonic causes of abnormal neck posture[4]

Psychogenic

Ocular causes
- Paresis of extraocular muscles
- Strabismus
- Hemianopia
- Oculomotor apraxia

Musculo-skeletal causes
- Atlanto-axial sublaxation
- Ankylosing spondylitis
- Cervical spondylosis
- Fracture of cervical spine
- Osteomyelitis of cervical spine
- Congenital torticollis due to fibrotic band or aplasia of sternocleidomastoid
- Fibrosis of subcutaneous tissue after local radiotherapy
- Stiff person syndrome

Local neck mass
- Cervical lymphadenopathy
- Goitre
- Soft tissue neck mass

Other neurological causes
- Syringomyelia
- Arnold–Chiari malformation
- Vestibular torticollis
- Posterior fossa mass

Many patients do well on combination treatments depending on severity of cervical dystonia. Physical therapies such as physiotherapy, acupuncture, osteopathy, chiropractic or the wearing of the neck collar are not consistently effective and collars can be counter productive as well[55]. Neck manipulation can be dangerous and there is a risk of vertebral or carotid artery dissection[59]. Relaxation therapies such as hypnosis, behaviour therapy, biofeedback and meditation may work[60]. Electromyographic (EMG) biofeedback is sometimes effective.

6.11 Pharmacologic therapy

Before the introduction of botulinum toxin therapy, oral medications were for many years the treatment of choice for cervical dystonia[61,62]. These included anticholinergic agents, GABA (gamma-aminobutyric acid) mimetic agents, dopamine receptor antagonists, dopamine-depleting agents, and dopamine receptor agonists. Nevertheless, these agents continue to play an important role in the management of this condition, particularly as many patients require combination treatment with oral drugs and chemodenervation to achieve acceptable results and concerns about development of immunoresistance to botulinum toxin therapy.

6.11.1   Anticholinergic agents

These agents have been the first line treatment of cervical dystonia for years. The benefits of anticholinergic agents have been documented in large series of patients evaluated in open-label and double-blind studies[62,63]. In a retrospective analysis of open-label trials of initial therapy with high dose anticholinergic agents[62], 39 per cent of cervical dystonia patients reported good response particularly for patients with a disease duration of less than five years, women and older age at onset.

These agents should be started at a very low dose, which should be titrated upwards slowly with weekly increments until there is either benefit or appearance of side effects. Using low initial doses and slow dose titration may reduce adverse effects. Effective doses vary widely between patients so the minimum dose that provides relief should be used. Side effects of these agents are related to their peripheral and CNS actions and include dry mouth, blurred vision, constipation, urinary retention, confusion, memory loss, hallucinations and behavioural changes.

6.11.2   GABA mimetic agents

Baclofen is a GABA receptor agonist that acts presynaptically to decrease the firing of motor neurons and interneurons in the CNS. It is less effective than anticholinergic agents[64,65] and in one study 11 per cent of patients with cervical dystonia treated with baclofen reported good response[62]. Dose related adverse effects include muscle weakness, drowsiness, lethargy, gastrointestinal complaints and urinary frequency. It is more useful in generalized dystonia and blepharospasm and is rarely used in isolated cervical dystonia.

Benzodiazepines act by potentiating the neural inhibition mediated by GABA. It has been reported that clonazepam is effective in about 21 per cent of patients with cervical dystonia[62]. Clonazepam is particularly effective in tiding over painful exacerbations of cervical dystonia and exacerbations of dystonia related to anxiety and social situations. Adverse effects of benzodiazepines include sedation, confusion and potential of addiction with prolonged treatment. Our practice is to prescribe clonazepam 0.5 mg TDS for three days during a painful exacerbation to ease the symptoms while adjusting treatment with other agents.

6.11.3 Dopamine-depleting agents, dopamine receptor antagonists and dopamine receptor agonists

Interestingly, patients with cervical dystonia may respond favourably to treatment that either increases or decreases dopaminergic neuro-transmission reflecting the heterogeneous nature of the disorder[66]. Results of treatment with dopamine receptor antagonists (e.g. haloperidol) and dopamine-depleting agents (e.g. tetrabenazine) have been less promising than anti-cholinergic agents[66] with a greater spectrum of adverse effects. Tetrabenazine has been found to be particularly helpful in the treatment of tardive dyskinesias[67] but troublesome adverse effects can occur with its use including parkinsonian features, hypotension, depression, drowsiness and fatigue. Clozapine, an atypical anti-psychotic agent, predominantly blocks the dopamine D4 receptor in addition to various other complex neuro-chemical effects. It has been found to be helpful in the treatment of tardive dyskinesia[68] although it has been found ineffective for cervical dystonia[69]. Levodopa and dopamine agonists are not useful in idiopathic cervical dystonia[66] except for rare cases of dopa-responsive dystonia[70,71].

6.11.4 Other oral medications

Mexiletine has been tried in one study with some benefit[72].

6.12 Role of surgery

The role of surgery is confined to patients in whom chemodenervation with botulinum toxin injections alone or in combination with traditional pharmacotherapy fail to provide adequate relief of symptoms[57]. As a proportion of patients (10–20 per cent) may experience spontaneous remission, surgical procedures should be reserved for those patients in whom disease duration is longer than 1 year. Both peripheral and central surgical approaches for the treatment of cervical dystonia have been tried and are important options for patients. The magnitude of the clinical benefit appears to be similar to that provided by botulinum toxin therapy, but the results are most reliable for less complex postures such as simple rotation. These techniques should be performed only at centres with significant experience and expertise in the surgical management of movement disorders.

6.12.1 Peripheral surgery

A variety of peripheral surgical procedures have been used for the treatment of cervical dystonia[73]. These include

1. Myotomy
2. Microvascular decompression

3. Spinal accessory nerve (SAN) section
4. Ventral rhizotomy combined with SAN section
5. Selective dorsal ramisectomy combined with SAN section.

The most common surgical procedure for cervical dystonia is selective dorsal ramisectomy combined with SAN section[74]. Several open-labelled and uncontrolled studies have yielded response rates ranging from 48 to 98 per cent[75-80]. In another retrospective analysis of 16 patients with botulinum toxin A resistance undergoing selective dorsal ramisectomy to treat cervical dystonia, clinical rating scales showed a mean objective improvement of 32 per cent. However, none of these patients was able to return to work[81]. Complications of surgery include almost complete sensory loss over the distribution of greater occipital nerve, dysphagia, occipital neuralgia and hyperaesthesia in the area governed by the greater occipital nerve[74-80].

6.12.2   Central surgical approaches

These include:
1. Stereotactic thalamotomy
2. Pallidal surgery
3. Deep brain stimulation (DBS)

Results of thalamotomy for the treatment of cervical dystonia have been variable[82]. Bilateral thalamotomy is more effective but is associated with 10–40 per cent risk of serious complications especially bulbar weakness resulting in speech impediment and dysphagia, and cognitive impairment[82].

After the resurgence of pallidotomy for the treatment of Parkinson's disease, considerable interest has developed in using this technique to treat primary dystonia. However, only a small number of patients have undergone this procedure for cervical dystonia, and data is insufficient to be conclusive. Previous reports showed variable results with placement of lesions in anterior pallidum[82]. However more recent reports have uniformly described striking benefits after unilateral or bilateral posteroventral pallidotomy in patients with primary generalized dystonia many of whom had cervical dystonia[83-86]. Bilateral pallidotomy has a greater effect than unilateral pallidotomy but is associated with more side effects as well including bulbar weakness and cognitive impairment.

Deep brain stimulation has been used extensively for the treatment of movement disorders and appears to provide efficacy comparable to that of lesioning procedures but with a more favourable safety profile, especially for bilateral procedures[87]. DBS of the thalamus has been used in a small number of patients with primary dystonia with mild improvement only[87]. DBS of globus pallidus interna in a small number of patients with idiopathic generalized, segmental, or cervical dystonia has been reported to provide benefits comparable to those obtained with pallidotomy[88-91]. These preliminary results are very promising and before this treatment can be recommended to treat resistant patients with severe cervical dystonia, we need the results of larger clinical trials. DBS seems to be safer than lesioning and it has the added advantage of adaptability of stimulation settings and reversibility should adverse effects appear or curative therapy is found in the future. On the other hand it is more expensive in the long run due to the extra cost of the device and follow up, and to the drawbacks of the chronically implanted device including infection, migration of leads and battery replacement, etc.

6.13   Treatment with botulinum toxin therapy

Chemodenervation with botulinum toxin therapy has now taken over as the treatment of choice for cervical dystonia. It has given hope and relief to many patients with this condition. It is one of the few conditions in which the FDA in the USA has approved treatment with both botulinum toxin A and botulinum toxin B. This injection therapy benefits the highest percentage of patients in the shortest time and has been proven effective in many double-blind placebo-controlled botulinum toxin trials[92]. It has fewer side effects than other pharmacological oral treatments[93].

6.13.1   Review and clinical evidence of therapeutic efficacy

In 1986, Tsui *et al.* were the first to show the efficacy of treatment with botulinum toxin injections in cervical dystonia in a report of a double-blind, placebo-controlled trial[94]. Subsequent to this initial trial, many studies confirmed the benefits of botulinum toxin injections for cervical dystonia[95-100]. There is also extensive evidence that suggests long-term benefit of this treatment[101,102]. Two of the largest trials are representative[101,102]. During a 12-week period, 55 patients who were not responsive to oral medications received either botulinum toxin or placebo in a double-blind fashion, followed by a 4-week open phase when all patients received botulinum toxin. Overall, 74 per cent of patients showed improvement with botulinum toxin therapy by the end of the study. Similarly, a retrospective review of 205 patients treated with botulinum toxin therapy over a 5-year period showed an improvement in posture in 71 per cent and improvement of pain in 76 per cent of patients.

Most of these initial trials used botulinum toxin A injections[95-97], while more recent studies have used botulinum toxin B with success in A-responders and A-resistant patients[103-106]. In view of overwhelming evidence, botulinum toxin therapy is now recognized and recommended as first line treatment for cervical dystonia[101,107-109].

Botulinum toxin therapy is not a cure but is a symptomatic treatment of cervical dystonia. The benefit of injections lasts for an average of 12 weeks with a range of 8–16 weeks but can vary between patients. The benefit from the botulinum toxin injections start generally within the first week but rarely may be delayed. In our experience patients generally need two to three visits to find the correct dose of toxin and site of injection so as to get the optimum benefit. The maximum or peak effect is seen after about 2 weeks. Patients continue to benefit from injections and may experience progressive improvement of dystonia with continued botulinum toxin injections[103,110,111].

6.13.2   Non-responders to botulinum toxin treatment

Non-responders to botulinum treatment can be broadly classified into two groups[10]. Primary non-responders are the patients who do not respond to this treatment from the very beginning. Secondary non-responders become resistant to treatment after initial response.

Important factors resulting in primary non-response include contractures due to long-standing disease, additional musculo-skeletal problems, injection at the wrong site, selection of incorrect muscles for injection, insufficient initial dose of the toxin or failure to properly prepare the toxin. About half of these will subsequently respond to botulinum toxin therapy[112]. It is for these reasons that we need to review a patient at least three times before labelling them as primary non-responders. EMG may be required to properly localize the muscles primarily responsible for dystonic posture. However, even after considering and correcting all these factors there are certain patients who still fail to benefit, for which no explanation is available. This is believed to result from involvement of deep neck musculature.

There can be several factors to account for secondary non-response. The two most important include a change in the pattern of muscle activity and development of neutralizing antibodies. It is therefore extremely important to make a careful assessment of the patient, their symptoms and dystonic posture on each visit to take into consideration any change in muscle involvement. The development of neutralizing antibodies is a serious problem as it obliterates any future response to botulinum toxin[113,114]. Neutralizing antibodies develop in at least 5–10 per cent of treated patients[115]. It has been suggested that any patient who loses responsiveness to injections and fails to develop atrophy in the injected muscles should be assumed to have developed neutralizing antibodies[116]. A short interval between treatments of less than 3 months[114,116], and high doses of botulinum toxin[116,117] are considered risk factors for development of these antibodies. In view of the above it is recommended that botulinum toxin injections be given no more frequently than every 3 months and minimum possible dose should be used[115]. If the clinical response remains inadequate adjunctive medication should be used[10]. Patients who become resistant to botulinum toxin A therapy due to development of neutralizing antibodies have been successfully treated with botulinum toxin B[104].

6.13.3 Botulinum toxin type B

Botulinum toxin B (NeuroBloc/Myobloc) is effective and safe in the treatment of cervical dystonia as shown by many double-blind, placebo-controlled studies[103–105]. It is shown to be effective in unselected patients with cervical dystonia[105], in responders to botulinum toxin A[103] and non-responders to botulinum toxin A[104]. It does seem that botulinum toxin type B has more side effects than type A and early open label studies suggest that botulinum toxin type B (Neurobloc/Myobloc) is not as efficacious as type A toxin and is less well tolerated[118]. However, it does have a role in the treatment of cervical dystonia in patients who have developed resistance to botulinum toxin A. There are important differences between botulinum toxin A and type B in terms of preparation, storage and adverse effects such as antibody formation. More research is needed to clarify these issues to determine its position in the management of cervical dystonia.

6.14   Side effects of botulinum toxin therapy

Most studies report side effects in 20–30 per cent of patients per treatment cycle and about 50 per cent of the patients experience such events sometime during therapy. The true incidence of these side effects is quite variable among patients and depends upon individual patients, expertise of the injector, total dose of the toxin used and pattern of injections. Dysphagia and neck weakness are the most important dose related side effects while local pain and flu-like syndrome seems unrelated to the dose. Studies employing the highest dosages reported side effects in nearly 100 per cent of patients[119], whereas the use of low dosages resulted in low incidence of side effects[110]. However, side effects are usually minimal and of little functional consequence in most people.

6.14.1 Dysphagia

Pharyngeal weakness resulting in dysphagia is an important and sometimes troublesome side effect. It should be taken seriously and actively enquired from the patients as it can lead to aspiration with serious consequences. Fortunately most of the time it is mild and only rarely requires the institution of a soft diet[120]. In one study 33 per cent of patients undergoing treatment with botulinum toxin therapy for cervical dystonia experienced dysphagia[121]. Dysphagia is dose related and most commonly occurs with injections of sternocleidomastoid muscles especially if both are injected at the same sitting. It occurs because of the local spread of the toxin to the underlying pharyngeal musculature[122,123].

Dysphagia usually starts about a week after the injections and lasts on average for 2 to 3 weeks. Other causes need to be excluded if it persists for more than 2 months. This complication can be reduced by avoiding bilateral sternocleido-mastoid injections and if multiple small-volume injections are used rather than a single large-volume bolus[122,124]. Patients should be warned of this possible complication and given full information and advice. They should also be given a contact point in case they need help and further advice. Care is needed if there is pre-existing bulbar or respiratory problems.

6.14.2   Local neck pain

The injection pain is mildly uncomfortable but is well tolerated by most patients. Sometimes this pain persists for longer than usual and is slightly more intense as well but usually settles with simple analgesia. On rare occasions patients report increased pain and dystonic posture after these injections. A short course of clonazepam is sometimes required to tide over this period which lasts a few days. However, botulinum toxin type B does seem to induce more pain at the injection site that may last for some days.

6.14.3   Neck muscle weakness

This is a dose-related side effect that occurs in less than 5 per cent of patients. Transient weakness of neck muscles can be very problematic and can last a few weeks. Avoiding high dose of toxin and careful selection of muscles can prevent this complication in most cases.

6.14.4   Dry mouth

Dry mouth is relatively more common with botulinum toxin B as compared to botulinum toxin A and is a dose-related side effect[104]. Dry mouth can aggravate dysphagia and sometimes may be confused with this symptom. It lasts for a few weeks and usually does not require any treatment.

6.14.5   Flu-like illness

Some patients (1–9 per cent) report flu-like symptoms for a few days after the injections with generalized lethargy. None of our patients has stopped treatment because of this symptom.

6.14.6   Other minor side effects

These include dysphonia, back pain after trapezius injections, dyspnoea and local allergic skin reactions. Rarely brachial neuritis has been reported[125,126].

6.14.7 Distant side effects

Distant effects of botulinum toxin on neuromuscular transmission have been demonstrated by single fibre EMG, although there were no clinical symptoms in these patients[127]. Severe and prolonged side effects have been reported in patients with underlying neuromuscular disease[128–130]. At the same time, with care, cervical dystonia can be treated successfully and safely in patients with myasthenia gravis[131,132].

6.15 Practical aspects of treatment with botulinum toxin

Treatment with botulinum toxin injections is a symptomatic treatment of cervical dystonia. Patients being considered for this treatment should be given all the relevant information regarding cervical dystonia and all the possible treatment options available to manage it. Before the commencement of the treatment, it is very important to establish the treatment objectives, discuss the various options available, discuss the efficacy of different treatment options and convey all the possible side effects of these injections. Patients should be provided with written information regarding the dystonia in general and cervical dystonia and botulinum toxin in particular. Treatment with botulinum toxin should only start after the patient's informed consent.

Various *indications* for botulinum treatment of cervical dystonia are:

- pain or spasms
- abnormal head or neck posture
- impairment of daily activities of life
- social embarrassment and loss of self confidence
- depression as a result of this condition
- head tremor

6.15.1 Optimum goals of treatment with botulinum toxin

The main aim of treatment with botulinum toxin therapy is to achieve a balance between inducing muscle weakness sufficient to reduce spasm but insufficient to interfere with function. Thus a combination of reduction in dystonia and pain with optimization of function should be sought.

6.15.2 Commencement of botulinum toxin treatment

Only trained specialists with experience in the treatment of movement disorders should administer botulinum toxin injections. They must also have a good understanding of both the anatomy of affected muscles and the resultant movement disorder.

6.15.3   Patient education and counselling

Patient education and counselling are essential components of a comprehensive therapeutic approach to all patients with dystonia. Before the first injection, patients should be informed about the process involved in the selection of muscles to be injected, possible number and sites of injections (preferably with the help of diagrams and posters), the frequency of these injections, nature and time course of its benefits and side effects and what to do and whom to contact if problems arise after the injections. Patients should also be informed that it usually takes a little time to get the dose and site of injections right for optimum benefit. It is also extremely important to inform patients that these injections do not work for everyone and a patient is usually considered a non-responder if there is no benefit after three injections.

6.15.4   Process of muscle selection

This is the most crucial aspect of treatment of cervical dystonia with botulinum toxin therapy. Both history and physical examination are important in making this judgement. Patients are naturally very anxious when attending this clinic for the first time and many are very reluctant to attend the hospital as they normally avoid public places because of abnormal head or neck posture and head tremor. It is extremely important to try to build rapport with them early on to gain their confidence. Muscle selection process starts as soon as a patient enters the consultation room. We feel that specialists working in the cervical dystonia clinics should have a system which they should develop and follow every time they see a patient in the clinic either for the first time or on a follow-up visit. This will ensure that proper assessment takes place and correct treatment is devised initially and then modified later on if required according to the feedback obtained from the patients. Some basic principles that can help to devise a system include the following important points.

- Make the patient feel comfortable in the consultation room and ask them if they would like to be seen with a relative or a friend.
- Make them sit in a comfortable chair and try to sit in front of the patient to get a good view of the head and neck.
- Make sure that you are able to see the neck and clothing does not cover it.
- Encourage the patient not to use compensatory tricks during the consultation and let him or her be seen with the dystonic posture.
- Take the help of the relative or a friend accompanying the patient in ascertaining the dystonic posture and the difficulties experienced by the patient in daily life.
- Ask the patient to demonstrate the most common neck posture.
- Identify the most common problems, discomforts and difficulties arising from these postures.

- Find out how this is impacting on the life of the patient. This includes their professional life, marital relationship, social life, leisure activities and activities of daily life.
- Ask about the mood of the patient as a result of this and their pattern of sleep.
- Take a detailed drug history.
- Get a feel for the patient's expectations of the botulinum toxin therapy.

6.15.5 Examination

Careful examination of the patient in different positions is indicated and required.
- Instruct the patient to position the head in an upright posture.
- Ask the patient to look both ways and flex and extend the neck and document the range of neck movements.
- Passively adjust the head and observe for additional extension, flexion, and rotation that may be compensated by the patient and note any contractures.
- Palpate for contracting and hypertrophied muscles and elicit any points of tenderness.
- The patient should be asked to walk and head position observed and recorded.
- Ask the patient to demonstrate sensory trick or geste if possible. The patient should try to keep his head straight for as long as possible and try to observe the first movement away from the midline.
- Always remember that some movements are compensatory in nature and therefore clarify that from history, accompanying relative or friend and effects of a geste.
- The head position that is most abnormal is used to select the muscles for injections.

In summary, we should aim to select muscles that cause dominant movements, that are painful and tender or that are visibly hypertrophied and hyperactive. It is not difficult to define the dystonic muscles in simple forms of cervical dystonia, but it requires an experienced specialist to identify the muscles involved in complex or fluctuating cervical dystonia. In more complex cases, EMG can be used to identify the muscles involved. Normally we should try to restrict the number of muscles injected in one sitting to a limited number. The pattern of muscles injected should be evaluated and reviewed on every follow-up visit keeping in view the feedback from the patient and physical examination. We should keep in mind that pattern of dystonia can vary with the passage of time.

6.15.6 Injection techniques

The most commonly injected muscles include sternocleidomastoid, trapezius, splenius capitus, levator scapulae and scalene complex. Muscles involved in the abnormal posturing are isolated using standard anatomic landmarks.

Table 6.3. Muscles commonly involved and injected in various types of cervical dystonia

Forward propulsion (anterior shift)
- Bilateral sternocleidomastoid

Head retraction (posterior shift)
- Bilateral splenius capitis
- Bilateral levator scapulae

Anterocollis (head tips forward)
- Bilateral sternocleidomastoid

Retrocollis (head tips back)
- Bilateral splenius capitis
- Bilateral semispinalis capitis
- Bilateral cervical part of trapezius

Laterocollis (tilt)
- Ipsilateral sternocleidomastoid
- Ipsilateral trapezius
- Ipsilateral splenius capitis
- Ipsilateral scalene complex

Torticollis (rotation)
- Contralateral sternocleidomastoid
- Ipsilateral splenius capitis
- Ipsilateral levator scapulae
- Ipsilateral trapezius

Muscles that are commonly involved in various types of cervical dystonia are listed in Table 6.3. Most of these muscles can be identified and injected without the help of EMG and therefore the majority of the centres treating cervical dystonia with botulinum toxin injections reserve the use of EMG for special circumstances, which will be discussed later. We recommend a 5–10 ml syringe and a 27-gauge hypodermic needle.

Toxin dose

There are three preparations of botulinum toxin that are available in the United Kingdom at present. Dysport and BOTOX® are type A toxins while NeuroBloc is type B. The dose of each preparation is measured in mouse units (mu), although 1 mu of Dysport is not equivalent to 1 mu of BOTOX® or NeuroBloc. Roughly 1 mu of BOTOX® is equivalent to 3–4 units of Dysport and 50 units of NeuroBloc. There is no clinical evidence at the moment to suggest clear advantage of one preparation over the other. It is therefore recommended to choose one preparation initially in clinics to avoid confusion of dosage and dilutions. Patients should be started with a minimum dose, as there is no way to predict the patient's response to these injections. The dose of the toxin should be adjusted in subsequent visits keeping in mind the response of the injected muscles to the toxin, patient's feedback regarding efficacy, side effects and findings on physical examination. Suggested initial dose for individual muscles is listed in Table 6.4. Total initial starting dose can vary from 200 mu to 400 mu of Dysport depending on severity of symptoms, type of cervical dystonia and build of the patient. The maximum dose in one sitting should probably not exceed 1000 mu Dysport.

Toxin dilution

Different centres use different dilutions of botulinum toxin for these injections. We recommend diluting 500 mu Dysport or 100 mu BOTOX® in 5 ml normal saline. There is no clinical evidence to suggest the best dilution to use in cervical dystonia. In our experience the higher concentrations reduce the incidence of side effects especially local pain and dysphagia.

Follow-up visits

Follow-up visits are as important as the initial visit. Feedback from the patient is crucial in determining the dose and sites of the next injections. Patients should be asked about the efficacy of the injections, duration of the benefit and severity and duration of the side effects. Patients should be observed and examined at each follow-up visit and on the basis of subjective feedback and objective observations, decisions should be made to continue with the treatment or any adjustments made in the dose or site of the injections (Table 6.5).

Table 6.4. Dose range recommendations for individual muscles in cervical dystonia

Muscles	Dysport® (mu)	BOTOX® (mu)	Neurobloc (mu)
Sternocleidomastoid	50–150	10–40	500–2000
Splenius capitis	50–150	10–40	500–2000
Semispinalis capitis	50–100	10–25	500–1250
Levator scapulae	50–200	10–50	500–2500
Trapezius	50–200	10–50	500–2500
Scalene complex	50–150	10–40	500–2000

Notes:
• Start with the lowest dose and gradually increase the dose to the maximum.
• Modify the above-recommended doses according to the clinical situation.

Table 6.5. Dose modifiers

Clinical situation	Decrease dose	Increase dose
Patient weight	Low	High
Muscle bulk	Small	Large
Severity of dystonia	Mild	Severe
Number of muscles being injected simultaneously	Many	Few
Results of previous therapy	Too much weakness	Inadequate response
SCM, splenius capitis injections	If bilateral injections	If unilateral injections

Cervical dystonia rating scales

These outcome assessments can be documented by using one of many cervical dystonia rating scales[133], but in our experience these are time consuming in busy clinics and difficult to score. Initial outcome measures were suggested by Swash *et al.*[134], Couch[135], Tolosa[136] and Lang *et al.*[137] Currently, rating scales as suggested by Tsui *et al.*[94] and the Toronto Western Spasmodic Torticollis Rating Scale (TWSTRS) are popular[138].

Injecting individual muscles

It is imperative to know the local anatomy of the neck before embarking on treatment of cervical dystonia with botulinum toxin injections. One should know the function of important neck muscles and their relationship with other important neck structures such as blood vessels and nerves. Some of the more important muscles involved in cervical dystonia are discussed below.

Sternocleidomastoid

The sternocleidomastoid arises from the mastoid process and lateral half of the superior nuchal line and is inserted below onto the manubrium sterni and the medial third of the clavicle. Its main action is to rotate the neck to the opposite side. It can also pull the head over towards the ipsilateral shoulder in laterocollis, propel the head forwards in propulsion and pull the chin directly downwards in anterocollis.

Normally it is very easy to identify a contracting and hypertrophied sternocleidomastoid. In difficult cases, especially obese patients, ask the patient to press his or her hand against the chin on the opposite side to activate the muscle. It is recommended to inject in the upper third of the muscle by identifying the muscle first and then holding it in your fingers to make sure that you inject the identified muscle only.

Trapezius

The trapezius is attached to the medial third of the superior nuchal line of the occipital bone, the external occipital protuberance and the ligamental nuchae above, and to the lateral third of the clavicle below. The middle and inferior fibres arise from the thoracic vertebrae and attach to the acromian and scapula.

The trapezius elevates the shoulder and is involved in ipsilateral laterocollis, ipsilateral retrocollis and ipsilateral torticollis. Being a superficial muscle, it is easy to palpate and inject. If in doubt ask the patient to elevate the shoulder and grasp the muscle between two fingers. Distribute the injection between two or three sites for optimum results.

Levator scapulae

The levator scapulae is attached superiorly to the transverse processes of the axis, atlas, third and fourth cervical vertebrae. Inferiorly, it is attached to the superior third of the medial border of the scapula.

Its main function is to elevate the ipsilateral shoulder and is involved in ipsilateral laterocollis and torticollis. It is easily felt anterior to the trapezius.

Splenius capitis

Superiorly the splenius capitis is attached to the mastoid process and rough surface of the occipital bone just below the lateral third of the superior nuchal line. It goes downwards, medially and posteriorly to attach to the lower half of the ligamentum nuchae, supine of the seventh cervical vertebra and spines of the upper thoracic vertebrae. It lies deeply in the neck beneath the trapezius for the most part but can be palpated just behind the upper posterior border of the sternomastoid.

Ipsilateral splenius capitis is involved in ipsilateral torticollis, ipsilateral laterocollis and tilts the head backwards in retrocollis. To inject this muscle ask the patient to activate the sternomastoid. This muscle lies behind the upper posterior border of the sternomastoid at the level of angle of jaw and can be palpated with fingers. Inject directly into the muscle at a depth of 1−2 cm. Branches of the lesser occipital nerve may course over the muscle and sometimes patients can experience severe neuralgic pain if these are irritated during the procedure.

Semispinalis capitis

This muscle, superiorly, is attached to the medial aspect of the area between the superior and inferior nuchal lines of the occipital bone. Inferiorly, it attaches to the lower cervical vertebrae and the upper thoracic vertebrae. It lies deep to trapezius and splenius capitus for the most part. It extends the neck in retrocollis and may be involved in ipsilateral laterocollis and torticollis. For injecting this muscle ask the patient to extend the neck against your hand to activate it and inject directly into the muscle after palpating it with your fingers.

Anterior neck muscles

This group of muscles along with both sternomastoid muscles is responsible for anterocollis or propulsion. This group includes longus colli, longus capitis, rectus capitis anterior and rectus capitis lateralis. Most of these muscles are deep seated and are difficult to inject in a clinic setting. For practical purposes, injecting both sternomastoids in anterocollis is sufficient to give reasonably good results. On occasions, dystonic spasms of platysma influence head posture. This muscle is superficial and thus is easy to identify as it stands out as thickened cords that can be easily injected.

Role of electromyographic (EMG) recordings

Electromyographic recordings are not routinely used for assisting botulinum toxin injections in the treatment of cervical dystonia in most centres in the world. EMG-assisted toxin injections do produce better results than injections based on clinical examination[139,140], but can be time consuming and adds to the discomfort and expense of the treatment. Indications for EMG-assisted toxin injections include

- Patients who are technically difficult to assess or inject (e.g. very obese patients).
- Patients who have not responded to clinically placed injections.
- Complex dystonic postures.
- Changing pattern of dystonia that is difficult to assess.

REFERENCES

1. Fahn, S., Marsden, C. D. and Calne, D. B. (1987). Classification and investigation of dystonia. In C. D. Marsden and S. Fahn, eds., *Movement Disorders 2*. London: Butterworths, pp. 332–58.
2. Chan, J., Brin, M. F. and Fahn, S. (1991). Idiopathic cervical dystonia: clinical characteristics. *Mov. Disord.*, **6**, 119–26.
3. Jankovic, J. and Van der Linden, C. (2000). Dystonia and tremor: predisposing factors. *J. Neurol. Neurosurg. Psychiatry*, **51**, 1512–19.
4. Stacy, M. (2000). Idiopathic cervical dystonia: an overview. *Neurology*, **55**, S2–S8.
5. Mathews, W. B., Beasley, P., Parry-Jones, W. and Garland, G. (1978). Spasmodic torticollis: a combined clinical study. *J. Neurol. Neurosurg. Psychiatry*, **41**, 485–92.
6. Jayne, D., Lees, A. J. and Stern, G. M. (1984). Remission in spasmodic torticollis. *J. Neurol. Neurosurg. Psychiatry*, **47**, 1236–7.

7. Lowenstein, D. H. and Aminoff, M. J. (1988). The clinical course of spasmodic torticollis. *Neurology*, **38**, 530–2.

8. Friedman, A. and Fahn, S. (1986). Spontaneous remissions in spasmodic torticollis. *Neurology*, **36**, 398–400.

9. Nutt, J. G., Muenter, M. D., Aronson, A., Kurland, L. T. and Melton, L. J. III. (1998). Epidemiology of focal idiopathic cervical dystonia. *Brain*, **121**, 547–60.

10. Dauer, W. T., Burke, R. E., Greene, P. and Fahn, S. (1991). Current concepts on the clinical findings and associated movement disorders. *Neurology*, **41**, 1088–91.

11. Duane, D. D. (1988). Spasmodic torticollis. *Adv. Neurol.*, **49**, 135–50.

12. Meares, R. (1971). Natural history of spasmodic torticollis, and effect of surgery. *Lancet*, **2**, 149–50.

13. Jankovic, J., Leder, S., Warner, D. and Schwartz, K. (1991). Cervical dystonia: clinical findings and associated movement disorders. *Neurology*, **41**, 1088–91.

14. Lowenstein, D. H. and Aminoff, M. J. (1988). The clinical course of spasmodic torticollis. *Neurology*, **38**, 530–2.

15. Jahanshahi, M., Marion, M. H. and Marsden, C. D. (1990). Natural history of adult onset idiopathic spasmodic torticollis. *Arch. Neurol.*, **47**, 548–52.

16. Chan, J., Brin, M. F. and Fahn, S. (1991). Idiopathic cervical dystonia: clinical characteristics. *Mov. Disord.*, **6**, 119–26.

17. Comella, C. L., Stebbins, G. T. and Miller, S. (1996). Specific dystonia factors contributing to work limitation and disability in cervical dystonia abstract. *Neurology*, **46** (Suppl. 2), A295.

18. Kutvonen, O., Dastidar, P. and Nurmikko, T. (1997). Pain in spasmodic torticollis. *Pain*, **69**, 279–86.

19. Papathanasiou, I., Macdonald, L., Whurr, R. and Jananshahi, M. (2001). Perceived stigma in spasmodic torticollis. *Mov. Disord.*, **16**, 280–5.

20. Jananshahi, M. (1991). Psychosocial factors and depression in torticollis. *J. Psychosom. Res.*, **35**, 493–507.

21. Comella, C. L., Tanner, C. M., Defoor-Hill, L. and Smith, C. (1992). Dysphagia after botulinum toxin injections for spasmodic torticollis: clinical and radiological findings. *Neurology*, **42**, 1307–10.

22. Camfiels, L., Ben-Schlomo, Y., Warner, T. and Warner, T. (2000). The impact of cervical dystonia on quality of life. *Mov. Disord.*, **15**, 143.

23. Naumann, M., Magyar, S., Reiners, K., Erbguth, F. and Leenders, K. (2000). Sensory tricks in cervical dystonia. Perceptual dysbalance of parietal cortex modulates frontal motor programming. *Ann. Neurol.*, **47**, 332–8.

24. Lekhel, H., Popov, K., Anastasopoulos, D. *et al.* (1997). Postural responses to vibration of neck muscles in patients with idiopathic torticollis. *Brain*, **120**, 583–91.

25. Grunewald, R. A., Yoneda, Y., Shipman, J. M. and Sagar, H. J. (1997). Idiopathic focal dystonia, a disorder of muscle spindle afferent processing? *Brain*, **120**, 2179–85.

26. Berardelli, A., Rothwell, J. C., Hallet, M. *et al.* (1998). The pathophysiology of primary dystonia. *Brain*, **121**, 1195–212.

27. Lenz, F. A., Suarez, J. I., Metman, L. V. *et al.* (1998). Pallidal activity during dystonia: somatosensory reorganization and changes with severity. *J. Neurol. Neurosurg. Psychiatry*, **65**, 767–70.

28. Bara Jimenez, W., Catalan, M. J., Hallett, M. and Georlff, C. (1998). Abnormal somatosensory homunculus in dystonia of the hand. *Ann. Neurol.*, **44**, 828–31.

29. Rome, S. and Grunewald, R. (1999). Abnormal perception of vibration-included illusion of movement in dystonia. *Neurology*, **53**, 1794–800.

30. Kaji, R. and Murase, N. (2001). Sensory function of basal ganglia. *Mov. Disord.*, **16**, 593–4.

31. Murase, N., Kaji, R., Shimazu, H., *et al.* (2000). Abnormal pre-movement gating of somatosensory input in writer's camp. *Brain*, **123**, 1813–29.

32. Tinazzi, M., Priori, A., Bertolasi, L., *et al.* (2000). Abnormal central integration of a dual somatosensory input in dystonia. Evidence for sensory overflow. *Brain*, **123**, 42–50.

33. Consky, E. S. and Lang, A. E. (1994). Clinical assessments of patients with cervical dystonia. In J. Jankovic and M. Hallett, eds., *Therapy with Botulinum Toxin*. New York: Marcel Dekker, pp. 211–37.

34. Jananshahi, M. (2000). Factors that ameliorate or aggravate spasmodic torticollis. *J. Neurol. Neurosurg. Psychiatry*, **68**, 227–9.

35. Anderson, T. J., Rivest, J., Stell *et al.* (1992). Botulinum-toxin treatment of spasmodic torticollis. *J. R. Soc. Med.*, **85**, 524–9.

36. Herz, E. and Glascer, G. H. (1949). Spasmodic torticollis. *Arch. Neurol. Psychiatry*, **61**, 227–39.

37. Chan, J., Brin, M. F. and Fahn, S. (1991). Idiopathic cervical dystonia: clinical characteristics. *Mov. Disord.*, **6**, 119–26.

38. Defazio, G., Livrea, P., Guanti, G., Lepore, V. and Ferrari, E. (1993). Genetic contribution to idiopathic adult-onset blepharospasm and cranial-cervical dystonia. *Eur. Neurol.*, **33**, 345–50.

39. Uitti, R. J. and Maraganore, D. M. (1991). Adult onset familial cervical dystonia: report of a family including monozygotic twins. *Mov. Disord.*, **8**, 489–94.

40. Ozelius, L., Krammer, P. L., Moskowitz, C. B. *et al.* (1989). Human gene for torsion dystonia located on chromosome 9q32–34. *Neuron*, **2**, 1427–34.

41. De Leon, D. and Bressman, S. B. (1999). *Early-onset Primary Dystonia (DYT1)*. University of Washington, Seattle, WA.

42. Jarman, P. R., del Grosso, N., Valente, E. M. *et al.* (1999). Primary torsion dystonia: the search for genes is not over. *J. Neurol. Neurosurg. Psychiatry*, **67**, 395–7.

43. Tarsy, D. (1998). Comparison of acute- and delayed-onset posttraumatic cervical dystonia. *Mov. Disord.*, **13**, 481–5.

44. Hallet, M. (1995). Is dystonia a sensory disorder. Editorial? *Ann. Neurol.*, **38**, 139–40.

45. Tempel, L. W. and Perlmutter, J. S. (1993). Abnormal cortical responses in patient with writer's camp. *Neurology*, **43**, 2252–7.

46. Tolosa, E., Montserrat, L. and Bayes, A. (1988). Blink reflex studies in focal dystonias: enhanced excitability of brainstem interneurons in cranial dystonia and spasmodic torticollis. *Mov. Disord.*, **3**, 61–9.

47. Panizza, M., Lelli, S., Nilsson, J. and Hallet, M. (1995). H-reflex recovery curve and reciprocal inhibition of H-reflex in torticollis. *Mov. Disord.*, **10**, 455–9.

48. Colebatch, J. G., Di Lazzaro, V., Quartarone, A., Rothwell, J. C. and Gresty, M. (1995). Click evoked vestibulocollic reflexes in torticollis. *Mov. Disord.*, **10**, 455–9.

49. Sculze-Bonhage, A. and Ferbert, A. (1995). Cervical dystonia as an isolated sign of a basal ganglia tumor. Letter. *J. Neurol. Neurosurg. Psychiatry*, **58**, 108–9.

50. Schwartz, M., De Deyn, P. P., Van den Kerchove, M. and Pickut, B. A. (1995). Cervical dystonia as a probable consequence of focal cerebral lesion. Letter. *Mov. Disord. Mov.*, **10**, 797–8.

51. Galardi, G., Perani, D., Grassi, F. *et al.* (1996). Basal ganglia and thalamo-cortical hyper metabolism in patients with spasmodic torticollis. *Acta Neurol. Scand.*, **12**, 704–8.

52. Magyar-Lehmann, S., Antonini, A., Roelcke, U. *et al.* (1997). Cerebral glucose metabolism in patients with spasmodic torticollis. *Mov. Disord.*, **12**, 704–8.

53. Naumann, M., Pirer, W., Reiners, K., Lange, K. W., Becker, G. and Brucke, T. (1998). Imaging the pre- and post-synaptic side of striatal dopaminergic synapes in idiopathic cervical dystonia: a SPECT study using ^{123}I epipride and ^{123}I beta-CIT. *Mov. Disord.*, **13**, 319–23.

54. Suchowersky, O. and Calne, D. B. (1988). Non-dystonic causes of torticollis. *Adv. Neurol.*, **50**, 501–8.

55. Benecke, R., Moore, P., Dressler, D. and Naumann, M. (2003). Cervical and axial dystonia. In P. Moor and M. Naumann, eds., *Handbook of Botulinum Toxin Treatment*. pp. 158–91.

56. Risvoll, H. and Kerty, E. (2001). To test or not? The value of diagnostic tests in cervical dystonia. *Mov. Disord.*, **16**, 286–9.

57. Adler, C. and Kumar, R. (2000) Pharmacological and surgical options for the treatment of cervical dystonia. *Neurology*, **55**, S9–S14.

58. Marchetti, A., Magar, R., Lau, H. *et al.* (2000). Treatment algorithm for cervical dystonia. *Mov. Disord.*, **15**, 150.

59. Sherman, D. G., Hart, R. G. and Easton, J. D. (1988). Abrupt change of head position and cerebral infraction. *Stroke*, **12**, 2–6.

60. Janhanshahi, M. and Marsden, C. (1989). Treatments for torticollis. *J. Neurol. Neurosurg. Psychiatry*, **52**, 1212.

61. Fahn, S. (1987). Systemic therapy for dystonia. *Can. J. Neurol. Sci.*, **14**, 528–32.

62. Greene, P., Shale, H. and Fahn, S. (1988). Analysis of open-label trials in torsion dystonia using high dosages of anticholinergics and other drugs. *Mov. Disord.*, **36**, 160–4.

63. Burke, R. E., Fahn, S. and Marsden, C. D. (1986). Torsion dystonia: a double-blind, prospective trial of high-dosage trihexyphenidyl. *Neurology*, **36**, 160–4.

64. Greene, P. (1992). Baclofen in the treatment of dystonia. *Clin. Neuropharmacol.*, **15**, 276–88.

65. Greene, P. E. and Fahn, S. (1992). Baclofen in the treatment of idiopathic dystonia in children. *Mov. Disord.*, **77**, 48–52.

66. Lang, A. (1988). Dopamine agonists and antagonists in the treatment of idiopathic dystonia. *Adv. Neurol.*, **50**, 561–70.

67. Jankovic, J. and Orman, J. (1988). Tetrabenzine therapy of dystonia, chorea, tics, and other dyskinesias. *Neurology*, **38**, 391–4.

68. Lieberman, J., Saltz, B., Johns, C., Pollack, S., Borenstein, M. and Kane, J. (1991). The effects of clozapine on tardive dyskinesia. *Br. J. Psychiatry*, **14**, 652–7.

69. Theil, A., Dressler, D., Kistel, C. and Ruther, E. (1994). Clozapine treatment of spasmodic torticollis. *Neurology*, **44**, 957–8.

70. Ichinose, H., Ohye, T., Takahashi, T. *et al.* (1994). Hereditary progressive dystonia with marked diurnal fluctuation caused by mutations in the GTP cyclohydrolase type I gene. *Nature Genet.*, **8**, 236–42.

71. Ludecke, B., Dworniczak, B. and Bartholome, K. (1995). A point mutation in the tyrosine hydroxylase gene associated with Segawa's syndrome. *Hum. Genet.*, **95**, 123–5.

72. Ohara, S., Hayashi, R., Momoi, H., Miki, J. and Yanagisawa, N. (1998). Mexiletine in the treatment of spasmodic torticollis. *Mov. Disord.*, **13**, 934–40.

73. Lang, A. E. (1998). Surgical treatment of dystonia. In S. Fahn, C. D. Marsden and M. DeLong, eds., *Dystonia 3: Advances in Neurology*. Philadelphia: Lippincott-Raven Publishers, pp. 185–98.

74. Bertrand, C. M. and Molina-Negro, P. (1988). Selective peripheral denervation in 111 cases of spasmodic torticollis: rationale and results. *Adv. Neurol.*, **50**, 637–43.

75. Arce, C. and Russo, L. (1992). Selective peripheral denervation: a surgical alternative in the treatment for spasmodic torticollis. Review of fifty-five patients. *Mov. Disord.*, **7**, 128. Abstract.

76. Bouvier, G. (1989). The use of selective denervation for spasmodic torticollis in cervical dystonias. *Can. J. Neurol. Sci.*, **16**, 242. Abstract.

77. Bertrand, C. M. (1993). Selective peripheral denervation for spasmodic torticollis: surgical technique, results and observations in 260 cases. *Surg. Neurol.*, **40**, 96–103.

78. Davis, D. H., Ahlskog, J. E., Litchy, W. J. and Root, L. M. (1991). Selective peripheral denervation for torticollis: preliminary results. *Mayo Clin. Proc.*, **66**, 365–71.

79. Braun, V. and Richter, H.-P. (1994). Selective peripheral denervation for the treatment of spasmodic torticollis. *Neurosurgery*, **35**, 58–63.

80. Braun, V., Neff, U. and Richter, H. P. (1996). Selective peripheral denervation for spasmodic torticollis in cervical dystonias. *Mov. Disord.*, **11**, 208. Abstract.

81. Ford, B., Louis, E. D., Greene, P. and Fahn, S. (1998). Outcome of selective ramisectomy for botulinum toxin resistant torticollis. *J. Neurol. Neurosurgery Psychiatry*, **65**, 472–8.

82. Vitek, J. L. (1998). Surgery for dystonia. *Neurosurg. Clin. North Am.*, **9**, 345–66.

83. Justesen, C. R., Penn, R. D., Kroin, J. S. and Egel, R. T. (1990). Stereotactic pallidotomy in a child with Hallervorden-Spatz disease. *J. Neurosurg.*, **90**, 551–4.

84. Lozano, A. M., Kumar, R., Gross, R. E. *et al.* (1997). Globus pallidus internus pallidotomy for generalized dystonia. *Mov. Disord.*, **12**, 865–70.

85. Lin, J.-J., Lin, G.-Y., Shih, G., Lin, S.-Z., Chang, D.-C. and Lee, C.-C. (1999). Benefit of bilateral pallidotomy in the treatment of generalized dystonia. *J. Neurosurg.*, **90**, 974–6.

86. Ondo, W. G., Desaloms, J. M., Jankovic, J. and Grossman, R. G. (1998). Pallidotomy for generalized dystonia. *Mov. Disord.*, **13**, 693–8.

87. Benabid, A. L., Pollack, P., Gao, D. *et al.* (1996). Chronic electrical simulation of the ventralis intermedius nucleus of the thalamus as a treatment of movement disorders. *J. Neurosurg.*, **84**, 203–14.

88. Brin, M. F., Germano, I., Dansai, F. O. *et al.* (1998). Deep brain stimulation (DBS) of pallidum in intractable dystonia. *Mov. Disord.*, **13**, 274.

89. Fogel, W., Tronnier, V., Krause, M., Schinippering, H. and Meinck, H. M. (1998). Bilateral pallidal stimulation in a case of idiopathic torsion dystonia: a new treatment option? *Mov. Disord.*, **13**, 199.

90. Krauss, J. K., Pohle, T., Webber, S., Ozodoba, C. and Burgunder, J. M. (1999). Bilateral stimulation of globus pallidus internus for treatment of cervical dystonia. *Lancet*, **354**, 837–8.

91. Kumar, R., Dagher, A., Hutchinson, W. D., Lang, A. E. and Lozano, A. M. (1999). Globus pallidus deep brain stimulation for generalized dystonia: clinical and PET investigation. *Neurology*, **53**, 1–4.

92. Marsden, C. D. and Fahn, S. (1994). *Movement Disorders 3*. Oxford: Butterworth-Heinemann.

93. Brans, J. W., Lindeboom, R., Snoek, J. W., Zwartz, M. J., van Weerden, T. W., Brunt, E. R. *et al.* (1996). Botulinum toxin versus trihexyphenidyl in cervical dystonia: a prospective, randomised, double-blind controlled trial. *Neurology*, **42**, 1066–72.

94. Tsui, J. K., Eisen, A., Stoesl, A. J., Calne, S. and Calne, D. B. (1986). Double-blind study of botulinum toxin in spasmodic torticollis. *Lancet*, **2**, 245–7.

95. Jankovic, J. and Orman, J. (1987). Botulinum A toxin for cranial-cervical dystonia: a double-blind, placebo-controlled study. *Neurology*, **37**, 616–23.

96. Gelb, D. J., Lowenstein, D. H. and Aminoff, M. J. (1989). Controlled trial of botulinum toxin injections in the treatment of spasmodic torticollis. *Neurology*, **39**, 80–4.

97. Lorentz, I. T., Subramanium, S. S. and Yiannikas, C. (1991). Treatment of idiopathic spasmodic torticollis with botulinum toxin A. A double-blind study on twenty-three patients. *Mov. Disord.*, **6**, 145–50.

98. Naumann, M., Yakovleff, A. and Durif, F. (2002). A randomised double-masked, crossover comparison of the efficacy and safety of botulinum toxin type A produced from the original bulk toxin source and current toxin source for the treatment of cervical dystonia. *J. Neurol.*, **249**, 57–63.

99. Jankovic, J., Schwartz, K. and Donovan, D. T. (1990). Botulinum toxin treatment of cranial-cervical dystonia, spasmodic dysphonia, other focal dystonias and hemifacial spasm. *J. Neurol. Neurosurg. Psychiatry*, **53**, 633–9.

100. Greene, P., Kang, U., Fahn, S., Brin, M., Moskowitz, C. and Flaster, E. (1990). Double-blind, placebo-conrolled trial of botulinum toxin injections for the treatment of spasmodic torticollis. *Neurology*, **40**, 1213–18.

101. Comella, C., Jankovic, J. and Brin, M. (2000). Use of botulinum toxin type A in the treatment of cervical dystonia. *Neurology*, **55**, S15–S21.

102. Jankovic, J. and Schwartz, K. S. (1999). Longitudinal experience with botulinum toxin injections for treatment of blepharospasm and cervical dystonia. *Neurology*, **43**, 8.

103. Brashear, A., Lew, M. F., Dyskstra, D. D. *et al.* (1999). Safety and efficacy of NeuroBloc (Botulinum toxin type B) in type A responsive cervical dystonia. *Neurology*, **53**, 1439−46.

104. Brin, M. F., Lew, M. F., Adler, M. D. *et al.* (1999). Safety and efficacy of NeuroBloc (Botulinum toxin type B) in type A resistant cervical dystonia. *Neurology*, **53**, 1431−8.

105. Lew, M. F., Adornateo, B. T., Duanne, D. D. *et al.* (1997). Botulinum toxin type B. A double-blind, placebo-controlled safety and efficacy study in cervical dystonia. *Neurology*, **49**, 701−7.

106. Cullis, P. A., O'Brian, C. F., Truong, D. D. *et al.* (1998). Botulinum toxin type B: an open-label, dose escalation safety and preliminary efficacy study in cervical dystonia patients. *Adv. Neurol.*, **78**, 227−30.

107. Adler, C. (2001). *Botulinum Toxin Treatment of Movement Disorders Neurobase*, 3rd edn. San Diego, CA: Arbor Publishing.

108. Williams, A. (1993). Consensus statement for the management of focal dystonias. *Br. J. Hosp. Med.*, **50**, 655−9.

109. Report of the therapeutics, and technology assessment subcommittee of the American Academy of Neurology (1994). Training guidelines for the use of botulinum toxin for the treatment of neurological disorders. *Neurology*, **44**, 2401−3.

110. Van den Bergh, P., Francart, J., Mourin, S., Kollmann, P. and Laterre, E. C. (1995). Five years experience in the treatment of focal movement disorders with low dose dysport botulinum toxin. *Muscle Nerve*, **18**, 720−9.

111. Green, P. (1994). Controlled trials of botulinum toxin for cervical dystonia: a critical review. In J. Jankovic and M. Hallet, eds., *Therapy with Botulinum Toxin*. New York: Marcel Dekker, pp. 279−87.

112. Poewe, W. and Wissel, J. (1994). Experience with botulinum toxin in cervical dystonia. In J. Jankovic and M. Hallet, eds., *Therapy with Botulinum Toxin*. New York: Marcel Dekker, pp. 211−37.

113. Hambleton, P., Cohen, H. E., Palmer, B. J. and Melling, J. (1992). Antitoxins and botulinum toxin treatment. *BMJ*, **304**, 959−60.

114. Zuber, M., Sebald, M., Bathien, N., de Recondo, J. and Rondot, P. (1993). Botulinum antibodies in dystonic patients treated with type A botulinum toxin: frequency and significance; see comments. *Neurology*, **43**, 1715−18. Comment in *Neurology*, 1995, **45**, 204.

115. Borodic, G. E., Johnson, E., Goodnough, M. and Schantz, E. (1996). Botulinum toxin therapy, immunological resistance, and problems with available materials. Review. *Neurology*, **46**, 26−9.

116. Greene, P., Fahn, S. and Diamond, B. (1994). Development of resistance to botulinum toxin type A in patients with torticollis. *Mov. Disord.*, **9**, 213−17.

117. Jankovic, J. and Schwartz, K. (1995). Response and immunoresistance to botulinum toxin injections. *Neurology*, **45**, 1743−6.

118. Barnes *et al.* (2005). The use of botulinum toxin type B in the treatment of patients who have become unresponsive to botulinum toxin type A, initial experiences. *Eur. J. Neurology*, (in press).

119. Moore, A. P. and Blumhardt, L. D. (1991). A double blind trial of botulinum toxin A in torticollis, with one year follow up. *J. Neurol. Neurosurg. Psychiatry.*, **54**, 813−16.

120. Anderson, T. J., Rivest, J., Stell, R., Steiger, M. J., Cohen, H., Thompson, P. D. *et al.* (1992). Botulinum toxin treatment of spasmodic torticollis, see comments. *J. R. Soc. Med.*, **85**, 524–9. Comment in: *J. R. Soc. Med.* (1995), **88**, 239–40.

121. Comella, C. L., Tanner, C. M., DeFoor-Hill, L. and Smith, C. (1992). Dysphagia after botulinum toxin injections for spasmodic torticollis; clinical and radiological findings. *Neurology*, **42**, 1307–10.

122. Blackie, J. D. and Lees, A. J. (1990). Botulinum toxin treatment in spasmodic torticollis. *J. Neurol. Neurosurg. Psychiatry*, **53**, 640–3.

123. Borodic, G. E., Joseph, M., Fay, L. Cozzolino, D. and Ferrante, R. J. (1990). Botulinum A toxin for the treatment of spasmodic torticollis: dysphagia and regional toxin spread. *Head Neck*, **12**, 392–9.

124. Borodic, G. E., Pearce, L. B., Smith, K. and Joseph, M. (1992). Botulinum A toxin for spasmodic torticollis: multiple Vs single injection points per muscle. *Head Neck*, **14**, 33–7.

125. Sampaio, C., Castro-Caldas, A., Sales-Luis, M. I. *et al.* (1993). Brachial plexopathy after botulinum toxin administration for cervical dystonia. Letter. *J. Neurol. Neurosurg. Psychiatry*, **56**, 220.

126. Glanzman, R. L., Gelb, D. J., Drury, I., Bromberg, M. B. and Truong, D. D. (1990). Brachial plexopathy after botulinum toxin injections. *Neurology*, **40**, 1143.

127. Girlanda, P., Vita, G., Nicolosi, C., Milone, S. and Messina, C. (1992). Botulinum toxin therapy: distant effects on neuromuscular transmission and autonomic nervous system. *J. Neurol. Neurosurg. Psychiatry*, **55**, 844–5.

128. Erbguth, F., Claus, D., Englehardt, A. and Dressler, D. (1993). Systemic effects of local botulinum toxin injections unmasks subclinical Lambert-Eaton myasthenic syndrome, letter. *J. Neurol. Neurosurg. Psychiatry*, **56**, 1235–6.

129. Claus, D., Druschky, A. and Erbguth, F. (1995). Botulinum toxin: influence on respiratory, heart rate variation. *Mov. Disorder*, **10**, 574–9.

130. Mezuki, T., Kaji, R., Kohara, N. and Kimura, J. (1996). Development of general weakness in a patient with amyotrophic lateral sclerosis after focal botulinum toxin injection. *Neurology*, **46**, 845–6.

131. Emmerson, J. (1994). Botulinum toxin for spasmodic torticollis in a patient with myasthenia gravis. *Mov. Disorder*, **9**, 367.

132. Duane, D., Stuart, S., Case, J. and LaPointe, L. (2000). Successful and safe use of botulinum toxin in a patient with sub-clinical myasthenia gravis and lingual/brachial/manual dystonia. *Mov. Disord.*, **15**, 149.

133. Lindeboom, R., Brans, J. W. M., Aramideh, M., Speelman, S. D. and De Haan, R. J. (1998). Treatment of cervical dystonia: a comparison of measures for outcome assessment. *Mov. Disord.*, **13**, 706–12.

134. Swash, M., Roberts, A. H., Zakko, H. and Heathfield, K. W. (1972). Treatment of involuntary disorders with tetrabenazine. *J. Neurol. Neurosurg. Psychiatry*, **35**, 186–91.

135. Couch, J. R. (1976). Dystonia and tremor in spasmodic torticollis. *Adv. Neurol.*, **14**, 245–58.

136. Tolosa, E. S. (1978). Modification of tardive dyskinesia and spasmodic torticollis by apomorphine. *Arch. Neurol.*, **35**, 459–62.

137. Lang, A. E., Sheehy, M. P. and Marsden, C. D. (1982). Anticholinergics in adult-onset dystonia. *Can. J. Neurol. Sci.*, **9**, 313–19.

138. Consky, E., Basinky, A., Belle, L., Ranawaya, R. and Lang, A. (1990). The Toronto Western Spasmodic Torticollis Rating Scale (TWSTRS). *Neurology*, **40**(Suppl.1), 445.

139. Jankovic, J. and Schwartz, K. S. (1991). Clinical correlates of response to botulinum toxin injections. *Arch. Neurol.*, **48**, 1253–6.

140. Dubinski, R. M., Grey, C. S., Vetere-Overfield, B. and Koller, W. C. (1991). Electromyographic guidance of botulinum toxin treatment in cervical dystonia. *Clin. Neuropharmacology*, **14**, 262–7.

The use of botulinum toxin in otolaryngology

Maurice Hawthorne[1] and Khalid Anwar[2]

[1] James Cook University Hospital, Middlesbrough, UK
[2] Hunters Moor Regional Neurological Rehabilitation Centre, Newcastle upon Tyne, UK

7.1 Introduction

In this chapter, the therapeutic use of botulinum toxin for disorders that predominately manifest themselves in the larynx and pharynx will be covered. The treatment of laryngeal dystonia with botulinum toxin remains the best documented use of botulinum toxin in this field but it has been successfully used to treat other laryngeal and pharyngeal disorders (Table 7.1).

7.2 Laryngeal dystonia/spasmodic dysphonia

The term dystonia is defined as a sustained, involuntary contraction of muscle that produces an abnormal posture and frequently causes twisting and turning[1]. It is a chronic neurological disorder of the central nervous system characterized by action induced muscle spasms and can be generalized or focal. Dystonia that affects the larynx is usually focal and mainly results in speech disorders but can also, albeit rarely, cause breathing difficulties.

Laryngeal dystonia begins in middle age and is more common in females than males[2]. Adductor dysphonia, which causes strangled voice quality, is much more common than abductor dysphonia, which results in breathy voice. Voice is obviously extremely important in social interactions and in spasmodic dysphonia, voice impairment can be long lasting, which has significant negative social consequences[3,4]. Patients with spasmodic dysphonia have a high incidence of anxiety and depression[5,6] and can suffer significant psychological problems. The condition can have a direct effect on their quality of life and work place performance[7].

Clinical Uses of Botulinum Toxins, eds. Anthony B. Ward and Michael P. Barnes. Published by Cambridge University Press. © Cambridge University Press 2007.

Table 7.1. Use of botulinum toxin injections for treatment of disorders of the larynx and pharynx

1. Dystonia
   - Laryngeal dystonia
   - Tongue dystonia
   - Jaw opening dystonia
   - Jaw closing dystonia
   - The slewed jaw
2. Other laryngeal disorders
   - Neurological disorders
     ◦ Essential voice tremor
     ◦ Stuttering blocks
     ◦ Vocal tics
   - Mucosal disorders
     ◦ Vocal fold granuloma
     ◦ Glottic synechia
   - Functional disorders
     ◦ Muscle tension dysphonia
3. Disorders of pharynx
   - Upper oesophageal sphincture spasm
   - Palatal myoclonus

Unfortunately, there is no cure for spasmodic dysphonia but it can be symptomatically treated with botulinum toxin injections and in recent years this treatment has emerged as the treatment of choice for this disorder[8–10].

7.2.1 Classification

The commonest form of laryngeal dystonia is the adductor type. Less common is abductor and finally there is the much more rare mixed type.

Adductor laryngeal dystonia

In this disorder there are involuntary movements of the vocal cords, which pull the cords together; the voice has a strangled quality. In severe cases there are periods of aphonia lasting a second or so when the cords are clamped together and therefore there is no mucosal wave. Vowel prolongations are common especially in those cases where fluency is not grossly disrupted.

Abductor laryngeal dystonia

The voice has a breathy quality and lacks power. There are periods of aphonia due to the fact that the vocal cords are pulled apart. Breath support can appear to be poor due to loss of air from the lungs secondary to the widely patent airway.

Mixed laryngeal dystonia

This is often difficult to diagnose. It often only becomes apparent when the patient has been treated for adductor dystonia and the anticipated outcome does not result. The patient may appear to be particularly breathy after treatment and a fibreoptic laryngoscopy may reveal that the cords are being actively pulled apart. Regrettably, treatment with botulinum toxin will often give poor results in this condition.

7.2.2   Assessment of speech disorders due to dystonia

Speech can be affected depending on which muscles are predominantly involved. Sometimes diagnosis is straightforward, but often it is difficult to determine the root cause of the problem. Involvement of the speech therapist can be essential in the early stages of diagnosis. The following table describes the type of speech and voice problems and the muscles usually involved (Table 7.2).

It is sometimes useful for the speech to be recorded on video or DVD in order to facilitate post-treatment comparison. Initial clinical assessment should be followed by fibreoptic examination.

Fibreoptic examination

The nose and throat are sprayed with a topical anaesthetic. Any nasal abnormality is noted such as a deviated nasal septum or nasal polyps. A flexible scope is passed into the nose until the soft palate can be inspected. The position of the palate

Table 7.2. Speech and voice problems, and the muscles usually involved

Name	Muscles usually involved	Description of voice
Adductor dystonia	Vocalis, thyroarytenoid, cricothyroid	Strangled quality, brief periods of aphonia due to the cords clamped shut; vowel prolongations.
Abductor dystonia	Posterior cricoarytenoid	Breathy voice, lacks power, aphonia due to cords being pulled apart
Bunched tongue	Tongue body	Sounds like speaking with a marble in the mouth. Poor articulation where the tongue needs to contact the front teeth
Protruding tongue	Tongue body and tip	Speech sounds as if the tongue is preventing the lips coming together.
Palatal tension		The palate is pulled excessively taut so that there is nasal escape
Palatal elevation		Hyponasality

is noted and any involuntary spasm observed. If the spasm is so intense that the scope will not pass into the oropharynx then the patient is asked to sniff, which usually facilitates the passing of the scope. Next, with the scope at the level of the palate and the patient breathing quietly, any involuntary movements are noted. In particular, the tongue, prevertebral muscles and the vocal cords are observed for at least one minute. The patient is then asked to say a sustained 'EE'. The patient then counts to ten and recites a piece of free speech such as a poem or nursery rhyme. Finally, a swallow is observed from the level of the soft palate and again within the nose, just to check that the palate rises and closes off the nose in the normal fashion.

7.2.3 Treatment of spasmodic dysphonia

Botulinum toxin was used for the first time in 1988 by Brin *et al.*[11] for the treatment of spasmodic dysphonia. Since then it has been recognized as the treatment of choice[12] and the gold standard of treatment for patients with spasmodic dysphonia. Over the last 20 years, a large number of studies have tried to document the effectiveness of botulinum toxin for the treatment of spasmodic dysphonia. Botulinum toxin acts by restricting acetylcholine release at the neuromuscular junction causing laryngeal muscle weakness and thereby relieving the symptoms of laryngeal dystonia

Numerous reports have confirmed the benefit of botulinum toxin injections for the symptomatic treatment of this disorder[8–10]. However, many of the studies have relied on patient self-reporting of symptoms or have been carried out on only a small number of patients over a short period of time. The largest study by Blitzer *et al.* in 1998[2] reported their experience treating almost 1000 patients over a 13-year period. The study shows impressive outcome but relied on patient's self-rating of symptoms.

Recently Watts and colleagues have published a Cochrane Review of the use of botulinum toxin injections in the treatment of spasmodic dysphonia[12]. The authors searched the Cochrane central register of controlled trials as well as other standard sources, including MEDLINE, EMBASE, CINAHL and PsycINFO. The authors looked for all studies in which participants were randomly allocated prior to intervention and in which botulinum was compared to an alternative treatment, placebo or non-treated control group. They only found one study in the literature that met these inclusion criteria. This was a study by Truong and colleagues[13]. This was a double-blind, placebo-controlled study to examine the effects of botulinum toxin (BOTOX®) on voice quality (via spectrographic analysis), perceived voice improvement and acoustic measures in subjects with adductor spasmodic dysphonia who either received drug or saline injection into the thyroarytenoid muscles. Thirteen subjects were randomly assigned to either botulinum toxin or saline treatment. The study showed that subjects injected with botulinum toxin exhibited significantly decreased perturbation and fundamental frequency range compared to subjects who received saline. The active treated subjects also exhibited significant improvement in ratings of speech quality.

Other studies were reported which did not meet the rather stringent criteria. The authors found approximately 77 articles published with regard to botulinum toxin treatment for spasmodic dysphonia, but only seven of these articles were randomized, controlled clinical trials. Only three of these published adequate data that could be further analysed through a systematic review. On further inspection only the Truong study allowed any conclusions to be drawn. However, the authors do point out there was a large body of data of non-randomized clinical studies which, taken altogether, suggested a positive clinical outcome for the use of botulinum toxin for spasmodic dysphonia. The authors made a number of recommendations regarding methodology that should be incorporated into future studies. These included subjective and objective measures of the degree and duration of effectiveness of vocal improvement and neuromuscular functioning as well as acoustic, aerodynamic and endoscopic measures of the effects of the injection on laryngeal function.

In summary, the authors did not find sufficient evidence from randomized controlled trials for firm conclusions to be drawn about the effectiveness of botulinum toxin for all types of spasmodic dysphonia, but this was largely due to lack of worthwhile studies rather than a demonstrated lack of efficacy. The conclusion of the Cochrane Review has also been recently reiterated in a review published in *Clinical Rehabilitation* in 2006[14].

Before the widespread use of botulinum toxin, treatment was mostly surgical and consisted of denervation of one vocal cord[15], but unfortunately with high rates of treatment failure[16]. Over the years various other surgical procedures have been tried, but without consistent results. Other authors have suggested the use of behavioural treatment for this condition, but overall it has not proven beneficial[17,18]. However, one study has shown the merit of combining pharmacological treatment with voice therapy[19]. Botulinum is by far the most successful form of treatment.

7.2.4   Treatment of adductor laryngeal dystonia with botulinum toxin

This is usually treated by injecting the vocalis muscle under EMG control and local anaesthetic. The EMG is used to locate the vocalis muscle. A Teflon® coated injecting needle is inserted through the cricothyroid membrane and angled to enter the thyroarytenoid muscle (vocalis part) as far anterior in the larynx as is possible. By placing the injection far forward there is a reduced risk of swallowing problems.

The usual dose that the authors use is 5 units of Dysport into each vocalis muscle. Other authorities have suggested using up to 60 units of Dysport as a unilateral injection and others have suggested the possibility of alternating the sides at each treatment session.

If the result is a breathy voice then it can be worth a trial of treatment of the cricothyroid muscle instead of the vocalis.

The commonest side effects are initial breathiness of the voice and temporary swallowing problems. The authors routinely prescribe a thickening agent to be added to drinks if swallowing problems occur.

Some authors have recommended the use of a flexible nasolaryngoscope for the injection technique[20]. Some authors have advocated the use of bilateral injections, but it is generally accepted that unilateral injections are safer and produce a similar result[21].

Recently, Boutsen and colleagues have undertaken a useful meta-analysis of botulinum treatment for this condition, but robust conclusions are difficult to draw given the paucity of the literature[22].

7.2.5   Treatment of abductor laryngeal dystonia with botulinum toxin

The authors favour a transcutaneous injection of the posterior cricoarytenoid muscle under EMG control. Local anaesthetic is not usually necessary. The Teflon® coated injecting EMG needle is inserted through the skin at the mid point of the sternomastoid muscle. The larynx is held with the other hand and rotated so as to present the posterior aspect of the larynx towards the needle. The needle is advanced until it strikes the back of the cricoid cartilage and then withdrawn slightly. The patient is asked to sniff which enhances the muscle activity recorded by the EMG machine.

There is not a clear consensus in the literature regarding dosages. The authors usually commence with a starting dose of 10 units of Dysport toxin. If necessary this can be increased to 25 units at subsequent treatments.

Fortunately, side effects from treatment of abductor dystonia are less common. Side effects with injection of the posterior cricothyroid muscle are unusual.

7.3   Tongue dystonia

This is usually seen as part of a more complex dystonia involving the mandible and muscles of facial expression. Rarely, it can occur on its own. It is crucial to try and determine if any associated jaw movement is due to the tongue moving the jaw or whether it is other muscles attached to the jaw, such as the pterygoids. If there is doubt, it may be wise to start treatment with tongue injections and reserve injections into the pterygoid muscles for later consultation.

7.3.1 Bunched tongue

In this recognizable subgroup of tongue dystonia the tongue appears to be bunched up in the mouth. On a videofluroscopy the tongue has a shortened anterior–posterior diameter. The tongue tends to lie at the back of the mouth and be in contact with the soft palate. Often there is difficulty in forming a bolus but usually there is an adequate ability to force the bolus into the oropharynx. This is often seen in jaw closing dystonia with spasm of the masseter and temporalis.

Once again there is no clear consensus in the literature with regard to dosage. The authors recommend an initial dose of 25 units of Dysport (around 6 units of BOTOX®). This is injected transcutaneously with a 23 gauge blue needle. The hyoid bone is palpated and the injection placed in the midline about 1 cm anterior to the hyoid, aiming at the vertex of the skull. The needle is inserted approximately 2 cm, depending on the amount of subcutaneous fat.

7.3.2 Tongue protrusion

The major feature of this distressing condition is the tongue's tendency to protrude from the mouth. In its mildest form this may only be a tendency for the tongue to flick out beyond the teeth for a moment during speech or mastication. In a severe case the tongue may protrude out so far that it touches the tip of the chin. It is associated with jaw opening dystonia, and often with mouth opening dystonia, in which the patient is unable to bring the lips together in a sustained manner. It is impossible to swallow a bolus without closing the lips together. In severe cases the patient loses weight due to the protruding tongue and the difficulties in closing the mouth.

In this condition the body of the tongue and the tongue tip usually require injecting. Occasionally, the extrinsic muscles of the tongue that pull the tongue forward towards the lower incisors require injecting, especially genioglossus. This muscle usually needs an EMG to accurately place the injection. If the body of the tongue is injected then the authors use about 15 units of Dysport (approximately 4 units of BOTOX®). This is injected through a transcutaneous route via a 23 gauge blue needle. The tip of the tongue can be injected with a similar gauge needle and using a similar dose of BOTOX® or Dysport. The authors usually start with such injections and at subsequent visits the technique can be modified to include 2–4 units of BOTOX® (or equivalent of Dysport) as required into each genioglossus.

7.3.3 Side effects from tongue injections

The main risk is inability to form a bolus and then clear it from the mouth into the oropharynx. Aspiration is most unusual, presumably due to the fact that the competence of the larynx is not at risk with tongue injection techniques.

7.4 Jaw opening dystonia

The muscles that open the jaw are the lateral pterygoids, assisted by the anterior belly of digastric. The lateral pterygoids cannot be effectively palpated and so the spasm in these muscles can only be inferred after palpation of the anterior belly of digastric. It is most unusual to find a jaw opening dystonia that is due to over activity in the anterior belly of digastric alone.

7.4.1 Injection technique

Some authors recommend an intraoral approach, but this does carry significant risk of affecting the palatal function. The authors favour an external approach. The neck of the mandible is identified just below the head. The needle is introduced with the jaw closed or just closed immediately anterior to the upper neck. A 23 gauge blue needle is used and advanced up to the hilt so that its tip is into the body of the lateral pterygoid muscle. This access is limited and contact with the bone is common and this can be painful. The patient should be warned that if the needle touches the periosteum then significant pain would be felt. In dystonia, a commencing dose of 40 units of Dysport (about 10 units of BOTOX®) is reasonable and unlikely to lead to significant side effects. The authors do not use EMG to locate the muscle and have not found a need for this, as the success rate of the injection in weakening the lateral pterygoid is virtually 100 per cent. However, those that are unfamiliar with injecting in this area may prefer the reassurance that EMG can give.

The anterior belly of digastric can be more difficult to inject. The greater cornu of the hyoid is easy to palpate but the depth of the muscle is much more difficult to estimate and so there is considerable risk of passing the needle right through the muscle and injecting the floor of the mouth musculature. Therefore, for accurate placing of the injection, EMG is recommended. A starting dose of 20–40 units of Dysport (about 5–10 units of BOTOX®) is reasonable.

7.4.2 Side effects

The principal risk with lateral pterygoid injections is weakness of the palate with nasal escape and regurgitation of food or drink into the nose. This appears to be more common with an intraoral technique.

There is a rich venous complex in the infratemporal fossa and therefore a direct venous injection can occur if the injector does not draw back on the syringe to check for position.

Side effects from injections of the anterior belly of digastric at the recommended doses are very unusual. The usual problem is a failure of the injection to produce a desired effect and this may be due to poor position of the needle.

7.5 Jaw closing dystonia

This condition is broadly as common as jaw opening dystonia. Often the tongue is involved and usually the bunched tongue variation is seen. The principle muscles involved are the masseter and the temporalis. These muscles are easily palpated and so history and palpation usually indicate whether one pair of muscles dominates. The patient may complain of excess dental wear, cheek and tongue biting and grinding of the teeth.

7.5.1 Injection technique

A simple transcutaneous injection is usually all that is required. A starting dose of 60 units of Dysport is effective but often after several injections the dose can be cut to 40 units. Occasionally, jaw clenching is seen as a spasticity problem after head injury and occasionally after a stroke. In these cases the dose required may have to be increased to 80–100 units of Dysport.

7.5.2 Side effects

These are unusual with injections for jaw clenching. Dry mouth can occasionally occur, but this is usually only a problem after a number of treatment cycles.

7.6 The slewed jaw

This presents more of a diagnostic problem than the jaw with simple jaw opening or jaw closing dystonia. It is sufficiently rare that when it is seen the diagnosis should be carefully considered. The possibility of a focal lesion involving the basal ganglia should be excluded and if there is a rhythmical slewing movement then the cerebellum should be imaged. The main issue is to determine whether the medial pterygoid is involved. Usually the slewing does not occur when the mouth is completely closed and the teeth are touching. Once the teeth part, the degree of slewing increases. At the initial assessment EMG of both pterygoid muscles can give information concerning relative over-activity of one muscle. Another clue as to the site of the problem can be a complaint of pain or discomfort. Usually, once the side has been determined, a unilateral injection into the medial pterygoid will produce a reduction in the tendency for the jaw to slew to one side.

7.7 Palatal myoclonus

There are very few studies with regard to this disorder. Most patients complain about the constant ticking noise in both ears. Some patients only get myoclonus when the mouth is open, whilst an unfortunate few have the condition all the time. The condition is covered later in Chapter 16.

REFERENCES

1. Fahn, S., Marsden, C. D. and Calne, B. D. (1987). Classification and investigation of dystonia. In Marsden, C. D. and Fahn, S., eds., *Movement Disorders 2*. Butterworths: London, pp. 332–58.
2. Blitzer, A., Brin, M. F. and Stewart, C. F. (1998). Botulinum toxin management of spasmodic dysphonia (laryngeal): a 12-year experience in more than 900 patients. *Laryngoscope*, **108**, 1435–41.
3. Izdebski, K. (1992). Symptomatology of adductor spasmodic dysphonia. *J. Voice*, **6**, 306–19.
4. Izdebski, K., Dedo, H. H. and Boles, I. (1984). Spastic dysphonia: a patient profile of 200 cases. *Am. J. Otolaryngol.*, **5**, 7–14.
5. Murray, T., Cannito, M. P. and Woodson, G. E. (1994). Spasmodic dysphonia: emotional status and botulinum toxin treatment. *Arch. Otolaryngol. Head Neck Surg.*, **120**, 310–16.
6. Liu, C. Y., Yu, J. M., Wang, N. M. *et al.* (1998). Emotional symptoms are secondary to the voice disorder in patients with spasmodic dysphonia. *Gen. Hosp. Psychiatry*, **20**, 255–9.
7. Smith, E., Taylor, M., Mendoza, M., Barkmeier, J., Lemke, J. and Hoffman, H. (1998). Spasmodic dysphonia and vocal fold paralysis; outcomes of voice problems on work related functioning. *J. Voice*, **12**, 223–32.
8. Ludlow, C. L., Naunton, R. F., Terada, S. *et al.* (1991). Successful treatment of selected cases of adductor spasmodic dysphonia using botulinum toxin injection. *Otolaryngol. Head Neck Surg.*, **104**, 849–55.
9. Castellanos, P. F., Gates, G. A., Esselman, G. *et al.* (1994). Anatomic considerations in botulinum toxin type A therapy for spasmodic dysphonia. *Laryngoscope*, **104**, 656–62.
10. Borodic, G. E., Ferrante, R. J., Pearce, L. B. and Elderson, K. (1994). Pharmacology and histology of the therapeutic application of botulinum toxin. In Jankovic, J. and Hallett, M. eds., *Therapy with Botulinum Toxin*. New York; Marcel Dekker, pp. 199–207.
11. Brin, M. F., Fahn, S., Moskowitz, C. *et al.* (1988). Localized injections of botulinum toxin for the treatment of focal dystonia and hemifacial spasm. *Adv. Neurol.*, **50**, 599–608.

12. Watts, C. C. W., Whurr, R. and Nye, C. (2004). Botulinum toxin injections for the treatment of spasmodic dysphonia (Review). *The Cochrane Database of Systematic Reviews*, Issue 3. Art. No.:CD004327.pub2. DOI: 10.1002/14651858.CD004327.pub2.

13. Truong, D., Rontal, M., Rolnick, M., Aronson, A. and Mistura, K. (1991). Double blind controlled study of botulinum toxin in adductor spasmodic dysphonia. *Laryngoscope*, **101**, 630–4.

14. Watts, C., Nye, C. and Whurr, R. (2001). Botulinum toxin for treating spasmodic dysphonia (laryngeal dystonia): a systematic Cochrane review. *Clin. Rehab.*, **20**, 112–22.

15. Dedo, H. H. (1976). Recurrent laryngeal nerve section for spastic dysphonia. *Ann. Otol. Rhinol. Laryngol.*, **85**, 451–9.

16. Aronson, A. E. and DeSanto, L. W. (1983). Adductor spastic dysphonia: 3 years after recurrent laryngeal nerve section. *Ann. Otol. Rhinol. Laryngol.*, **93**, 1–8.

17. Boone, D. and Macfarlane, S. (2000). *The Voice and Voice Therapy*. Boston: Allyn and Bacon.

18. Cannito, M. (2001). Neurological aspects of spasmodic dysphonia. In Voel, D. and Cannito, M. eds., *Treating Disordered Speech Motor Control*. Austin: Pro-Ed.

19. Stemple, J. (2000). *Voice Therapy: Clinical Studies*. San Diego: Singular.

20. Rhew, K., Fiedler, D. A. and Ludlow, C. L. (1994). Technique for injection of botulinum toxin through the flexible nasolaryngoscope. *Otolaryngol. Head Neck Surg.*, **111**(6), 787–94.

21. Bielamowicz, S., Stager, S. V., Badiloo, A. and Godlewski, A. (2002). Unilateral versus bilateral injections of botulinum toxin in patients with adductor spasmodic dysphonia. *J. Voice*, **16**, 117–23.

22. Boutsen, F., Cannito, M. P., Taylor, M. and Bender, B. (2002). Botox treatment in adductor spasmodic dysphonia: a meta-analysis. *J. Speech Lang. Hear Res.*, **45**(3), 469–81.

Spasticity

Anthony B. Ward

North Staffordshire Rehabilitation Centre, Stoke-on-Trent, UK

8.1 Introduction

Spasticity is a physiological consequence of an insult to the brain or spinal cord, which can lead to life-threatening, disabling and costly consequences. This typically occurs in the following patients following stroke, brain injury (trauma and other causes, e.g. anoxia, post-neurosurgery), spinal cord injury, multiple sclerosis and other disabling neurological diseases, and cerebral palsy. Its current management has been advanced considerably over the last ten years by new thinking and by new drugs and technology. Lance's definition[1] of 1980 is still relevant and the impairment is classified as one of the movement disorders. It is important therefore to stress when teaching on this topic, in order to highlight the need for patients' spasticity to be assessed while they are functioning. The fact that many attempts have been made to define it shows the degree of its complexity, but Young[2] described spasticity as part of the upper motor neuron syndrome and gave a definition as *a velocity-dependent increase in muscle tone with exaggerated tendon jerks resulting in hyper-excitability of the stretch reflex in association with other features of the upper motor neuron syndrome.*

He also described spastic dystonia and spastic paresis, which are somewhat contentious terms, but do highlight the positive and negative features of the upper motor neuron syndrome and these are set out in Table 8.1. Essentially, if left untreated following damage to the brain or spinal cord, it is characterized by muscle overactivity and high-tone spasms and will lead to muscle and soft tissue contracture.

Applying this definition to patients in clinical settings has been difficult because upper motor neuron lesions produce an array of responses. The pattern depends on the age and onset of the lesion, its location and size. Patients with diffuse lesions produce, for instance, different characteristics to those with localized pathology and the speed of onset changes this again[3]. More recently, the SPASM

Clinical Uses of Botulinum Toxins, eds. Anthony B. Ward and Michael P. Barnes. Published by Cambridge University Press. © Cambridge University Press 2007.

Table 8.1. Upper motor neuron symptoms

Positive	Negative
Increased muscle tone	Paresis
Hyper-reflexia	Loss of fine control
Repetitive stretch reflexes (clonus)	Loss of dexterity
Extensor stretch reflexes	Fatiguability
Released flexor reflexes	Early hypotonia
(Babinski, mass synergy pattern)	

Consortium in Newcastle upon Tyne, UK has tried to adapt the accepted definition to a more practical base and make it more relevant to clinical practice and to clinical research[4]. Its definition is as follows.

Assuming that all involuntary activity involves reflexes, spasticity is an intermittent or sustained involuntary hyperactivity of a skeletal muscle associated with an upper motor neurone lesion.

It takes as read, that there are a number of different syndromes seen following an injury to the brain or spinal cord and that the assessment and management of spasticity is one of a number of events that occurs. Its treatment should be planned whatever the other features of the upper motor neuron syndrome.

Spasticity is also frequently classified by its presentation and divided into generalized, regional and focal categories. The term focal spasticity is imprecise, for it is not the spasticity that is focal, but that spasticity is producing a focal problem that may be treated by local means. In this respect, botulinum toxin is one of the pharmacological interventions of first choice and this will be discussed in further detail below. In addition, its place in the overall management of spasticity will be discussed.

8.2　Pathophysiology

The pathophysiology of spasticity will only be described here as it relates to therapy with BoNT. Spasticity is not the only result of a damaged upper motor neuron. Its definition is a velocity-dependent increase in stretch reflex[1], but although patients are easily recognized from their clinical picture, they are usually impaired by weakness, muscle shortening, spastic co-contractions and spastic dystonia. The pathophysiology is thus complex and while the actual problem of spasticity of increased resistance to passive movement is part of a bigger picture, the other aspects are fortunately also amenable to treatment with agents such as botulinum toxin. Muscle overactivity occurs in two scenarios. The first involves high-stretch sensitivity when excessive motor unit recruitment occurs with recruitment of stretch receptors and forms the stretch sensitive forms of muscle overactivity, which includes spasticity itself, spastic dystonia and co-contraction. These are distinguished by their primary triggering factor, phasic muscle stretch, tonic muscle stretch or volitional command. The second scenario is found in muscles that are not particularly stretch sensitive. They include associated reactions, when there is extra-segmental co-contraction due to cutaneous or nociceptive stimuli, or inappropriate muscle recruitment during autonomic or reflex activities, such as yawning.

The definition of *spasticity* has been given above, but presents with muscle overactivity in the absence of a volitional command[1]. It is thus measured in resting muscles. *Spastic dystonia* is a tonic muscle contraction in the absence of a phasic stretch or volitional command[5]. It is primarily due to abnormal supraspinal descending drive, which causes a failure of muscle relaxation (despite efforts to do so) and is sensitive to the degree of tonic stretch imposed on that muscle[6]. There is inappropriate recruitment of antagonist muscles in *spastic co-contraction* upon triggering of the agonist under volitional command. This occurs in the absence of phasic stretch and is sensitive to the degree of tonic stretch of the co-contracting antagonist[7]. For instance, triceps will be recruited during volitional action of biceps and will lead to elbow stiffness.

The resultant pattern is determined by the age, size and location of the lesion and knowing this helps with management. Supra-bulbar lesions present predominantly with flexor patterns of spasticity, whereas spinal cord lesions produce extensor patterns predominately. Patients with partial lesions, where sensation is intact or partially intact, are typically bombarded by nociceptive inputs and display greatly increased α-motor neuron activity. Different patterns emerge early on after the neurological insult and later, when patients may find themselves in a rehabilitation unit. Figure 8.1 shows the effects of the different scenarios.

Immediately after injury, a period of neuronal shock occurs and spinal reflexes are lost, which include stretch reflexes. A flaccid weakness is seen, but even during this, the positive features of hypertonia can start to be seen. Limbs are not sufficiently stretched and may be immobilized is shortened positions. Rheological changes occur within muscles in the form of loss of proteins and sarcomeres and accumulation of connective tissue and fibroblasts[8,9]. Unless treated, tendon and soft tissue contracture and limb deformity are established. Altered sensory inputs, such as pain, recurrent infection and poor posture, maintain a further stimulus to lead to yet further shortening and this cycle is difficult to break.

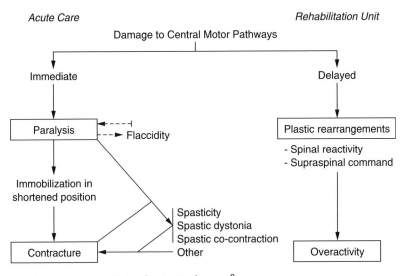

Figure 8.1   Development of spasticity after UMN damage[8].

Spasticity is set up later on, as plastic rearrangement occurs within the brain, spinal cord and muscles. This attempt at restoration of function through new neuronal circuitry creates movement patterns based on existing damaged pathways. Neuronal sprouting occurs at many levels with interneuronal endings moving into unconnected circuits from decreased supraspinal command through the vestibular, rubrospinal and reticulospinal tracts[10]. The end-effect is muscle overactivity and exaggerated reflex responses to peripheral stimulation[11]. This process occurs at anytime, but is usually seen between 1 and 6 weeks after the insult. Muscle overactivity declines over time and the following are suggested as possible causes:

• Structural and functional changes due to plastic rearrangement
• Axonal sprouting
• Increased receptor density

In reality, biomechanical stiffness takes over and tends to diminish exaggerated α-motor neuronal activity.

The upper motor neuron syndrome covers a range of impairments, which are also governed by the pathways damaged (Figure 8.2). In addition to afferent drive changes affecting the spinal reflex, there are problems with *efferent reflexes* (non-afferent drive) and *disordered control of voluntary movement*. Both tend to occur as a result of plastic rearrangement and efferent drive problems are linked with associated reactions and spastic dystonia, whereas motor control problems include reciprocal inhibition, co-contractions, mass movements and phasic stretch reflexes (Table 8.2).

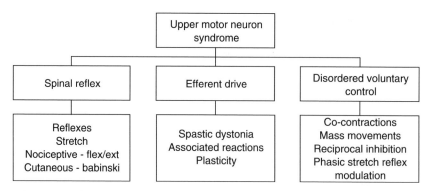

Figure 8.2   Schematic of the features of the upper motor neuron syndrome.

Table 8.2. Features of the upper motor neuron syndrome

	Impairment	Description
Afferent drive	Stretch reflexes	Type 1a afferent active in shortened muscle; as limb progressively stretched, type II inhibition over-rides type 1a facilitation and clasp knife effect occurs — tonic stretch reflex plus length dependent inhibition from flexor reflex afferents — not Golgi organ inhibition
	Nociceptive and cutaneous stimuli	Failure to inhibit increased α-motor neuron activity. γ-neurons possibly not as overactive as α, but α–γ linkage held to near-normal degree.
Efferent drive	Associated reactions	Segment movements occur involuntarily during unrelated activity
	Spastic dystonia	Tonic muscle contraction[12] in the absence of phasic stretch or voluntary command. Muscles do not relax despite antagonist action and relaxation. Sensitive to amount of tonic stretch on muscle.
Disordered voluntary	Reciprocal inhibition	Agonist muscle action inhibits antagonist. May lead to co-contractions (decreased) or contribute to weakness (increased), e.g. spastic foot drop
Motor control	Co-contractions mass movements phasic muscle stretch (4)	Inappropriate recruitment of antagonist following voluntary agonist action. Mainly due to abnormal supraspinal motor drive and can be brought on by overactive muscle stretch Failure to inhibit motor activity spread

8.3   Why treat spasticity and prevent complications?

Spasticity is in itself disabling and leads to complications. There are therefore very good clinical, humanistic and economic reasons to treat it effectively and judiciously. As it leads to muscle shortening and limb deformity, the following can occur:

- Contractures
- Pressure sores
- Limb deformity
- Pain
- Muscle spasms
- Loss of function
- Inability to participate in rehabilitation

The misery of painful spasms or of tendon traction from bones is well known and the complications will prevent patients achieving their optimal functioning. Deconditioning from ill-health and pain will also have a negative effect and patients and their carers may find reduced quality of life. Untreated or sub-optimally treated spasticity will go on to give the following consequences (Table 8.3).

In addition to the human cost, it is important to highlight the economic cost to payers and health service managers. The cost of treating a Grade III/IV pressure sore was estimated at £63 000[13] and the cost of treating a contracture is thought to be £21 000[14] (estimated cost, £4000–6000). This puts into perspective the potential costs of inadequate treatment of patients with upper motor neuron syndrome.

8.4   Epidemiology

The prevalence of spasticity is not known, as there are many patients with mild spasticity for whom little or no treatment is required for their condition. However, 18 per cent of patients with severe traumatic brain injury, 16 per cent

Table 8.3. Impact of spasticity on health

- Unremitting pain from muscle spasms, limb deformity and pressure on pressure points
- Treatment for pressure sores and other tissue viability problems
- Contractures leading to abnormal body segment loading and sensory change
- Limb deformity and altered body mechanics
- Need for special wheelchairs and seating and pressure-relieving equipment
- Progression to degenerative joint disease
- Altered body image
- Mood problems

---

of patients following stroke and 60 per cent of patients moderately and severely disabled by multiple sclerosis (30 per cent of the total population of multiple sclerosis patients) require specific treatment[15]. In a hospital catchment population, such as that of the University Hospital of North Staffordshire, 600 new strokes occur annually and there is a prevalence of 3000[16]. In addition, there is a prevalence of patients with traumatic brain injury[17] and with multiple sclerosis[18]. The burden on health care in any district could therefore be quite considerable. The pharmacological budget for spasticity has traditionally not been the subject of controversy, as oral antispastic agents have been relatively cheap. However, this has changed with the arrival of new technologies, such as botulinum toxin and intra-thecal baclofen and health payers have become concerned at a potential rise in costs in a market, where there has traditionally been a small budget. As the number of patients requiring spasticity treatment is unknown, there was considerable fear in the potential for patients requiring these new technologies. As a result, it has become important to inform policy makers and payers of the likely costs of treatment to a population, as not all patients with an upper motor neuron syndrome require spasticity treatment, let alone botulinum toxin.

There are no incidence and prevalence figures for spasticity, but our early brain injury study estimates that 16 per cent and 18 per cent of first time stroke sufferers and patients following traumatic brain injury respectively require spasticity treatment[15]. A third of these (in each group) require botulinum toxin treatment. Sixty per cent of severely disabled patients from multiple sclerosis and 25 per cent of adults with cerebral palsy also require spasticity treatment, but the figures for those requiring botulinum toxin are unknown.

Put in terms of a 250 000 UK population, this equates to:
- 320 new first time strokes with a prevalence of 1675 people
- 48 people with severe traumatic brain injury with a prevalence of 260 people
- 500 people with multiple sclerosis, of whom 100 are severely disabled
- 31 adults with cerebral palsy
- Plus other conditions affecting the upper motor neuron

About 500 patients require spasticity treatment at some time and approximately a third of these require botulinum toxin treatment for focal spasticity, which is becoming increasingly used in rehabilitation medicine, neurology, geriatric medicine (stroke medicine), paediatric orthopaedic surgery and, in certain places, neuropsychiatry.

8.5 Management principles

Spasticity requires treatment when it is causing harm and this is the sole indication. Some patients early on after their stroke or brain injury are helped by their spasticity. For example, patients may start to support their weight by using their spastic lower limb when the degree of weakness in the leg would not otherwise allow it. Clearly, for these patients, reducing muscle tone would not be helpful, but it requires treatment when it causes problems or symptoms. Successful treatment strategies have now been developed and there is good evidence of treatment effectiveness. Physical management (good nursing care, physiotherapy, occupational therapy) through postural management, exercise, stretching and strengthening of limbs, splinting and pain relief is the basis of spasticity management[18]. The aim of treatment in all cases is to reduce abnormal sensory inputs, in order to decrease excessive α-motor neuron activity[8]. All pharmacological interventions are adjunctive to a programme of physical intervention. 'A Guide to Clinical Practice for the Treatment of Adults with Spasticity using Botulinum Toxin' (supported by the Royal College of Physicians of the London Clinical Effectiveness and Evaluation Unit and by specialist societies in neurology, rehabilitation medicine, geriatric medicine, physiotherapy, occupational therapy) was produced in April 2001[20] and is currently the most useful document highlighting clinical practice and the evidence base for treatment with this agent. Stretching plays an important part in physical management, but needs to be applied for several hours per day[21]. This is of course impossible to do on a one-to-one basis with a therapist and limb casting has been developed in this field to provide a prolonged stretch.

Clinicians in practice have to become used to being more specific about their treatment aims than they have perhaps been used to before. Payers and the health care economy are demanding greater clarity about its use and clinicians have therefore to be clear about why they are treating patients with BoNT. It is essential to discuss the treatment aims and expected outcomes with the patient, carer and the treating team and everyone must be clear on what is to be done and what the expected outcomes are. To achieve this a management strategy is adopted (Figure 8.3), which shows the treatment principles adopted in specialist units. This system recognizes the educational element of spasticity management.

Following an injury to the brain or spinal cord (whatever the cause), an individual develops features of the upper motor neuron syndrome. These are for life and therefore their management is for life. Any medical intervention, be it pharmacological or surgical, is an intermittent episode in the overall life of that 'upper motor neuron syndrome'. Therefore one has to look at the long-term picture when treating patients. The only long-term treatments are those stretching and mobilizing exercises that patients do themselves and any medical intervention should aim to see a sustained benefit from treatment over time. In other words, clinicians should wish to see a long-term improvement in the functioning (be it active or passive) of the patient.

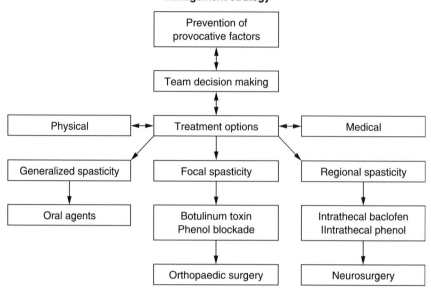

Figure 8.3   A management strategy for adults with spasticity[20].

Successful spasticity management is a multidisciplinary activity. Clinicians working in isolation should not be treating patients without the support of a multidisciplinary team. It is first necessary to manage any underlying provocative factors such as nociceptive stimulus, e.g. poor posture, constipation, incontinence, limb pain, and skin or tissue damage. Even tight clothing can cause an increase in sensory stimulation and the role of the nurse in managing these factors is crucial. Once they have been dealt with, spasticity may still require more active management and the team can then discuss with the patient and carer the available options. Some will be physical treatments and some will be pharmacological or medical/surgical interventions. A management plan is therefore devised for each patient. Management is not a question of moving from one treatment to another when the first fails. Patients should be exposed to the appropriate choice of treatments to meet their needs.

The pharmacological options depend on the pattern of the presenting problem. Figure 8.3 shows the drugs of choice for generalized, regional and focal spasticity and these are guides. One does not see focal spasticity as such. One sees a focal problem in the context of a generalized impairment. Managing spasticity involves dealing with the patient's problems and not simply the impairments seen. However, oral drugs are more useful for generalized problems than focal problems, for which BoNT is the pharmacological treatment of choice.

8.6 Planning treatment

It is important to develop a treatment plan as soon as possible, so as to be clear about the intended outcomes. To reiterate, the underlying principles are that:

1. Antispastic drugs treat spasticity. They do not treat contractures and they will not make hemiplegic limbs function, unless it is the spasticity that prevents a functional improvement.
2. The management of spasticity is physical and all pharmacological interventions are adjunctive to that.

With this in mind, the treatment plan follows a standard pathway (Table 8.4).

It is therefore important to develop a system of assessment and of clinical examination for spasticity. The first point to find out is what the patient wants and their view of what is wrong. Outcome expectations can be discussed and the team can evaluate any unrealistic goals.

8.6.1 Patient assessment

Spasticity is a movement disorder and patients cannot be adequately assessed unless they are observed during movement and function. Physiotherapists and occupational therapists contribute to the observation and examination process, but some patients with complex movement patterns need assessing in a gait laboratory. The assessment process highlights the differences in patterns of limb posture and movement following an upper motor neuron lesion. Where there is no movement, the assessment process is fairly straightforward, but where there is loss of motor control rather than a spastic dystonia, one has to attempt to identify the different aspects of motor impairment. Patients with longstanding problems also develop compensatory movements, which may or may not require treatment and the clinician has to be clear about the underlying pathophysiological processes.

One can then identify how function is impaired and whether the problem is generalized, focal, or more regional. This will then point to the options for treatment, but, if BoNT is planned, then more specific detail is required about

Table 8.4. Principles of treatment

Assessment
Define goals for treatment
Identify expected outcomes
Measurement
Treat patient according to guidelines
Review and record details of treatment outcomes

which muscles are contributing to the functional impairment. The clinician therefore has to learn about functional anatomy as well as surface anatomy, when therapeutic injections are planned (Table 8.5).

Traditionally, BoNT has not been used early on following a stroke or brain injury, but there is now evidence of its safety within a few days of the event, even during the patient's stay in the intensive care unit[15]. The indication for pharmacological treatment therefore is *when spasticity is causing the patient harm*. Some patients early on in their rehabilitation following a stroke or brain injury use their spasticity to walk on, when their weakness would otherwise not allow it. Clearly, treating the spasticity here would not be helpful and physical measures to utilize the developing movement patterns would be the treatment of choice, but where the spasticity gives rise to problems for either the patient or the carer, then treatment is required.

It is sometimes quite difficult to distinguish between severe spasticity and contracture formation, but it is important to do so. The clinicians and the patient/carer can then know what anti-spastic treatment can or cannot achieve and realistic expectations can then be identified. Severe, inadequately-treated spasticity will go on to develop a limb contracture through shortening the muscle and tendons, as described above. A contracture may be fixed and will require serial splinting or surgery to correct it, but before it becomes fixed, the spasticity contributes to a dynamic contracture and treating the underlying spasticity may allow easier treatment of the contracture. One way to do that is to sedate patients with a short-acting benzodiazepine, such as midazolam. This can be done quite safely in the ward and a pulse oximeter is used to ensure an adequate and safe oxygen saturation. Four milligrams of midazolam is injected intravenously and a further 1 mg is injected every 30 s until the patient falls asleep and loses their corneal reflex. This relaxes spastic muscles and allows the range of passive joint movement to be assessed. The sedation is quickly reversed by injecting 200 µg of flumazenil. This too is titrated by injecting 100 µg every 30 s until the patient wakes up and can be further assessed while functioning. The anti-spastic effects of the midazolam will last for an hour or two thereafter. It is advisable to use a general anaesthetic for children, as the midazolam may not sedate sufficiently to achieve the desired effect and will, in some cases, simply disinhibit the child! A local anaesthetic nerve block can also be used equally well, but is perhaps more time-consuming. One particular use is in assessing patients who externally rotate their leg during walking. The adductor muscles can compensate for weak hip flexors and the patient can rotate the leg accordingly. Blocking the obturator nerve reduces the function of the adductors and it is then possible to see the degree of hip flexor weakness, so that a programme of muscle strengthening can be started rather than of BoNT injections which weaken the adductors.

8.6.2 Aims of treatment

There has to be a guide to defining the aims of treatment because patients have individual programmes of rehabilitation. As spasticity covers a range of clinical scenarios, it is tempting to use BoNT in a random manner, which may thus diminish its value. Although there are a wide number of reasons to treat spasticity with antispastic drugs and botulinum toxin in particular, the actual indications are quite specific and clinicians should follow these closely[20]. Patients may fulfil more than one indication, e.g. pain relief and care management, but it is inappropriate to give BoNT simply to 'see its effect'. There are many other ways, as described above.

The five indications are shown in Table 8.6.

Table 8.5. Patient selection checklist

What are the problems and will BoNT help?
Is there a significant component of muscle overactivity to treat effectively with BoNT?
Is the problem localized to a number of muscles?
Is there a clear aim for treatment?
Are the advantages of BoNT treatment clear?
Are there any contraindications to BoNT injection?
How will treatment outcomes be evaluated and are there appropriate measures to use?

Table 8.6. Indications for antispastic treatment

Indication	Example
Functional improvement	Mobility: enhance speed, quality or endurance of gait or wheelchair propulsion
	Improve transfers
	Improve dexterity and reaching
	Ease sexual functioning
Symptom relief	Relieve pain and muscle spasms
	Allow wearing of splints/orthoses
	Promote hygiene
	Prevent contractures
Aesthetic improvement	Enhance body image
Decrease carer burden	Help with dressing
	Improve care and hygiene
	Positioning for feeding, etc.
Enhance service responses	Prevent need for unnecessary medication and other treatments
	Facilitate therapy
	Delay or prevent surgery

In essence the assessment process for BoNT treatment aims to answer the questions shown in Table 8.6.

The assessment process determines the most appropriate treatment and the outcome measures that should be employed. These will be discussed later.

8.7   Medical interventions in the treatment for spasticity

These are well known and this section will only give a brief overview in relation to the place of BoNT in patient management. To reiterate, all medical interventions are adjunctive to a programme of physical treatment. All the medical interventions described can be given with BoNT and the assessment process should determine the management plan with the whole range of interventions in mind.

Table 8.7 gives a brief description of the available treatments that have been proven to be effective. There are others, but most people will be initially subject to an oral antispastic agent, such as baclofen or dantrolene sodium. Most clinicians will feel reasonably comfortable with using these two drugs and much has been

Table 8.7. Current proven effective treatments

Treatment	Value	Problems
Oral agents	Baclofen and Dantrolene cheap Tizanidine (seven times cost) Gabapentin/Pregabalin	40 per cent of patients unable either to tolerate oral agents because of side effects or unable to produce an adequate antispastic effect before side effects occur
Botulinum toxin	Effective for focal spasticity Simple to prescribe Simple intramuscular injection Need trained clinician to treat	Seen as expensive, but good value over the four-month effect of the drug budgetary limits. Reversible effects. Considerable benefit to management
Phenol nerve and motor point block	Cheap drug Time consuming to give	Expensive to give in clinical time. Painful to give. Potential for severe complications
Intrathecal baclofen	Expensive hardware Seven and a half year guaranteed life	Need for prolonged inpatient assessment required. Requires patient compliance and education. Need proper contract to deal with pump renewals
Intrathecal phenol	Technically more difficult Lumbar puncture required Cheap product	Only indicated for very severely disabled patients with limited life expectancy. Must be incontinent
Surgery	Neurosurgical and orthopaedic procedures expensive, but valuable Limited indications and patients	Painful, irreversible, invasive Variable results and effectiveness Paraesthesiae, bowel/bladder changes

written about them in other texts[21,22]. They tend to be used as first-line treatments, but there are occasions when this is ill-advised. Both these drugs can harm the brain's ability to repair after injury and should only be given after serious consideration of all the factors in the patient's care[23].

Most drugs alter chemical neurotransmitter action in the central nervous system (CNS), but some like tizanidine and the benzodiazepines also have a peripheral muscle action. Neurotransmission is stimulated by glutamate inhibited by gamma-aminobutyric acid (GABA) and modulated by serotonin (5HT). Drugs acting on these, such as the oral agents, can therefore modulate the response of the brain or spinal cord. BoNT is therefore quite different in its action and only works peripherally at the neuromuscular junction by blocking the release of acetyl-choline at presynaptic nerve terminals[24,25]. This gives only a local result and does not control generalized spasticity. As a result, pharmacological agents should be used in as a specific way as possible within the management principles described above. For example, if the problem is a spastic hand in a functionless limb after a stroke, the treatment of choice will be BoNT followed by physical therapy and splinting to maintain the benefit, whereas the management of generalized spasms will be best tackled by an oral antispastic drug.

8.7.1   Oral agents

The use of baclofen and dantrolene sodium has not changed much over the years[6,21], but some newer products have emerged. However, most give trouble-some side effects or idiosyncratic problems and care must be used when they are given. An audit of the patients attending the North Staffordshire Rehabilitation Centre in 1999 showed that 40 per cent of them could not tolerate oral agents because they either developed side effects or could not achieve an optimal dose to treat their spasticity effectively before side effects appeared[8].

Baclofen

Baclofen is a structural analogue of gamma-amiobutyric acid (GABA) and binds to GABA-B receptors both pre- and post-synaptically[26,27]. After oral administra-tion, it is rapidly and completely absorbed from the gastro-intestinal tract, with peak plasma levels occurring 1–2 hours after administration. Its plasma half-life is approximately 3.5 hours (range 2–6.8 hours). The serum protein binding rate is approximately 30 per cent. Seventy to eighty per cent of baclofen is excreted in unchanged form through the kidneys within 72 hours and a small proportion (about 10 per cent) is metabolized in the liver[28]. It can cross the placenta and only a small amount can cross the blood–brain barrier[29].

Baclofen has been used as an anti-spastic drug for over 30 years and most of the clinical trials in several countries involving patients mostly with multiple sclerosis and spinal cord lesions, has proved that baclofen is quite effective in reducing spasticity and sudden painful flexor spasms[30]. However, most of the studies failed to demonstrate improvement of mobility and activities of daily living[31]. There have been very few studies investigating the effect of baclofen in the treatment of spasticity of cerebral origin and the results described suggest a more limited benefit than that achieved among patients with multiple sclerosis and spinal cord lesions[32]. The recommended oral dosage range from 40 to 100 mg daily and begins with small doses, which gradually titrate to achieve an optimal clinical response with minimal side effects. If the therapeutic effects are not evident in 6 weeks, it may not benefit the patient to continue with the therapy. Elderly patients are more susceptible to side effects and small initial doses with gradual increments under careful supervision are advised. In children, dosages in the range of 0.75 to 2.5 mg^{-1}kg body weight should be used and treatment usually initiates with 2.5 mg four times daily with gradual increments at approximately three day intervals until a therapeutic response is achieved.

Dantrolene sodium

Dantrolene acts peripherally on muscle fibres, where by suppressing the release of calcium ions from the sarcoplasmic reticulum, it dissociates excitation–contraction coupling and diminishes the force of muscle contraction[33]. Placebo-controlled trials of dantrolene have demonstrated that it is superior to placebo in spasticity due to a variety of conditions and this is shown by muscle and reflex responses to mechanical and electrical stimulation and by clinical assessment of disability and activities of daily living[34]. It tends to be generally preferred for spasticity due to supraspinal lesions such as stroke, traumatic brain injury or cerebral palsy and some workers have suggested that stroke patients are more likely to improve with dantrolene[35,36]. Others have found that it neither altered muscle tone clinically or functional outcome in patients with hemispheric stroke when commenced within 8 weeks of onset of stroke[37]. It was reported that patients with spinal cord injury also responded well to dantrolene[38], but was somewhat less effective in patients with multiple sclerosis (MS)[39,40].

Dantrolene may cause side effects, such as drowsiness, dizziness, weakness, general malaise, fatigue and diarrhoea at the start of therapy, but these are generally mild. Muscle weakness may be the principal limiting side effect in ambulant patients, particularly in those with multiple sclerosis with pre-existing bulbar or respiratory muscle weakness[40]. Dantrolene is associated with idiosyncratic symptomatic hepatitis, which may rarely be fatal in 0.1 to 0.2 per cent of patients[41,42]. The risk occurs at all doses, but is more frequent in patients taking over 400 mg per day and in women over 35 years with concomitant medication such as oestrogen. Hence, liver function tests should be checked periodically during dantrolene therapy. Pleuro-pericardial reactions with eosinophilia have been reported[43].

Tizanidine

Tizanidine has a long history of use in continental Europe, which has more recently extended to the UK and USA. A number of studies have clearly demonstrated its benefit in spasticity due to multiple sclerosis and spinal cord injured patients, but definite functional improvements have not been shown[44−46]. It is also comparable to baclofen in efficacy in multiple sclerosis or spinal cord injured patients[47−50]. It was similarly efficacious in comparison with diazepam in hemiplegia due to stroke and traumatic brain injury and allowed significantly better walking distance ability[51]. Tizanidine also had a favourable adverse effects profile, although sedation remained a prominent side effect[52].

The dose is titrated over a 2 to 4 week period to a maximum of 36 mg per day, divided in three or four doses. Anecdotally, and certainly at higher dosages, sedation is still a limiting factor, and dryness of mouth, drowsiness, somnolence, insomnia, dizziness, postural hypotension and muscle weakness are all reported. Visual hallucinations and liver function test abnormalities also occur with clinically significant increases in liver enzymes in 5−7 per cent of patients[53]. In particular, liver problems have been reported with concomitant administration of baclofen, diazepam, flurazepam and diclofenac[54]. An assessment of the liver function test is therefore recommended before starting tizanidine and then after a month of treatment.

Benzodiazepines

The antispastic effect of benzodiazepines is mediated via $GABA_A$ receptors, which consists of a GABA recognition site, a benzodiazepine binding site and a chloride ion channel[55]. Among benzodiazepines, diazepam was the earliest antispasticity medication used in clinical practice, but is not much used now because of its daytime sedation. It is effective and compares well to baclofen in multiple sclerosis and spinal cord injured patients[56]. Other benzodiazepine analogues such as clonazepam, are used in epilepsy and have been compared to baclofen in mainly multiple sclerosis patients[57]. It was found to be equally effective as diazepam, but it was less well tolerated due to adverse effects such as sedation, confusion and fatigue, resulting in more frequent discontinuation of the drug. It is thus used mainly for suppression of nocturnal painful spasms.

Gabapentin

Gabapentin is useful when there is pain and particularly when there is cortical dysaesthesia giving rise to abnormal sensory inputs. Like other oral agents, it is poorly tolerated in a significant proportion of patients and its use is therefore limited. Clinicians are now also using pregablin in this context too.

Cannabis

There has also been a lot of interest in the use of cannabinoids following the identification and cloning of cannabinoid receptors located in the central nervous system and by the discovery of the endogenous cannabinoid ligands. Cannabinoids are also efficacious in animal models of MS. However, there have been only ten published clinical reports on the use of cannabis in MS, involving 78 individuals worldwide, and the results have been equivocal. Researchers encounter a number of difficulties in designing clinical studies that use cannabinoids. From the studies reporting the use of cannabinoids in MS patients with spasticity, the somewhat better designed studies failed to demonstrate objective improvement. Therefore, convincing evidence that cannabinoids are effective in MS is still lacking[58].

Much of the evidence that cannabinoids could help spasticity symptoms is anecdotal. The recent CAMS study in multiple sclerosis patients compared oral cannabis extract and Δ^9-tetrahydrocannabinol with placebo in 667 patients with stable multiple sclerosis and muscle spasticity in 33 UK centres over a 15 week period. The primary outcome measure was a change in the Ashworth scale. Treatment with cannabinoids did not have a beneficial effect on spasticity, but there was evidence of a treatment effect on patient-reported spasticity and pain[59].

8.7.2   Intrathecal baclofen

The technique of placing baclofen at its site of action in the spinal cord has really taken off in the last ten years with the introduction of programmable electronic pumps. The main indication is for people with paraplegia and tetraplegia, who are unable to tolerate or respond adequately to oral antispastic drugs. The development of intrathecal baclofen has followed that of intrathecal morphine for unremitting cancer pain[60]. The treatment consists of the surgical fitting of a pump in the anterior abdominal wall attached to a subcutaneous catheter tunnelled around the trunk and inserted into the spinal canal at about the L2/3 level. The catheter is then placed up to a level between D8 and D10. This allows baclofen to be delivered in the spine at higher concentrations than would be possible with oral administration and without the expected CNS side effects[61].

It is particularly useful in both brain and spinal cord injured patients, who do not have residual functioning, but the pump settings can also deliver doses in a highly specific manner to allow ambulant people to balance the weakening effect of baclofen against the spasticity required for weight support and joint mobility. The appearance of electronic programmable pumps has made a great difference to the ease of pump management for both patients and their medical attendants by allowing the delivery of the drug in one of many ways. They can deliver a single bolus or provide a continuous infusion of baclofen throughout the day. A phasic response may also be employed to deliver a different dose at different times of day by programming the pump's built-in computer. This gives a very precise antispastic control to achieve patient functioning, but some degree of compliance is required for this, as potential complications exist. Mechanical faults and human error in setting up the pump are known and baclofen is a CNS depressant and thus overdosage can lead to respiratory depression and coma, which may be fatal unless rapidly treated[62]. Deaths have also been reported due to overdosage due to faulty dosing calculation[63]. Mechanical pump failure has been reported, but this is now improving with better technology[64]. Complications of the surgery are also becoming less common, but CSF collection and leaks and headaches are occasionally seen[65].

8.7.3 Chemodenervation

Phenol nerve blockade

Chemical neurolysis describes a destructive process of a nerve. Both alcohol and phenol have been used in this way, but the former is not greatly employed in the UK or USA. It is different from the ion channel blockade of local anaesthetics[66]. Intrathecal 2–5 per cent phenol was first described to carry out regional blockade[67,68] and has enjoyed a little revival. Motor point injections were then used to reduce the morbidity associated with spinal injections, but were time consuming and had a variable effect. As a result, a perineural injection was developed using a 3–6 per cent aqueous solution, which has allowed groups of muscles to be blocked, when more proximal nerves are injected. This provides an initial local anaesthetic effect, which is later followed by blockade 1 hour later as protein coagulation and inflammation occur[69]. Wallerian degeneration then occurs later on before healing by fibrosis starts after about 4–6 months. This leaves the nerve with about 25 per cent less function than before, but does not disadvantage people with little or no residual function, as a mild progressive denervation can be beneficial in reducing spasticity[70]. Khalili *et al.* first pioneered nerve blockade[71] and re-growth of most axons is seen with preservation of γ-neurons[70]. This means that, unlike BoNT, phenol can reduce spasticity without reducing strength to the same extent. The effect is concentration and volume dependent[72] and concentrations above 3 per cent are more likely to result in histological change[73].

The indications for use are as an alternative to BoNT or surgery in the treatment of focal problems and has about the same efficacy as BoNT[74]. The effect can last for 4−6 months, which is slightly longer than that of BoNT and the renewal of muscle overactivity is probably due to nerve regeneration[75]. It can also be a useful addition to BoNT in allowing a wider distribution of chemodenervation, as described above. It is not really a first line alternative because of its potential for harm. The main problems are that it takes time to give and therefore can only be done where suitable facilities exist. As it can cause tissue necrosis, great care is required to give as little phenol as possible. Placement of the needle is therefore critical. Nerves are located by stimulation at 1−2 Hz and a muscle twitch responds to it. When the stimulus intensity is <1 mA, the needle is optimally placed and the smallest amount of phenol is injected perineurally so that the muscle stimulation ceases. The patient feels a burning sensation, which may be unpleasant[76]. The main problems occur later with vascular problems, reported as producing local oedema and venous thrombosis[77]. This can produce a localized tissue necrosis, which may take considerable efforts to treat. Dysaesthesia is perhaps one of the most distressing complications and will occur if the phenol is placed in proximity to sensory nerve fibres. As a result, only certain nerves are recommended for phenol chemoneurolysis. These are the obturator nerve (purely a motor nerve), which will treat adductor and gracilis spasticity and the musculocutaneous nerve, which supplies the biceps brachii, brachialis and coracobrachialis muscles. It has a small sensory component, for which gabapentin is very effective in treating. It is worth giving the patient a prescription for this drug, as one gives the phenol, so that patients can start treatment the moment they notice the complication. The tibial nerve may also be treated in experienced hands for triceps surae spasticity by blocking the nerve in the popliteal fossa. The nerve has separate sensory and motor bundles and the latter can be isolated after training. Although phenol is cheap and a lot cheaper than BoNT, its total cost is about the same as that of BoNT, if the clinician's time (it may take up to 45−60 minutes to perform a nerve block compared to a few minutes for a BoNT injection) and the need for more specialized facilities are taken into account. To this must be added the considerable cost of gabapentin and the potential cost of ulcer treatment. On top of this is, of course, the human misery of these complications.

Five per cent intrathecal phenol in glycerin is given on infrequent occasions for the management of paraplegia. With the patient lying on one side and with the foot of the bed down, 1−2 ml are instilled via a lumbar puncture needle. Afterwards, the patient lies on his or her side for 2−4 hours. The phenol is heavier than CSF (specific gravity 1.25 compared to 1.007 for CSF) and the phenol will sink distally. The patient may notice a tingling sensation. One to two days later, the procedure is repeated with the patient lying on the other side. Alcohol, on the other hand, is lighter than CSF and the foot of the bed should be raised to an angle of 25°. The procedure is only indicated for people with progressive disease, who are refractory to other antispastic treatments and who have no ambulatory function. It is also only indicated for those already rendered incontinent, as the phenol will otherwise lead to permanent urinary and faecal incontinence. Terminally-ill MS patients are the main group of patients for whom this treatment is given, when they have severe spasticity and do not have the ability or resilience to cope with intrathecal baclofen treatment. In addition, the surgical placing of a pump designed to last for 8 years has to be counterbalanced by the risks to the patient and logistics of living with a pump. The block is usually painless, as the phenol exerts a local anaesthetic effect and the procedure can be repeated as required.

8.7.4 Botulinum toxin

Doctors who wish to inject BoNT must be trained, as gaining the necessary skills requires time and commitment. The placing of the injection accurately is straightforward, but to get good results does require careful thought and planning. BoNT has a great propensity to seek neuromuscular junctions, but placing the toxin as near as practical to them may achieve better results and may possibly allow a smaller dose of the drug to achieve the same clinical outcome. A sound knowledge of anatomy is therefore necessary. Dilution is also an important factor and more dilute solutions have a greater ability to be taken up in neuromuscular junctions. A recent study showed a good response in the neuromuscular junction uptake of BOTOX® when 5 ml dilutions $(20\,U\,ml^{-1})$ were injected in a four point pattern in biceps brachii muscle compared to 1 ml dilutions $(100\,U\,ml^{-1})$. These were both compared to motor point injections of 1 ml dilutions $(100\,U\,ml^{-1})$[79]. Three preparations of botulinum toxin are commercially available in clinical practices in Europe and the USA and their differences have been highlighted in Chapter 5. These differences are perhaps most easily seen in spasticity and dystonia treatment and some studies have highlighted the inappropriateness of trying to find a fixed dosage ratio. It is better for a clinician to learn the effect of a 100 U BOTOX® or 400 U Dysport® or 5000 U Myo/Neurobloc on, say, a biceps brachii muscle. A muscle chart is shown in Appendix 8.1.

In addition, the drug should be placed in different locations of the muscle to obtain an optimal effect. It is unwise to inject more that 50 U BOTOX® or 200 U Dysport® or 2500 U Myo/Neurobloc in any one site, as too much local denervation may occur with saturation of the nearest neuromuscular junctions[78]. Appendix 8.1 gives a list of dosages for individual muscles.

8.7.5 Muscle location

Electromyography and muscle stimulation

The use of electromyography (EMG) guidance and muscle stimulation is generally favoured to locate muscles accurately for injection. This is not necessary for large, superficial, easily visible muscles, but is advisable for smaller and deep muscles and particularly applies to arm and forearm and lower leg muscles and small inaccessible muscles around the jaw. The aim is to record muscle action potentials and their interference pattern on muscular activation. This can sometimes be difficult to interpret in view of mass synergies in spasticity and either active contraction of the muscle or passive movements will inform the injector of correct placement. EMG guidance is particularly useful in flexor digitorum profundus and extensor digitorum communis muscles, which are organized in muscular fascicles supplying each digit. Correct placement of the needle can therefore allow neuromuscular blockade for each fascicle and thereby a very accurate result. Observing muscle action potentials ensures that the needle is in a muscle, but cannot always correctly identify which muscle. This is particularly so in small muscles. The combination of this with muscle stimulation makes for a more accurate assessment and gives the injector confidence of the actual location of the needle.

The procedure is carried out using a hollow Teflon-coated EMG needle with a sideport for syringe attachment. Motor point stimulation can also be carried out to activate small intramuscular fascicles, but this is time-consuming. Its advantage, however, is that it places the toxin as closely as possible to the motor end plate, the binding area, but increased effectiveness has not been shown in human studies. Animal studies would support a relationship between dose-related diffusion and the muscle response[80] and it is now important to study humans. At the present time the avid binding of toxin to a presynaptic nerve terminal would not necessarily make this vital for clinical practice. Motor stimulation has been used primarily for nerve blockade and the immediate expected response can authenticate the accuracy of the procedure. It is possible that accurate localization through EMG guidance and muscle stimulation can reduce the dose of toxin. This is obviously important for patients with progressive disorders, such as MS, and for patients requiring repeated injections. In this way, costs will be contained and the chance of antibody-mediated non-responsiveness will be decreased. Again there is no direct evidence of this and opinions for and against the technique have been based on a small number of patients in an uncontrolled situation[81,82]. However, motor point injection with phenol takes longer to do and the increased procedure time taken should be included in the comparison of costs.

8.7.6   Computerized tomography and ultrasonography

Routine computerized tomographic (CT) radiography location of muscles is not justifiable from a safety point of view in view of the accuracy of the above techniques. Ultrasound, on the other hand, has a useful place in locating both superficial and deep muscles. It is safe, non-invasive and does not distress patients. It is accurate, but does require the injector to learn the technique and to orientate him or herself to the expected findings. Alternately, a radiographer/radiologist is required, which increases both the cost and technical organization of the procedure.

8.7.7   Clinical scenarios for botulinum toxin treatment

A description of some common injected muscles with their points of origin and insertion and action are now studied.

Spastic shoulder and upper arm

The typical hemiplegic arm is adducted and internally rotated at the shoulder, flexed at the elbow, pronated in the forearm and flexed at the wrist and hand. Treatment should therefore be aimed at reversing this pattern. With increasing spasticity, contractures occur at the shoulder and elbow and difficulties arise in maintaining axillary hygiene. The clinical findings are due to overactivity in all groups, but particularly the subscapularis muscle, the pectoralis group and to a lesser extent the latissimus dorsi muscle. Injection of these muscles is indicated followed by physical therapy. Pronator teres and pronator quadratus muscles are responsible for the pronation deformity, but one should not forget the contribution of brachialis muscle. Elbow flexors are powerful and are essentially three in number. The first action of biceps brachii is to supinate the forearm before flexing the elbow. Brachioradialis flexes in a neutral position and brachialis has a pronatory contribution in flexion. If biceps alone is injected with BoNT, the tendency to supinate will be reduced and the forearm will be more likely to pronate, which of course is the reverse of the rehabilitative aim. Therefore, injecting both biceps and brachialis is useful and will take 80–120 U and 60–100 U BOTOX® respectively. Alternately, a musculo-cutaneous nerve block with phenol will achieve as good a result.

The clawed hand and flexed wrist

The flexor muscles in this deformity exert a greater influence than the extensors, which results in flexion deformities of the wrist and small joints of the hand, as well as pronation of the forearm. Flexor carpi radialis and ulnaris muscles are responsible for flexion of the wrist and the lumbrical muscles for flexion of the fingers at the metacarpophalangeal joints. The flexor digitorum superficialis muscle flexes the fingers at the proximal interphalangeal joints and the flexor digitorum profundus muscle is responsible for flexion of the terminal phalanges. It is important to differentiate between the action of these muscles as the first step in planning accurate treatment. Thereafter, getting to know the surface anatomy is helpful. Good hand function is impossible with a thumb in palm deformity, i.e. an adducted flexed thumb in the palm and it is important to assess this. The deformity is caused by overactivity in the opponens pollicis muscle and thumb flexion is due to a combination of flexor pollicis longus and brevis muscle shortening. Referral to Appendix 8.1 will help the injector find the right muscle to inject, its location and the range of dosage for adults. In patients with coarse hand function, it is sometimes better to leave a flexed stiff thumb terminal digit, as this will assist pincer grip.

Hip flexor and thigh adductor spasticity

Scissoring of the legs is a common feature in non-ambulant severely disabled people with paraplegia, due either to MS or spinal cord injury. Those affected, usually obligate wheelchair users, are not able to stretch their legs sufficiently to overcome hip flexor and adductor muscle shortening. With time, they become flexed at the hip and knee and may develop windswept deformities, where one leg becomes adducted and the other abducts. This is due to flexion deformities exerting a gravitational influence and gives rise to difficulties with perineal hygiene, dressing and with transfers. Patients often have considerable pain. Injecting the adductor muscles with BoNT is useful in patients with true adductor spasm, but is not the sole treatment of choice for many people. It is necessary to address hip flexor spasticity and shortening in addition. The psoas major and rectus femoris muscles are the two main flexors responsible for this. It also prevents patients being unable to stand erect and it is most important to deal with either of these muscles prior to the adductor group. Testing psoas is carried out by the Thomas test, where fully flexing of one hip anteverts the pelvis. If the contralateral psoas is shortened, the knee on that side will also flex and the degree of fixed flexion deformity can be measured by the principle of parallel angles. This manoeuvre is then carried out on the other leg. The length of the rectus femoris can be measured through the Duncan–Elie test with the patient lying prone. If the muscle is short, the patient will be unable to flex the knee fully without the bottom rising off the bed and the angle at the greater trochanter can be measured. However, many paraplegic patients find prone lying impossible and one can feel the tension of the shortened upper tendon of the muscle when the hip is extended. If one then abducts the leg and flexes the knee over the side of the couch, the lower leg would normally drop to 90°. If it cannot, then the shortening can be similarly measured.

The psoas major muscle arises from the lateral aspect of the vertebral bodies from T12 to L5, but the muscle is thin at T12 and L1 and lies posterior to the kidney. It is thus wise to avoid injecting here, but the muscle is thick and well rounded between L2−5. The lumbo-sacral plexus is closely applied at the L5 level and it is probably advisable to steer clear from this area as well. The muscle is thus injected with 50 U BOTOX® (200 U Dysport®) at L2, L3 and L4 to a total of 150 U BOTOX® (600 U Dysport®) per muscle. Below L5, the muscle joins the iliacus muscle at the pelvic brim and the two form the iliopsoas tendon to insert into the lesser trochanter. The psoas rather than the iliacus is responsible for providing the power to hip flexion. A considerable effect is achieved by injecting at L2, L3 and L4, which deals with hip flexor spasticity more than adequately. The most sensitive outcome measures for hip and thigh spasticity treatment are hip flexion deformity angle changes (as demonstrated by the Thomas test) and the stride length and walking speed (tested by a 10 m walking time) in ambulant patients and by a modified Ashworth scale in non-ambulant patients. Injecting the rectus femoris muscle is straightforward, as the muscle is easily identified. The muscle arises from the anterior inferior iliac spine and passes down the middle of the anterior thigh in front of the vastus intermedius muscle. It joins the other components of the quadriceps femoris muscle to insert into the tibial tubercle via the quadriceps and patellar tendons. About 100 U BOTOX® (400 U Dysport®) is a reasonable dose, but the patient should be warned that knee stability may be transiently altered for a couple of weeks after the procedure. This is due to mild weakening of the muscle.

Talipes equino-varus foot

A common feature of a spastic lower limb is an inverted plantar-flexed foot and it is important to demonstrate that this is due to spasticity rather than to imbalance between plantar flexor/inverter and dorsiflexor/everter muscles before treating it. BoNT will not be effective if the deformity is simply due to weakness. Where spasticity is the major feature, injecting the tibialis posterior and the posterior calf muscles is used to achieve a straight foot for weight bearing or to fit an orthosis. It thus facilitates standing transfers and allows the patient to stand on a flat foot, which is essential for safe walking. If the patient cannot achieve proper base of support, because the foot itself is flexed and inverted, it is necessary to inject the short toe flexors (flexor digitiorum and hallucis brevis muscles). The best outcome measures are the range of active and passive dorsi- and plantar-flexion at the ankle and walking speed in ambulant patients. It is often necessary to inject all the muscles, but differentiation between the contribution from the gastrocnemius and soleus muscles and the achilles tendon contracture is easy clinically and electromyographically and expertise comes with practice. Because the gastrocnemius muscle arises for the posterior aspect of the femoral condyles, flexing the knee effectively lengthens the muscle. One would therefore expect to see a greater dorsiflexion at the ankle. If the angle of passive dorsiflexion remains the same, either the soleus or the achilles tendon is short. In the case of the latter, the soleus feels soft and relaxed and the tendon can be palpated. The muscles can be found electromyographically or through ultrasound. Muscle action potential patterns are different in the type I fibres of the soleus and the mixed type I and II fibres seen in the gastrocnemius.

8.8   Post-injection care

The treatment of spasticity is enhanced by a programme of physical treatment after BoNT injections or nerve blockade[83] and physiotherapy in the form of stretching and strengthening is thus required for a period following the procedure. It has also been noted anecdotally, that the effect of a single dose of BoNT-A can be prolonged beyond its action duration and repeat injections, which are necessary for MS patients, can be reduced to a minimum. Limbs should be stretched to a functional position, but should not be traumatized, as this will provide a nociceptive stimulus to increase spasticity in non-injected muscles. Therapy should be given every day for a period of at least 4 weeks, but the benefit, duration and optimal regimen require scientific evaluation. Similarly, there is anecdotal information, that, to be effective, stretching should be carried out for several hours every day. Clearly, this cannot be done on a one-to-one basis and splinting/casting can provide a stretch for several hours. Occupational therapists have taken responsibility for this treatment. Night resting casts are particularly valuable, as they achieve this purpose, but do not interfere with daily activities.

Follow-up is important to identify whether or not the treatment objectives have been met and to plan further treatment. As has been stated above, it is important to identify those muscles requiring injection at the start of the treatment episode and to re-inject 3 to 4 months, if necessary, after the first. At each follow-up, the relevant outcome measures should be recorded and it is worth having a separate page in the clinical notes for this purpose, noting the date of the injection, the muscles injected and the outcome measures used. Multiple sclerosis patients, like others with chronic spasticity, may require repeated injections and it is important to have at a glance clear documentation of what has been previously done. A trend may thus be observed to aid further management. Good documentation is important to make the best of follow-up assessments and an example is attached in Appendix 8.2.

8.8.1   Organization of services for botulinum toxin treatment in spasticity

The optimal configuration of services will vary in different places, and flexibility is important. They will usually revolve around specialist rehabilitation units, neurology or stroke services or departments of medicine for the elderly. Requirements include:

1. Clinician(s) trained in spasticity management in general, with specific additional training in botulinum toxin treatment. This is probably best achieved by a combination of specific courses and apprenticeships with direct instruction and supervised practice.

2. An active physiotherapy and occupational therapy service, with roles in selecting patients for treatment and arranging or delivering targeted physiotherapy after injection, and ensuring appropriate provision of orthoses. There should be good links with physical therapy departments in referring units elsewhere.

3. Orthopaedic advice should be available.

4. Many injections can be performed in dedicated outpatient clinics. These allow more convenient and cost-effective assessment and follow-up by multidisciplinary teams, minimal wastage of BoNT, and easier access to equipment such as EMG to help with injections, plus availability of nursing staff trained to assist in the sometimes awkward patient manoeuvring required.

5. A ward or even a roaming service may be needed: many patients with spasticity are difficult to transfer to a clinic. A portable EMG device may be required.

6. Services should consider avoiding or minimizing the use of more than one of the available BoNT preparations in order to avoid the risk of confusion over doses.

7. Many patients like to have their next appointment for review and usually treatment at a pre-arranged interval, especially if their response is fairly predictable. Those with an unpredictable or long-lasting response may prefer self-referral when their last injections are wearing off. BoNT clinics should attempt to accommodate both: although patient-initiated appointments may be difficult to fit in, this strategy generally acts to reduce the number of injection sessions.

8. In future it may be possible for predictable injections to be given in the community by trained staff.

9. A clearly defined mechanism for paying for the toxin and the service. Ad hoc arrangements can be financially risky for host institutions.

8.8.2   Outcome measures

Outcome measurement in spasticity is controversial because of the huge array of available tools. Most clinicians do not actually measure the outcomes of their interventions in terms of the change to the neurogenic component of the upper motor neuron lesion. They more often measure the change in either the biomechanical consequence of the spastic limb (at impairment level) or the functional change (activity) of the goal of treatment. The main problem here is that the accepted measure of spasticity, the Ashworth score, does not actually measure what it purports to do. It does not follow Lance's definition and measures limb stiffness rather than velocity-dependent resistance[84]. The Tardieu Scale[85] and the Wartenburg Pendulum Test[86], on the other hand, do a better job, but are more unwieldy to use in clinical practice. Figure 8.4 demonstrates the complexity of the resistance to passive motion and increased tone.

Clinicians seek validation of the scales that they use and end up employing a mixture of neurophysiological and mechanical measures to quantify the resistance to passive stretch, which is the sum of the neurophysiological change and altered muscle properties and function.

Ashworth scale

This scale is based on the assessment of resistance to stretch when a limb is passively moved (Table 8.8). It was originally validated for patients with MS and was validated by Ashworth[88]. Its reliability is questioned by the subjectivity required by the observer to carry out the test and by the fact that it measures multiple aspects of limb stretch. However, it is in general use and has good inter- and intra-rater reliability[89]. Its validity in its general application to spasticity assessment, however, is not. The original Ashworth scale is only validated for measuring spasticity in the lower limb[90]. In addition, it does not distinguish between increased neurogenic muscle tone and mechanical limb stiffness. Despite this, it has nonetheless become the measure against which all other measures are compared. Based on the fact that resistance to passive movement (as performed during the Ashworth scale) is influenced by various factors, Lance's definition is not addressed despite the validity of the scale as a measure of that resistance. Measures of resting posture and

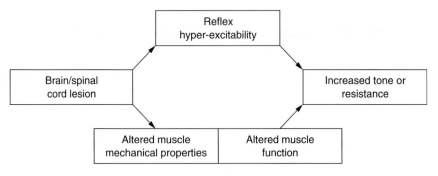

Figure 8.4   Resistance to passive motion (after Johnson[87]).

Table 8.8. Description of the Ashworth and Modified Ashworth Scales

Score	Ashworth (Ashworth 1964[88])	Modified Ashworth (Bohannon and Smith 1987[92])
0	No increase in tone	No increase in tone
1	Slight increase in tone giving a catch when the limb is moved in flexion/extension	Slight increase in tone giving a catch, release and minimal resistance at the end of range of motion (ROM) when the limb is moved in flexion/extension
1+		Slight increase in tone giving a catch, release and minimal resistance throughout the remainder (less than half) of ROM
2	More marked increase in tone, but the limb is easily moved through its full ROM	More marked increase in tone through most of the ROM, but limb is easily moved
3	Considerable increase in tone — passive movement difficult and ROM decreased	Considerable increase in tone — passive movement difficult
4	Limb rigid in flexion and extension	Limb rigid in flexion and extension

passive range of motion do not depend on stretch reflex activity, which is the element that needs to be measured[91]. The major modification was proposed to differentiate between mild and moderate spasticity, as discrepancies appeared in clinical judgement at the lower end of the original scale. Bohannon validated the scale in elbow flexion in post-stroke patients and attempts have been made to widen the validity[92]. A grade 1+ was added and the top of the scale was reduced from 5 to 4. The essential weakness in the scale remains that Grade 0 is not a floppy limb and that there is no reference to normality.

Further examination of this area of clinical practice has prompted new directions[91,93]. Gregson et al. showed good inter-rater and intra-rater reliability of the Ashworth scale with the Medical Research Council (MRC) scale for muscle power for wrist, elbow and knee flexor function, but less good association for the ankle[94]. They quite rightly warn of making assumptions about the scale when measuring foot dorsi- and plantar flexion. A straight comparison between the modified Ashworth and MRC scales is somewhat difficult, as the former behaves as a nominal measure, whereas the latter is ordinal. A better comparison may have been between the original scale, which does not have the difficulties in the context of differences between grades 1 and 1+. One of the difficulties is that neither scale covers the whole range of tonus. Normal is zero and neither takes hypotonia into account as a calculation and both are at best ordinal measures. In addition, there is no definition of what constitutes a slow stretch, although a maximum angular velocity of 80 per cent has been proposed before reflex activity alters muscle resistance[95].

Tardieu scale

The measurement of the velocity-dependent catch or the clasp-knife effect is demonstrated by other means. Tardieu described one such in 1954, which went somewhat unnoticed, but interest in it has recently been resurrected[85]. Its modification[96] was later validated and measures the angle at the point of resistance to a rapid velocity stretch when the overactive stretch reflex produces a 'catch' appears[97]. Both the dynamic and static muscle length and joint range of movement are assessed and the technique is described below (Table 8.9). Inter- and intra-rater reliability studies are already underway in order to define the best conditions under which to carry out the examination[98].

It is carried out by stretching a limb passively and the angle at the point of resistance is noted. This is performed during as slow a movement as possible (V1), under gravitational pull (V2) and at a fast rate (V3). The examiner will feel a catch in a muscle under the influence of an overactive stretch reflex. Five levels have been described at the point of this catch to capture the quality of the muscular reaction. In essence the scale assesses dynamic and static muscle length as well as joint range of motion. The inter- and intra-rater reliability is generally good[98], but the technique does require training to achieve this.

Other measures of spasticity

So why are we measuring tone and why is it important? In clinical practice, measures of disability are the most useful to quantify and relate to the patient's rehabilitation aims. Spasticity is but one component that has to be dealt with and the outcomes of rehabilitation depend on issues relating to other impairments, to activity and to participation. Clinicians must be clear about what they are doing and realize that global disability scores, such as the Functional Independence

Table 8.9. The Tardieu Scale[85]

Stretch velocity		Y angle (dynamic range of motion)		Quality of muscle reaction course of passive movement	
V1	Slow as possible	R2	Slow velocity	0	No resistance
V2	Speed of limb falling under gravity		Passive joint range of motion or muscle length	1	Slight resistance
				2	Clear catch at precise angle, then release
V3	Fast as possible	R1	Fast velocity Movement through full range of motion	3	Fatiguable clonus at precise angle
				4	Unfatiguable clonus at precise angle
				5	Rigid limb and joint

Measure, are unlikely to change following a BNTX injection into forearm flexors for a spastic hand in a stroke patient, in which there is no intrinsic function. An easy-to-measure tool is needed, whereas in research a standardized testing protocol is required to follow the definition of the condition as closely as possible. The Ashworth scale fails in this, but remains a useful bedside clinical measure. Pandyan *et al.* thus support the use of this scale as an ordinal measure of resistance to passive movement[85]. For research purposes the Wartenburg pendulum test follows the definition and gets round the complex variables that occur in the alpha motor neurons of agonist and antagonist muscles during passive movements. In this, the leg moves under gravity and the observer measures the pendular activity of a spastic limb as it relaxes. It is best carried out on the lower limb, for it is not so reliable for other limb segments. Rymer and Katz conclude, however, that biomechanical measures correlate most closely with the clinical state, as extending a limb against passive resistance may be related more to the visco-elastic properties of the soft tissues than to spasticity[99]. EMG activity and the motor unit magnitude correlate well with the torque and ramp and hold displacement around the elbow[100].

Clinical measures

Many scales bear little resemblance to what is happening to the patient, which is of course most relevant to clinical practice. Several studies have reported a decrease in spasticity (as measured by the Ashworth scale), pain, muscle spasms, carer burden, etc[101–104]. Most health services, however, wish to see a more tangible benefit in functional terms from what is regarded as expensive unproven treatment and look to see functional changes in patients. This is somewhat fallacious in view of individual characteristics and efforts have now been made to find a suitable outcome measure to demonstrate functional change, which is more applicable to this treatment. Bhakta *et al.* described some change in their functional assessment tool[102], but Brashear *et al.* devised a new scale in an attempt to show a more specific functional change in relation to BoNT treatment in upper limb spasticity[105]. They described a Disability Assessment Score (DAS), which looked at four domains (pain, hygiene, dressing and limb position), each with a four point subjective assessment of degree of difficulty for the patient and patients chose the item that most reflected their treatment aims. This was termed the Principal Intervention Target and a significant change was seen following treatment with BoNT. Physiotherapy was not assessed in these patients and more prolonged changes may have accrued. This highlights one of the difficulties in spasticity studies. Spasticity demands multi-facet treatment strategies, which have to be abandoned in randomized controlled studies. The DAS was later validated and represents a useful additional tool in this area. Unfortunately, it is difficult to apply to anywhere but the upper limb[106]. A number of other clinical tools are available and goal attainment is most relevant. If a patient is being treated with BoNT for pain in a clawed hand after a stroke, the best outcome in that patient is to see a reduction in pain. There are a number of validated measures for this in the visual analogue and the Likert Scales[107].

Functional aspects are therefore important to measure, but one of the problems is that functional change with treatment may be dependent on factors other than the spasticity. Few studies have shown a global correlation with the Ashworth score and the measurement of function, as in the Rivermead or Fugl−Meyer Motor Assessment scores[107], is best correlated with other impairment measures, like the spasm frequency score, adductor tone, pain score, etc. Therein lies the dilemma. We will probably have to keep on using the Ashworth scale in the clinical setting, but realize its limitations and always combine management of the patient with a functional outcome measure in relation to the rehabilitation goal.

The Action Research Arm Test has been used to measure functional activity in the arm in response to BoNT treatment[108] and has allowed researchers to make some sense of the part played by BoNT. Although there is a large placebo effect in receiving an injection of BoNT, it does reduce spasticity. It does not necessarily reduce the force-generating capabilities at the joint. The (modified) Ashworth scale is unable to measure clinically important changes in spasticity. Improvements in function observed in a chronic stroke population raises the question whether the effects of BoNT in treating spasticity are underestimated and whether early intervention using the toxin may augment its efficacy[109]. We also know that BoNT is effective and safe in treating acute muscle shortening and preventing contracture formation, even in the most ill patients[15]. This will undoubtedly lead to further confidence in its use.

Other measures have a particular use in physiotherapy practice and contribute to the overall picture of change following treatment. The walking speed (measured by a 10 m walking time), the stride length and joint goniometry are useful in measuring change in hip and thigh spasticity in spastic diplegics[110]. Pain has been addressed above and the Jebsen Taylor Hand test demonstrates improvement in dexterity and isolated finger movement, whereas the Berg Balance scale evaluates what it suggests[107]. The final thought is that clinicians tend to measure what they feel is the most relevant aspect of treatment. Just as we need to ask the patient and family their view of the goal, we probably ought to involve more in the measurement process too. The patient satisfaction score on a 10 cm visual analogue scale is very useful in identifying whether the targets were met in the patient's perspective and is useful when everyone is sure on expectations. The patient and physician global scores also address this aspect.

8.8.3   Evidence for the use of BoNT in spasticity

Many publications have gone over the scientific basis for using BoNT in spasticity management[111,112] and this section will simply update them rather than go over the subject again. In most randomized controlled trials (RCTs), the effects of BoNT are compared with placebo over a single injection cycle. The outcomes are generally positive and support the use of the drug, but they do not necessarily reflect what is important in clinical practice. In addition, data from RCTs are less convincing than those from open studies for a variety of technical reasons, which perhaps reflects the difficulties in finding good outcome measures for spastic patients[113]. Clinical experience tells us that BoNT can reduce spasticity and improve voluntary movement and active function in selected patients. Again, RCTs have had difficulty showing active functional improvement, despite the clear ability of BoNT to reduce spasticity and this is, to a large extent, due to poor methodology, especially in patient selection and injection protocols and the choice of outcome measures. Motor dysfunction is usually caused by weakness (and other 'negative' features of upper motor neuron syndrome) rather than by muscle overactivity. Clinical trials therefore need to take this into account in designing trials[114,115].

There is good evidence that BoNT has clinical benefit in treating the mechanical effects of spasticity. Future research strategies should now concentrate on its longer-term use, the as yet unresolved technical issues of how to get the best out of this new treatment and, of course, its cost-effectiveness. Brashear *et al.* showed very well the benefits of BoNT over a 12-week cycle in terms of Ashworth score, Disability Assessment score and patient and physician global rating scale[105]. Of the 126 patients (64 in the treatment group and 62 in the placebo group), 122 completed the study. Of these patients, 111 then entered an open-label phase and were followed up for 42 weeks[106]. This was the first long-term study of BoNT in a stroke population. One patient did not receive BoNT and the 110 who did, carried on treatment under clinical conditions. They had up to four further treatments and the value of this study is clear. All 110 were entered for the first cycle, 96 were entered for the second, 81 for the third and 26 for the fourth. First, there were significant improvements from baseline across all the measures at each treatment cycle and this remained constant, whether the patient was injected only once or four times. Second, there was considerable variation in the length of response to the injection and a beneficial effect lasted for over 24 weeks in 7.4 per cent of patients. The average number of treatments was 2.72 in this 42-week period. Overall, the patients were observed for 54 weeks and the safety profile of the drug remained, no matter how many treatments were given. This not only supports previous short-term work[101−103], but sets the scene for further long term studies to look more at the overall impact on patients' activity, functioning and participation, as well as on the impact to service provision.

There has been some work in studying the combination of BoNT and physical treatments, but most have run into problems standardizing treatments. However, some have produced evidence to show the increased benefit of BoNT to the physical management of spasticity. Muscle stretching may improve the therapeutic effect of BoNT and vice versa[116], but this needs to be established in a RCT. Standing and walking have improved following BoNT[19,117]. BoNT was compared to casting and to standard physiotherapy within a few days of a brain injury. Active treatment (BoNT ± casting) had a better outcome than standard treatment and there were no adverse events in the BoNT patient group[15]. Biomechanical changes may thus be prevented in the longer term by treating patients enthusiastically at such an early stage. Further studies will need to be done to show these benefits in functional terms, but BoNT and casting in combination has real potential.

There is now evidence for the effect of BoNT in all acute and chronic spastic conditions and the common thread is that the drug has a peripheral action, thereby negating the different effects of the aetiology. In summary, it is now certain that BoNT does reduce spasticity, as measured by the Ashworth score, pain, spasms and the symptoms associated with all of these. These include some local functional goals, such as hygiene and relieving carer burden for dressing, positioning, etc. as measured by the Disability Assessment score. One of the real beneficial aspects of BoNT is its safety profile and all of the RCTs and open studies make specific comment on this. Adverse events are small in number and only minor. Even in very ill patients, it was safe and it also contributed to a protective effect of anti-spastic treatment in preventing the immediate effects of limb deformity early on after severe brain injury[15].

Collecting evidence for the effectiveness of BoNT in managing spasticity is necessary[112] and the UK Department of Health recently called for applications for a longer-term study of the effectiveness and cost-effectiveness of BoNT in post-stroke spasticity. Studies are currently underway to demonstrate the place of the drug in comparison to oral agents in stroke and brain injury and this correlates with the reality of physicians making the choice between these two treatment strategies for their patients[118]. This placebo-controlled double-blind study of BoNT vs. tizanidine vs. placebo tablets and placebo injection will attempt to define a strategy for antispastic treatment early on in stroke and brain injury rehabilitation. This also needs to be done for chronic neurological disease to support the initial attempt by Hyman et al.[119]

Table 8.10. Advantages and disadvantages with BoNT treatment

Advantages	Disadvantages
• Efficacy whatever cause of spasticity	• Cannot treat widespread spasticity
• Effectively treats focal problems	• Requires a combined approach
• Specific treatment	• Reversible, needs repeating
• Very safe drug — reversible effects	• Not a long-term solution
• Easy to use	• Difficult to estimate cost-effectiveness
• May reduce need for systemic drugs	• Assessment of muscles to be injected
• Few drug interactions	can be difficult
• Role in prevention	• Potential cost implications

8.9   Conclusion

The contribution of BoNT in spasticity management is now well recognized. The trick in clinical management is to use it intelligently and know when and when not to use it. Table 8.10 highlights some of the advantages and disadvantages.

It must be remembered that BoNT is a useful short-term means of improving patients' function and the distressing features of spasticity. This is against the background of a long term condition, for which a long term management strategy is required.

REFERENCES

1. Lance, J. W. (1980). Symposium synopsis. In R. G. Feldman, R. R. Young, and W. P. Koella, eds., *Spasticity: Disordered Control.* Chicago: Yearbook Medical, pp. 485–94.
2. Young, R. R. (1994). Spasticity: a review. *Neurology,* **44,** 512–20.
3. Mayer, N. H. (2002). Clinicophysiologic concepts of spasticity and motor dysfunction in adults with an upper motoneuron lesion. In *Spasticity: Etiology, Evaluation, Management and the Role of Botulinum Toxin.* New York: We Move, pp. 1–10.
4. A European Thematic Network to Develop Standardised Measures of Spasticity (SPASM). CREST – Centre for Rehabilitation and Engineering Studies, University of Newcastle, Stephenson Building, Claremont Road, Newcastle upon Tyne, NE1 7RU, UK.
5. Denny-Brown, D. (1966). *The Cerebral Control of Movement.* Liverpool: Liverpool University Press, pp. 124–43.
6. Gracies, J. M., Elovic, E., McGuire, J. R. and Simpson, D. M. (2002). Traditional pharmacological treatments for spasticity. Part I: Local treatments. In *Spasticity: Etiology, Evaluation, Management and the Role of Botulinum Toxin.* New York: We Move, pp. 44–64.

7. Gracies, J. M., Wilson, L., Gandevia, S. C. and Burke (1997). Stretched position of spastic muscle aggravates their co-contraction in hemiplegic patients. *Annals of Neurology*, **42**(30), 438.

8. Ward, A. B. (1999). Botulinum toxin in spasticity management. *British Journal of Therapy and Rehabilitation*, **6**(7), 26—34.

9. Tardieu, J. C., Tabary, C., Tardieu, C., Tardieu, G. and Goldspink, G. (1972). Physiological and structural changes in cat soleus muscle due to immobilization at different lengths by plaster casts. *Journal of Physiology*, **224**, 231—44.

10. Krenz, N. R. and Weaver, L. C. (1998). Sprouting of primary afferent fibres after spinal cord transection in the rat. *Neuroscience*, **85**, 443—58.

11. Farmer, S. E., Harrison, L. M., Ingram, D. A. and Stephens, J. A. (1991). Plasticity of central motor pathways in children with hemiplegic cerebral palsy. *Neurology*, 15045—110.

12. Denny-Brown, D. (1966). In *The Cerebral Control of Human Movement*. Liverpool: Liverpool University Press, pp. 124—43.

13. New standards for nurses to boost patient care. Department of Health Report 0096 (2001). HMSO, London.

14. Fully Equipped: The Provision of Equipment to Older or Disabled People by the NHS and Social Services in England and Wales Audit Commission (2000). HMSO, London.

15. Verplancke, D., Snape, S., Salisbury, C. F., Jones, P. W. and Ward, A. B. (2005). A randomized controlled trial of the management of early lower limb spasticity following acute acquired severe brain injury. *Clinical Rehabilitation*, **19**(2), 117—125.

16. Wade, D. T. and Langton-Hewer, R. (1987). Epidemiology of some neurological diseases, with special reference to work load in the NHS. *International Rehabilitation Medicine*, **8**, 129—37.

17. Rehabilitation after traumatic brain injury: a Working Party Report of the British Society of Rehabilitation Medicine (1998). London: British Society of Rehabilitation Medicine.

18. Neurological rehabilitation — a working party report (Chairman, Barnes M. P.) of the British Society of Rehabilitation Medicine and the Neurological Alliance (1992). London: British Society of Rehabilitation Medicine.

19. Richardson, D., Sheean, G., Werring, D., Desai, M., Edwards, S., Greenwood, R. and Thompson, A. (2000). Evaluating the role of botulinum toxin in the management of focal hypertonia in adults. *Journal of Neurology, Neurosurgery and Psychiatry*, **69**, 499—506.

20. Ward, A. B. (Chairman) *et al.* (2001). Working party report on the management of adult spasticity using botulinum toxin type A — a guide to clinical practice. Byfleet: Radius Healthcare.

21. Tardieu, C., Lespargot, A., Tabary, C. and Bret, M. D. (1988). For how long must the soleus muscle be stretched each day to prevent contracture? *Developmental Medicine and Child Neurology*, **30**, 3—10.

22. Ward, A. B. and KoKo, C. (2001). Pharmacological management of spasticity. In M. P. Barnes and G. R. Johnson, eds., *Chapter in Clinical Management of Spasticity*. London, Cambridge: Cambridge University Press, pp. 165—87.

23. Dobkin, B. H. (2000). Functional rewiring of brain and spinal cord after injury: the three Rs of neural repair and neurological rehabilitation. *Current Opinion in Neurology*, **13**(6), 655–8.

24. Evans, M., Williams, R. S., Shone, C. C., Hamblton, P., Melling, J. and Dolly, O. (1986). Botulinum type B. Its purification, radio-iodination, and interaction with rat brain synaptosomal membranes. *European Journal of Biochemistry*, **154**, 409–16.

25. Kozachi, S. and Sakaguchi, G. (1982). Binding to mouse brain synaptosomes of *Clostridium botulinum* type E derivative toxin before and after tryptic activation. *Toxicon*, **20**, 841–6.

26. Hwang, A. S. and Wilcox, G. L. (1989). Baclofen, gamma-aminobutyric acid B receptors and substance P in the mouse spinal cord. *Journal of Pharmacology and Experimental Therapy*, **248**, 1026–33.

27. Price, G. W., Wilkin, G. P., Turnbull, M. J. and Bowery, N. G. (1984). Are baclofen-sensitive GABA-B receptors present on primary afferent terminals of the spinal cord? *Nature*, **307**, 71–3.

28. Aisen, M. L., Dietz, M. A., Rossi, P., Cedarbaum, J. M. and Kutt, H. (1993). Clinical and pharmacokinetic aspects of high dose baclofen therapy. *Journal of American Paraplegia Society*, **15**, 211–16.

29. Pederson, E., Arlien-Soborg, P. and Mai, J. (1974). The mode of action of the GABA derivative baclofen in human spasticity. *Acta Neurologica Scandinavia*, **50**, 665–80.

30. Hudgson, P. and Weightman, D. (1971). Baclofen in the treatment of spasticity. *British Medical Journal*, **4**, 155–7.

31. From, A. and Heltberg, A. (1975). A double blind trial with baclofen (Lioresal) and diazepam in spasticity due to multiple sclerosis. *Acta Neurologica Scandinavia*, **51**, 158–66.

32. Whyte, J. and Robinson, K. M. (1990). Pharmacologic management. In M. B. Glenn and J. Whyte, eds., *The Practical Management of Spasticity in Children and Adults*. Philadelphia: Lea & Febiger, pp. 201–26.

33. Pinder, R. M., Brogden, R. N., Speight, T. M. and Avery, G. S. (1977). Dantrolene sodium: a review of its pharmacological properties and therapeutic efficacy in spasticity. *Drugs*, **13**, 3–23.

34. Pinder, R. M., Brogden, R. N., Speight, T. M. and Avery, G. S. (1977). Dantrolene sodium: a review of its pharmacological properties and therapeutic efficacy in spasticity. *Drugs*, **13**, 3–23.

35. Chyatte, S. B., Birdsong, J. H. and Bergman, B. A. (1971). The effects of dantrolene sodium on spasticity and motor performance in hemiplegia. *Southern Medical Journal*, **64**(2), 180–5.

36. Ketel, W. B. and Kolb, M. E. (1984). Long-term treatment with dantrolene sodium of stroke patients with spasticity limiting the return of function. *Current Medical Research and Opinion*, **9**(3), 161–8.

37. Katrak, P. H., Cole, A. M. D., Poulos, C. J. and McCauley, J. C. K. (1992). Objective assessment of spasticity, strength, and function with early exhibition of dantrolene sodium after cerebrovascular accident: a randomized double-blind controlled study. *Archives of Physical Medicine and Rehabilitation*, **73**, 4–8.

38. Weiser, R., Terenty, T., Hudgson, P. *et al.* (1978). Dantrolene sodium in the treatment of spasticity in chronic spinal cord disease. *Practitioner*, **221**, 123−7.

39. Gelenberg, A. J. and Poskanzer, D. C. (1973). The effect of dantrolene sodium on spasticity in multiple sclerosis. *Neurology*, **23**, 1313−15.

40. Tolosa, E. S., Soll, R. W. and Loewenson. (1975). Treatment of spasticity in multiple sclerosis with dantrolene. *Journal of American Medical Association*, **233**(10), 1046.

41. Utili, R., Boitnott, J. K. and Zimmerman, H. J. (1979). Dantrolene-associated hepatic injury: incidence and character. *Gastroenterology*, **72**, 610−16.

42. Wilkinson, S. P., Portmann, B. and Williams, R. (1979). Hepatitis from dantrolene sodium. *Gut*, **20**, 33−6.

43. Miller, D. H. and Haas, L. F. (1984). Pneumonitis, pleural effusion and pericarditis following treatment with dantrolene. *Journal of Neurology, Neurosurgery and Psychiatry*, **47**(5), 553−4.

44. Smith, C., Birnbaum, G., Carter, J. L. *et al.* (1994). Tizanidine treatment of spasticity caused by multiple sclerosis: results of a double-blind, placebo-controlled trial. *Neurology*, **44**(Suppl. 9), S34−S43.

45. Nance, P. W., Bugaresti, J., Shellengerger, K. *et al.* (1994). Efficacy and safety of tizanidine in the treatment of spasticity in patients with spinal cord injury. *Neurology*, **44**(Suppl. 9), S44−S52.

46. The United Kingdom Tizanidine Trial Group. (1994). A double-blind, placebo-controlled trial of tizanidine in the treatment of spasticity caused by multiple sclerosis. *Neurology*, **44**(Suppl. 9), S70−S78.

47. Hassan, N. and McLellan, D. L. (1980). Double-blind comparison of single doses of DS103−282, baclofen, and placebo for suppression of spasticity. *Journal of Neurology, Neurosurgery and Psychiatry*, **43**, 1132−6.

48. Smolenski, C., Muff, S. and Smolenski-Kautz, S. (1981). A double-blind comparative trial of a new muscle relaxant, tizanidine and baclofen in the treatment of chronic spasticity in multiple sclerosis. *Current Medical Research and Opinion*, **7**, 374−83.

49. Newman, P. M., Nogues, M., Newman, P. K. *et al.* (1982). Tizanidine in the treatment of spasticity. *European Journal of Clinical Pharmacology*, **23**, 31−5.

50. Stein, R., Nordal, H. J., Oftedal, S. I. and Slettebo, M. (1987). The treatment of spasticity in multiple sclerosis: a double-blind clinical trial of a new anti-spasticity drug tizanidine compared with baclofen. *Acta Neurologica Scandinavia*, **75**, 190−4.

51. Bes, A., Eyssette, M., Pierrot-Deseilligny, E. *et al.* (1988). A multi-centre, double-blind trial of tizanidine, a new antispastic agent, in spasticity associated with hemiplegia. *Current Medical Research and Opinion*, **10**, 709−18.

52. Wagstaff, A. J. and Bryson, H. M. (1997). Tizanidine: a review of its pharmacology, clinical efficacy and tolerability in the management of spasticity associated with cerebral and spinal disorders. *Drugs*, **53**(3), 435−52.

53. Wallace, J. D. (1994). Summary of combined clinical analysis of controlled clinical trial with tizanidine. *Neurology*, **44** (Suppl. 9), S60−8.

54. De Graaf, E. M., Oosterveld, M. and Tjabbes, T. (1996). A case of tizanidine-induced hepatic injury. *Journal of Hepatology*, **25**, 772−3.

55. Davidoff, R. A. (1985). Antispasticity drugs: mechanisms of action. *Annals of Neurology*, **17**, 107−16.

56. Ketelaer, C. J. and Ketelaer, P. (1971). The use of Lioresal in the treatment of muscular hypertonia due to multiple sclerosis: spasticity: a topical survey. In Birkmayer, ed., *An International Symposium, Vienna*. Vienna: Huber, pp. 128−31.

57. Cendrowski, W. and Sobczyk, W. (1977). Clonazepam, baclofen and placebo in the treatment of spasticity. *European Journal of Neurology*, **16**, 257−62.

58. Killestein, J., Uitdehaag, B. M. and Polman, C. H. (2004). Cannabinoids in multiple sclerosis: do they have a therapeutic role? *Drugs*, **64**(1), 1−11.

59. Zajicek, J., Fox, P., Sanders, H., Wright, D., Vickery, J., Nunn, A. and Thompson, A. (2003). UK MS Research Group. Cannabinoids for treatment of spasticity and other symptoms related to multiple sclerosis (CAMS study): multi-centre randomized placebo-controlled trial. *Lancet*, **362**(9395), 1517−26.

60. Penn, R. D., Paice, J. A., Gottschalk, W. and Ivankovich, A. D. (1984). Cancer pain relief using chronic morphine infusion; early experience with a programmable drug pump. *Journal of Neurosurgery*, **61**(2), 302−6.

61. Penn, R. D. and Kroin, J. S. (1985). Continuous intrathecal baclofen for severe spasticity. *Lancet*, **ii**(8447), 125−7.

62. Rominjn, J. A., van Lieshout, J. J. and Velis, D. N. (1986). Reversible coma due to intrathecal baclofen. *Lancet*, **i**(8508), 696.

63. Penn, R. D. and Kroin, J. S. (1987). Long-term intrathecal baclofen infusion for treatment of spasticity. *Journal of Neurosurgery*, **66**(2), 181−5.

64. Campbell, W. M., Ferrel, A., McLaughlin, J. F., Grant, G. A., Loeser, J. D., Graubert, C. and Bjornson, K. (2002). Long-term safety and efficacy of continuous intrathecal baclofen. *Developmental Medicine and Child Neurology*, **44**(10), 660−5.

65. Levin, A. B. and Serling, K. B. (1995). Complications associated with infusion pumps implanted for spasticity. *Stereotactic and Functional Neurosurgery*, **65**(1−4), 147−51.

66. Baker, M. D. (2000). Selective block of late Na (+) current by local anaesthetics in rat large sensory neurons. *British Journal of Pharmacology*, **129**(8), 1617−20.

67. Nathan, P. W. (1959). Intrathecal phenol to relieve spasticity in paraplegia. *Lancet*, **ii**, 1099−102.

68. Kelly, R. E. and Gautier-Smith, P. C. (1959). Intrathecal phenol in the treatment of reflex spasms and spasticity. *Lancet*, **ii**, 1102−5.

69. Nathan, P. W., Sears, T. A. and Smith, M. C. (1965). Effects of phenol solution on the nerve roots of the cat: an electrophysiological and histological study. *Journal of Neurological Science*, **2**, 7−28.

70. Burkel, W. E. and McPhee, M. (1970). Effect of phenol injection on peripheral nerve of rat: electron microscope studies. *Archives of Physical Medicine and Rehabilitation*, **51**, 391−7.

71. Khalili, A. A., Harmel, M. H., Forster, S. and Benton, J. G. (1964). Management of spasticity by selective peripheral nerve block with dilute phenol solutions in clinical rehabilitation. *Archives of Physical Medicine and Rehabilitation*, **45**, 513−18.

72. Okazaki, A. (1993). The effects of 2 per cent and 5 per cent aqueous phenol on the cat tibial nerve in situ. *Masui*, **42**(6), 819−25.

73. Halpern, D. (1977). Histological studies in animals after intramuscular neurolysis with phenol. *Archives of Physical Medicine and Rehabilitation*, **58**, 448–53.

74. Kirazli, Y., On, A. Y., Kismali, B. and Aksit, R. (1998). Comparison of phenol block and botulinum toxin type A in the treatment of spastic foot after stroke: a randomized double-blind trial. *American Journal of Physical and Rehabilitation Medicine*, **77**(6), 510–15.

75. Bodine-Fowler, S. C., Allsing, S. and Botte, M. J. (1996). Time course of muscle atrophy and recovery following a phenol-induced nerve block. *Muscle and Nerve*, **19**(4), 497–504.

76. Glenn, M. B. (1990). Nerve blocks. In M. B. Glenn and Whyte, eds., *The Practical Management of Spasticity in Children and Adults*. Philadelphia: Lea & Febiger, pp. 227–58.

77. Macek, C. (1983). Venous thrombosis resulting from phenol injections *Journal of the American Medical Association*, **249**(14), 1807.

78. Gracies, J. M. (2004). Physiological effects of botulinum toxin in spasticity. *Movement Disorders*, **19**(Suppl. 8), S120–8.

79. Brin, M. F. (1997). Dosing, administration, and a treatment algorithm for use of botulinum toxin A for adult-onset spasticity. Spasticity Study Group. *Muscle and Nerve*, **20**(Suppl. 6), S208–20.

80. Borodic, G. E., Ferrante, R., Pearce, L. B. and Smith, K. (1994). Histologic assessment of dose related diffusion and muscle fibre response after therapeutic botulinum A toxin injections. *Movement Disorders*, **9**, 31–8.

81. Finsterer, J., Fuchs, I. and Mamoli, B. (1997). Automatic-guided botulinum toxin treatment of spasticity. *Clinical Neuropharmacology*, **3**, 195–203.

82. Childers, M. K., Stacy, D. O. M., Cooke, D. L. and Stonnington, H. H. (1996). Comparison of two injection techniques in spastic hemiplegia. *American Journal of Physical Medicine and Rehabilitation*, **75**, 462–8.

83. Edwards, S. (1996). In eds., *Neurological Physiotherapy: a Problem Solving Approach*. London: Churchill Livingstone, pp. 45–7.

84. Pandyan, A. D., Johnson, G. R., Price, C. I. M., Curless, R. H., Barnes, M. P. and Rodgers, H. (1999). A review of the properties and limitations of the Ashworth and modified Ashworth scales as measures of spasticity. *Clinical Rehabilitation*, **13**, 373–83.

85. Tardieu, G., Shentoub, S. and Delarue, R. (1954). A la recherche d'une technique de mesure de la spasticité. *Revue Neurologique*, **91**, 143–4.

86. Wartenburg, R. (1951). Pendulousness of the legs as a diagnostic test. *Neurology*, **1**, 18–24.

87. Johnson, G. R. (2001). Measurement of spasticity In M. P. Barnes and G. R. Johnson, eds., *Upper Motor Neuron Syndrome and Spasticity: Clinical Management and Neurophysiology*. Cambridge: Cambridge University Press, pp. 79–95.

88. Ashworth, B. (1964). Preliminary trial of carisprodal in multiple sclerosis. *Practitioner*, **192**, 540–2.

89. Sloan, R. L., Sinclair, E., Thompson, J., Taylor, S. and Pentland, B. (1992). Inter-rater reliability of the modified Ashworth scale for spasticity in hemiplegic patients. *International Journal of Rehabilitation Research*, **15**, 158–61.

90. Lee, K., Carson, L., Kinnin, E. and Patterson, V. (1989). The Ashworth scale: a reliable and reproducible method of measuring spasticity. *Journal of Neurological Rehabilitation*, **3**, 205–8.

91. O'Dwyer, N. J., Ada, L. and Neilson, P. D. (1996). Spasticity and muscle contracture following stroke. *Brain*, **119**, 1737—48.

92. Bohannon, R. W. and Smith, M. B. (1987). Inter-rater reliability of a modified Ashworth scale of muscle spasticity. *Physical Therapy*, **67**, 206—27.

93. Pomerory, V., Dean, D., Sykes, L., Faragher, E. B., Yates, M., Tyrrell, P., Moss, S. and Tallis, R. (2000). The unreliability of clinical measures of muscle tone: implications for stroke therapy. *Age and Ageing*, **29**(3), 229—33.

94. Gregson, J. M., Leathley, M. J., Moore, A. P., Smith, T. L., Sharma, A. K. and Watkins, C. L. (2000). Reliability of measurements of muscle tone and muscle power in stroke patients. *Age and Ageing*, **29**(3), 223—8.

95. Lamontagne, A., Malouin, F., Richards, C. L. and Dumas, F. (1998). Evaluation of reflex and non-reflex induced muscle resistance to stretch in adults with spinal cord injury using hand-held and isokinetic dynamometry. *Physical Therapy*, **78**, 964—77.

96. Held, J. P. and Pierrot-Deseilligny, E. (1969). *Rééducation motrice des affections neurologiques*. Paris: J B Bailière et Fils, pp. 31—42.

97. Boyd, R. N. and Graham, H. K. (1999). Objective measurement of clinical findings in the use of botulinum toxin type A in the management of spasticity in children with cerebral palsy. *European Journal of Neurology*, **6**(4), S23—S36.

98. Gracies, J. M. (2001). Evaluation de la spasticité. *Apport de l'echelle de Tardieu. Motricité Cérébrale*, **22**, 1—16.

99. Rymer, W. Z. and Katz, R. T. (1994). Mechanism of spastic hypertonia. *Physical Medicine and Rehabilitation*, **8**, 441—54.

100. Katz, R. T., Rovai, G. P., Brait, C. and Rymer, W. Z. (1994). Objective quantification of spastic hypertonia: correlation with clinical findings. *Archives of Physical Medicine and Rehabilitation Medicine*, **73**(4), 339—47.

101. Simpson, D. M., Alexander, D. N., O'Brien, C. F., Tagliati, M., Aswad, A. S., Leon, J. M., Gibson, J., Mordaunt, J. M. and Monaghan, E. P. (1996). Botulinum toxin type A in the treatment of upper extremity spasticity; a randomised, double-blind, placebo-controlled trial. *Neurology*, **46**, 1306—10.

102. Bakheit, A. M. O., Thilmann, A. F., Ward, A. B. et al. (2000). A randomised, double-blind, dose ranging study to compare the efficacy and safety of three doses of botulinum toxin type A (Dysport) in the treatment of upper limb spasticity after stroke. *Stroke*, **31**(10), 2402—6.

103. Bhakta, B. B., Cozens, A. A., Chamberlain, M. and Bamford, J. M. (2000). Impact of botulinum toxin type A on disability and carer burden due to arm spasticity after stroke: a randomised, double-blind, placebo-controlled trial. *Journal of Neurology, Neurosurgery and Psychiatry*, **69**, 217—28.

104. Smith, S. J., Ellis, E., White, S. and Moore, P. (2000). *Clinical Rehabilitation*, **14**, 5—13.

105. Brashear, A., Gordon, M. F., Elovic, E., Kassicieh, V. D., Marciniak, C., Do, M., Lee, C. H., Jenkins, S. and Turkel, C., Botox Post-Stroke Spasticity Study Group (2002). Intramuscular injection of botulinum toxin for the treatment of wrist and finger spasticity after a stroke. *New England Journal of Medicine*, **347**(6), 395—400.

106. Brashear, A., Zafonte, R., Corcoran, M., Galvez-Jimenez, N., Gracies, J. M., Gordon, M. F., McAfee, A., Ruffing, K., Thompson, B., Williams, M., Lee, C. H. and Turkel, C. (2002). Inter- and intra-rater reliability of the Ashworth Scale and the Disability Assessment Scale in patients with upper-limb post-stroke spasticity. *Archives of Physical Medicine and Rehabilitation*, **83**(10), 1349−54.

107. Wade, D. T. (1992). *Measurement in Neurological Rehabilitation*, Oxford: Oxford University Press.

108. Lyle, R. C. (1981). A performance test for assessment of upper limb function in physical rehabilitation treatment and research. *Int. J. Rehabil. Res.*, **4**, 483−92.

109. Pandyan, A. D., Vuadens, P., van Wijck, F. M., Stark, S., Johnson, G. R. and Barnes, M. P. (2002). Are we underestimating the clinical efficacy of botulinum toxin (type A)? Quantifying changes in spasticity, strength and upper limb function after injections of Botox® to the elbow flexors in a unilateral stroke population. *Clinical Rehabilitation*, **16**(6), 654−60.

110. Ward, A. B. (1999). Use of botulinum toxin type A in spastic diplegia resulting from cerebral palsy. *European Journal of Neurology*, **6**(Suppl. 4), S46−S48.

111. Simpson, D. (2002). Clinical trials of botulinum toxin in the treatment of spasticity. In *Spasticity: Etiology, Evaluation, Management and the Role of Botulinum Toxin*. New York: We Move, pp. 125−30.

112. Turner-Stokes, L. and Ward, A. B. (2002). The management of adult spasticity using botulinum toxin type A − a guide to clinical practice. *Clinical Medicine*, **2**(2), 128−30.

113. Moore, A. P. (2002). Botulinum toxin A (BoNT-A) for spasticity in adults. What is the evidence? *European Journal of Neurology*, **9**(Suppl. 1), 42−7.

114. Sheean, G. L. (2001). Botulinum treatment of spasticity: why is it so difficult to show a functional benefit? *Current Opinion in Neurology*, **14**(6), 771−6.

115. Shakespeare, D. T., Young, C. A. and Boggild, M. (2000). Anti-spasticity agents for multiple sclerosis. *Cochrane Database of Systematic Reviews*, **4**, CD001332.

116. Reiter, F., Danni, M., Lagalla, G., Ceravalo, G. and Provinciali, L. (1998). Low dose botulinum toxin with ankle taping for the treatment of spastic equinovarus foot after stroke. *Archives of Physical Medicine and Rehabilitation*, **79**, 532−5.

117. Burbaud, P., Wiart, L., Dubos, J. L., Gaujard, E., Debelleix, X., Joseph, P. A., Mazaux, J. M., Bioulac, B., Barat, M. and Lagueny, A. (1996). A randomised double-blind placebo-controlled trial of botulinum toxin in the treatment of spastic foot in hemiparetic patients. *Journal of Neurology, Neurosurgery and Psychiatry*, **61**, 265−8.

118. Simpson, D. *et al.* Placebo-controlled double-blind trial of BOTOX® (botulinum toxin type A) versus Zanaflex® (tizanidine) for the treatment of upper limb spasticity. Personal communication.

119. Hyman, N., Barnes, M., Bhakta, B., Cozens, A., Bakheit, M., Kreczy-Kleedorfer, B., Poewe, W., Wissel, J., Bain, P., Glickman, S., Sayer, A., Richardson, A. and Dott, C. (2000). Botulinum toxin (Dysport) treatment of hip adductor spasticity in multiple sclerosis: a prospective, randomised, double blind, placebo controlled, dose ranging study. *Journal of Neurology, Neurosurgery and Psychiatry*, **68**(6), 707−12.

Appendix 8.1.

Muscle	Origin	Insertion	Action	**BOTOX® Dose Dysport®	Injection point
TRUNK MUSCLES					
Psoas major	Transverse process and vertebral bodies of T12–L5	Lesser femoral trochanter	Flexes hip	150–200 600–800	Approach posteriorly advancing needle under U/S guidance
Iliacus	Ilium – floor of iliac fossa	Joins psoas muscle to insert into lesser femoral trochanter	Flexes hip		Anterior approach under lateral third of inguinal ligament.
Quadratus lumborum	Ilio-lumbar ligament and iliac crest	12th rib and L1–L5 tranverse processes	Laterally flexes trunk	100 400	Posterior approach lateral to vertebral column
LOWER LIMB THIGH ABDUCTORS					
Gluteus maximus	Posterior aspect ilium, sacrum, coccyx, sacrotuberous ligament	Greater trochanter	Extends thigh and laterally rotates hip	150 600	Four points in buttock under U/S guidance
Gluteus medius	Large area of sacrum below iliac crest	Posterior superior angle of greater trochanter	Abducts and internally rotates leg	100 400	Two points in buttock under U/S guidance
Gluteus minimus	Ilium between anterior and inferior gluteal lines	Lower lateral part greater trochanter	Abducts leg	Rarely injected	
THIGH–KNEE EXTENSORS					
Rectus femoris	Anterior inferior iliac spine (straight head), ilium (reflected head)	Tibial tubercle via quadriceps and atella ligaments	Flexes hip and extends knee	100–150 400–600	Four points along middle of muscle mass

Appendix 8.1. (*Cont.*)

Muscle	Origin	Insertion	Action	**BOTOX®** Dose *Dysport®*	Injection point
Vastus lateralis, intermedius and medialis	Large area of sacrum below iliac crest	Tibial tubercle via quadriceps and patellar ligaments	Knee extension	100–150 400–600	Two points in lateral thigh, one deep centrally in lower half thigh and one to two medially
THIGH ADDUCTORS AND KNEE FLEXORS					
Pectineus	Superior pubic ramus	Posterior aspect of femur below lesser trochanter	Adducts thigh and assists hip flexion	50–100 200–400	Difficult to inject because of overlying neuromuscular bundle below inguinal ligament medial to femoral vein
Adductor magnus	Ischial tuberosity	Posterior two-thirds of femur down to adductor tubercle on medial femoral condyle	Adducts and laterally rotates thigh. Main action while sitting	100–200 400–750	Large muscle in upper medial thigh. Inject into upper half of thigh
Adductor longus	Body of pubis below pubic crest and symphysis	Posterior aspect of middle of femur into linea alba	Adducts thigh. Main action on standing	Into whole	Anteromedial aspect of thigh one hand's breadth below inguinal ligament medial to femoral vein
Adductor brevis	Below pubic crest in superior pubic ramus	Upper femur posteriorly between lesser trochanter and linea aspera	Adducts and laterally rotates thigh	Adductor group	Behind adductor longus and pectineus and in front of adductor magnus
Gracilis	Inferior pubic ramus			80–120	Posteromedial edge of thigh. Four point down thigh

Muscle	Origin	Insertion	Action	Dose	Location
	Ischial tuberosity	Pes anserinus on posterior aspect of medial tibial condyle	Adducts thigh and flexes knee. Medially rotates fixed leg	300–400	Four points in medial posterior thigh
Semi-membranosus	Ischial tuberosity	Pes anserinus on posterior aspect of medial tibial condyle	Flexes knee. Medially rotates flexed leg and extends hip	100–150 / *400–600* Inject	Four points in posterior thigh
Semi-tendinosus	Common origin with biceps femoris	Pes anserinus on posterior aspect of medial tibial condyle	Same as semimembranosus	With semi-membranosus	Four points in lateral muscle in posterior thigh
Biceps femoris	Long head: Ischial tuberosity Short head: Linea aspera on back of femur	Head of fibula	Flexes knee, externally rotates leg and extends hip	100–150 / *400–600*	Deep over back of medial tibial condyle in popliteal fossa.
Popliteus	Popliteal groove on lateral epicondyle anteriorly	Pierces joint capsule to posterior aspect of upper medial tibia	Flexes knee, internally rotates lower leg in early flexion	30 / *120*	

LOWER LEG – ANTERO-LATERAL COMPARTMENT

Muscle	Origin	Insertion	Action	Dose	Location
Tibialis anterior	Upper half of lateral surface of tibia and interposseous membrane	Medial cuneiform bone	Dorsiflexes and inverts foot	75–120 / *300–500*	Front of shin, lateral to tibia
Extensor digitorum longus	Upper three-fourths of anterior surface of fibula	Bases of 2nd–5th middle and terminal phalanges	Dorsiflexes toes and foot	50–80 / *200–300*	Lateral to tibialis anterior in front of fibula
Extensor hallucis longus	Anterior surface of middle two-thirds of fibula and interosseous membrane	Base of distal phalanx of great toe	Extends great toe	50–60 / *200–250*	Between tibialis anterior and extensor digitorum longus in middle of shin
Peroneus longus	Upper two-thirds of lateral surface of tibia	Under base of 5th metatarsal and groove in cuboid to	Everts and plantarflexes foot	50–80 / *200–300*	Lateral aspect of shin anterior to fibula

Appendix 8.1. (*Cont.*)

Muscle	Origin	Insertion	Action	**BOTOX® Dose	*Dysport®*	Injection point
		medial cuneiform and to base of 1st MT				
Peroneus brevis	Lower two-thirds of fibular shaft	Base of 5th metatarsal	Everts foot	30–40	*120–160*	Lower half of lateral shin anterior to peroneus longus
LOWER LEG – POSTERIOR COMPARTMENT						
Gastrocnemius – medial head	Back of femoral condyle	Via Achilles tendon (AT) to calcaneum	Plantarflexes foot and flexes knee	75–100	*300–400*	Superficial muscle of medial aspect of calf
Gastrocnemius – lateral head	Back of femoral condyle	Via AT to calcaneum	Plantarflexes foot and flexes knee	75–100	*300–400*	Superficial muscle of lateral of calf
Soleus	Posterior surface of shaft of fibula and medial border of tibia	Via AT to calcaneum	Plantarflexes foot	100–150	*400–600*	4 points of back of calf deep to gastrocnemius
Flexor hallucis longus	Posterior surface of fibula	Through groove in posterior talus to terminal phalanx great toe	Flexes great toe (IP and MTP joints) – maintains longitudinal arch	50	*200*	Approach behind medial border of tibia, ½–⅔ way down shin. Extend needle through tibialis posterior
Flexor digitorum longus	Posterior surface of tibia	Terminal phalanges of 2nd–5th toes	Flexes toes 2–5 (IP and MTP joints) – maintains longitudinal arch	50	*200*	Approach behind medial border of tibia, ½–⅔ way down shin. Most medial muscle
Tibialis posterior	Interosseous membrane and adjoining surfaces of tibia and fibula	Tuberosity of navicular bone	Plantarflexes foot and inverts foot	50–80 U	*200–320 U*	Approach behind medial border of tibia, ½–⅔ way down shin.

Muscle	Origin	Insertion	Action	Dose (U)	Notes
Abductor hallucis	Medial aspect of calcaneum and flexor retinaculum	Medial aspect base of great toe proximal phalanx	Abducts and plantarflexes great toe	10–20 U 40–80 U	Medial aspect 1st metatarsal
Flexor hallucis brevis	Cuboid bone and flexor retinaculum	Two bellies inserted into each side of the base of the 1st proximal phalanx	Flexes 1st MTP joint	10–20 U 40–80 U	Plantar aspect of foot under 1st metatarsal
Flexor digitorum brevis	Medial aspect of calcaneum and septal fascia	Middle phalanges of toes 2–5	Flexes 1st IP joint and lateral four MTP joints	10–20 40–80 U	Plantar aspect of foot at base of metatarsals
PECTORAL GIRDLE					
Trapezius	Occiput down median line to last thoracic vertebra	Lateral third of clavicle, acromion and scapular spine	Scapular elevation and rotation	50–75 200–300	Large muscle between neck and shoulder
Rhomboid	Spinous processes C7–T5	Medial border of scapula	Scapular extension	50–60 200–250	Superficial between scapula and spine
Supraspinatus	Supraspinatus fossa	Greater tubercle of humerus	Abducts arm ≤15° and ≥90°	40–60 160–240	Supraspinous fossa on scapula
Infraspinatus	Posterior aspect of scapula below scapular spine	Greater tubercle of humerus	External rotation of arm	50–75 200–300	Infraspinous surface of scapula
Subscapularis	Posterior aspect of scapula	Lesser tubercle of humerus	Internal rotation of arm	60–80 240–320	Lateral border of scapula at spinous process and medial border at spine origin
Deltoid	Scapular spine, acromion and clavicle	Deltoid tuberosity of humerus	Fibres: Posterior – Arm extension Middle – Arm abduction Anterior – Arm flexion	50–100 200–400	Inject anterior, middle and posterior fibres as necessary

Appendix 8.1. (Cont.)

Muscle	Origin	Insertion	Action	**BOTOX® Dose** Dysport®	Injection point
Teres major	Dorsum of scapula at inferior angle	Crest of lesser humeral tuberosity	Adducts, internally rotates and extends arm	40–60 160–240	Lateral aspect of lower scapula
Teres minor	Upper half of lateral border scapula	Posterior aspect of greater tuberosity of humerus	Adducts and laterally rotates arm	30–40 120–160	Lateral aspect of upper scapula
Latissimus dorsi	Tips of lower six thoracic spines, thoracolumbar fascia and iliac crest	Floor of intertubercular groove of humerus	Adducts, retracts and internally rotates arm	80 320	Find in posterior axillary fold, while patient pulls down elevated arm
Serratus anterior	Upper eight ribs in three parts	Medial border scapula	Protracts arm limb	60–75 240–300	Lateral aspect of upper eight ribs
Pectoralis major	Clavicle and 3rd–8th anterior ribs	Greater tubercle of humerus	Adducts and internally rotates arm	100 400	Anterior axillary fold and between clavicle and arm for clavicular head
Pectoralis minor	3rd, 4th and 5th ribs at costochondral cartilages	Coracoid process	Draws scapula down and forwards depressing shoulder	40 160	Deep to upper part of pectoralis major
ARM					
Coracobrachialis	Coracoid process	Middle medial border humerus	Flexes and adducts arm	50 200	Medial to upper humerus between it and neurovascular bundle
Triceps brachii	Scapula and posterior humerus	Olecranon	Elbow extension and shoulder retraction	75–125 300–500	Three heads in posterior upper arm

Muscle	Origin	Insertion	Action		Location
Biceps brachii	Heads: Short: Coracoid process; Long: Supra-glenoid tubercle scapula	Bicipital aponeurosis	Supination and elbow flexion	75–125 / 300–500	Two points in each head in a line just under half way up muscle
Brachialis	Anterior aspect lower humerus	Coranoid process on ulna	Flexes elbow and assists in forearm pronation	80 / 320	Lower anterior humerus medial and lateral to bicipital tendon

EXTENSOR ASPECT OF FOREARM

Muscle	Origin	Insertion	Action		Location
Brachioradialis	Lateral supracondylar ridge of humerus	Lateral surface distal radius	Elbow flexion	60 / 180	Radial side upper forearm
Supinator	Radial notch of ulnar	Shaft of proximal radius	Supinates forearm	40–50 / 120–200	Deep in extensor aspect of forearm below radial neck
Extensor carpi radialis longus	Distal third of lateral supracondylar ridge of humerus	Base of 2nd metacarpal (MC)	Extends and abducts hand at the wrist	40–50 / 120–200	Posterior to brachioradialis in forearm
Extensor carpi radialis brevis	Common extensor origin (lateral humeral epicondyle)	Base of 3rd MC	Extends and abducts hand at the wrist	40–50 / 120–200	Posterior and medial to ECR longus
Extensor carpi ulnaris	Common extensor origin	Base of 5th MC	Extends wrist and elbow and adducts hand	40–50 / 120–200	Half way down most medial muscle of extensor compartment
Extensor digitorum communis	Common extensor origin	Bases of middle and distal phalanges	Extends wrist and fingers	40–50 / 120–200	Middle of back of forearm distal to radial tuberosity
Extensor digiti minimi	Common extensor origin	Bases of middle and distal phalanges of 5th finger	Extends 5th finger	40–50 / 120–200	Medial to extensor digitorum communis
Extensor pollicis longus	Posterior surface middle third ulna	Base of distal phalanx of thumb	Extends all joints of thumb	20–30 / 75–120	Midway down back of forearm

Appendix 8.1. (Cont.)

Muscle	Origin	Insertion	Action	**BOTOX® Dose** *Dysport®*	Injection point
Extensor pollicis brevis	Posterior surface radius and interosseous membrane	Base of proximal phalanx of thumb	Extends CMC and MCP joint of thumb	20–30 *60–120*	Distal third of forearm. Palpate by moving CMC and MCP joints
Abductor pollicis longus	Back of interosseous membrane and radius and ulna	Base of 1st MC	Abducts thumb and hand	20–30 *80–120*	Proximal to extensor pollicis brevis on back of forearm
Extensor indicis	Back of distal ulna and interosseous membrane	Extensor expansion of dorsum of 2nd phalanx	Extends forefinger	20–30 *80–120*	Medial to lateral aspect of extensor digitorum communis
FLEXOR ASPECT OF FOREARM					
Pronator teres	Heads: Humeral – Medial humeralepicondyle (MHE) Ulnar – Medial border ulnarcoronoid	Middle of lateral surface of radius	Pronates forearm and flexes elbow	40–60 *160–240*	Medial border anterior cubital fossa medial to brachial artery
Flexor carpi radialis	Medial humeral epicondyle	Base of 2nd MC	Flexes wrist and elbow	40–50 *120–200*	Upper forearm just below bicipital aponeurosis and medial to pronator teres
Flexor carpi ulnaris	Heads: Humeral: MHE Ulnar: Olecranon and upper-posterior border ulna	Pisiform bone in wrist	Flexes and adducts hand at wrist	40–50 *120–200*	Upper half of medial forearm
Flexor digitorum superficialis	Heads: Ulnar: MHE Ulnar: Olecranon and upper-posterior border ulna	Middle phalanges medial four fingers	Flexes PIP and MCP joints in fingers	40–50 *120–200*	Middle of forearm either side of palmaris tendon

Flexor digitorum profundus	Proximal two-thirds ulna	Distal phalanges of fingers	Flexes all finger joints	40–50	120–200	Medial approach through flexor carpi ulnaris
Flexor pollicis longus	Lateral border of upper two-thirds anterior radius	Distal phalanx of thumb	Flexes all thumb joints	20–30	75–120	Mid-forearm over anterior aspect of radius
Pronator quadratus	Anterior aspect distal ulna	Front of distal radius	Pronates forearm	20–30	75–120	Approach from extensor aspect proximal wrist and advance needle through interosseous membrane
HAND						
Abductor pollicis brevis	Lateral part of flexor retinaculum and scaphoid	Lateral side of base of 1st proximal phalanx	Abducts at 1st CMC joint drawing thumb anteriorly	10	40	Medial to APB
Flexor pollicis brevis	Lateral part of flexor retinaculum and trapezium	Lateral side of base of 1st proximal phalanx	Flexes thumb at 1st MCP joint	10	40	Medial to APB
Opponens pollicis	Lateral part of flexor retinaculum and trapezium	Lateral half of palmar aspect of 1st metacarpal and rotates medially at 1st CMC joint	Pulls thumb into centre of palm and rotates at CMC joint (opposition)	10	40	Medial to FPB and deep to it and to APB
Adductor pollicis	Heads: Oblique: Bases of 2nd and 3rd MCs and adjacent carpal bones Transverse: Front of 3rd MC	Medial side of base of proximal phalanx of thumb	Draws thumb posteriorly towards palm and acts as MCP joint in fully opposed thumb	10	40	Middle of forearm either side of palmaris tendon
Lumbricals	Radial side of four flexor digitorum profundus tendons in palm	Dorsum of terminal phalanges 2–5	Flexes fingers at MCP joint	10 × 4	40 × 4	Dorsal approach between fingers. Pierce inter-osseous membrane and locate muscle close to MCs

U/S = Ultrasound

Appendix 8.2.

SPASTICITY TREATMENT SHEET - INITIAL

| DATE OF ASSESSMENT..................... | Doctor: .... | Sheet No. [ ] |

NAME: .... Date of Birth: .... Age: ....   Hospital No. ....

DIAGNOSIS: .... Date of Onset: ....

Main Deficits: Physical ☐ Cognitive ☐ Communicative ☐
Physical Deficit: Right Hemiplegia/paresis   ☐   Left Hemiplegia/paresis   ☐
                        Paraplegia/paresis   ☐   Tetraplegia/paresis ☐   Diplegia ☐

Residual Active Function: Yes ☐   No ☐   Referrer: ....

Current & Previous Spasticity Treatment

Physical Therapy   Continuing Yes ☐ No ☐   *Activity*: Stretching ☐ Strengthening ☐ Pain Relief ☐
                        Last Treatment
                        F.E.S ☐
                        Splinting/Casting ☐

Oral Drugs ☐ (Baclofen ☐   Tizanidine ☐   Dantrolene ☐ Gabapentin ☐ Benzodiazepines ☐   Other ☐)

Botulinum Toxin ☐   U/Limb ☐ L/Limb ☐ Trunk ☐   Date: .... Documentation Yes ☐ No ☐

Phenol Nerve Block ☐   Nerve ....   Date(s) ....

Intrathecal Phenol ☐   Date(s) ....

Intrathecal Baclofen ☐   Date of Pump Insertion Placed (s) .... Refill Date ......
                           Dose.......µg/day. Continuous ☐ Phasic ☐

Surgery ☐   Date(s) .... Operation ....

Reason for Referral: ....

Patient's Aims: ....

Carer'(s) Aims: ....

Problem: Spasticity ☐ Spasms ☐ Dystonia ☐ Other ☐
                    Description ....
                              ....

                    Where

            ....

                    Contracture Yes ☐ No ☐ Fixed ☐ Dynamic ☐ Where ....

SPASTICITY TREATMENT SHEET – REVIEW

| DATE OF ASSESSMENT .... | Sheet No. ☐ |

NAME:......................... Date of Birth: .... Hospital No. ....

Current Spasticity Treatment

Physical Therapy   Continuing Yes ☐ No ☐   *Activity*: Stretching ☐ Strengthening ☐ Pain Relief ☐
   Last Treatment
   F.E.S ☐   Splinting/Casting ☐ Date ....

Oral Drugs   Baclofen ☐   Tizanidine ☐   Dantrolene ☐   Gabapentin ☐   Benzodiazepines ☐   Other ☐
   Dose: ....

Chemodenervation   (Document Sheet No....)
   Botulinum Toxin ☐   U/Limb ☐ L/Limb ☐ Trunk ☐   Date: ....
   Phenol Nerve Block ☐   Nerve ....   Date(s) ....

Intrathecal   Phenol ☐   Date(s)...........................
   Baclofen ☐   Date of Pump Insertion Placed (s) .... Refill Date ....
                   Dose ....μg/day.   Continuous ☐ Phasic ☐

Surgery ☐   Date(s) .... Operation ....

TREATMENT OUTCOME-Primary ☐   Secondary ☐

Measure	Score	Measure	Score
Patient Satisfaction	VAS ... cm	Measure 2	
Measure 1		Measure 3	

Likert/ Global Score	Much Worse	Worse	Same	Better	Much Better
Patient					
Carer					
Physician					

FURTHER TREATMENT REQUIRED   Yes ☐   NOT AT PRESENT ☐   *REASON*
                ....

Patient's Aims: ....

Problem: Spasticity ☐   Spasms ☐   Dystonia ☐   Other ☐
      Where ....

....

....
             Contracture Yes ☐ No ☐ Fixed ☐ Dynamic ☐ Where ....

Aim of Treatment (Mark Primary Aim with **)

Domain	Function	Goal	1°/2°	Measure	Score
Functional Gain	Mobility Dexterity	....		10M Walk Time Stride Length 9HPT Other	
Symptom Control	Pain Hygiene Orthotic Wear Other	....		10cm VAS Angle of R.o.M Other	
Posture/ Positioning		....		Pt Satisfaction VAS	
Carer Relief	Dressing Hygiene Other	....		Hygiene Score NWPCS Other	
Service Issues	Therapy Benefit Complication Rx Surgery	State:			
Global	Physician Rating Patient Satisfaction	....		Global Rating Score 10cm VAS	

TREATMENT

PT   □   Start Date .... Activity ....
Splinting   □   Date: .... Description of Splint ....
F.E.S.   □   Date: Site: ....
Medication   □ ....
ITB □ (Refer to ITB Assessment)   Surgery □ (Referral to Surgeon Yes □)

Botulinum Toxin Treatment–Date: .... **BOTOX**® □ **Dysport**® □ **Neurobloc**™ □

SIDE & MUSCLE	Dose	Dilution	No of Sites	SIDE & MUSCLE	Dose	Dilution	No. Sites Injected

Phenol Aqueous Soln 6% □, Glycerine 5% □   Date: .... Doctor: ....

Side	Site	Dose

DATE OF REVIEW: ....

Hyperhidrosis

DeeAnna Glaser[1] and Stephanie Benson[2]

[1]Department of Dermatology, Saint Louis University School of Medicine, St Louis, MO, USA
[2]University of Colorado, School of Medicine, Denver

9.1 Introduction

Sweating is a normal physiological response to increasing body temperature and is an important mechanism in releasing heat produced from endogenous and exogenous sources. The heat regulatory center is located in the brain within the hypothalamus, particularly involving the pre-optic and anterior nuclei. These sections of the brain monitor core body temperature through the blood stream, and the body's response to increasing temperature is to release heat through sweat.

Sweating is controlled by the sympathetic nervous system through its preganglionic and postganglionic pathways. Nerve fibers exit the pre-optic or anterior nuclei and descend ipsilaterally through the spinal cord until they reach the intermediolateral column, where they leave the cord and enter the sympathetic chain. The postganglionic fibers leave the chain and join the peripheral nerves until they reach the sweat gland[1]. The neurotransmitter for the sympathetic nervous system is generally norepinephrine; however, the neurotransmitter mainly involved in the sweating process is acetylcholine. Other chemical mediators found in the neuromuscular junction during sweating include vasoactive intestinal peptide, atrial natriuretic peptide, galanin, and calcitonin gene related peptide[2].

Three glands are important in the creation of sweat: the eccrine, apo-eccrine, and apocrine glands. They are located superiorly in the subcutaneous fat at the junction of the dermis and subcutaneous fat. Between two and four million eccrine glands are found within the skin, and their function is to secrete water while conserving sodium chloride for electrolyte maintenance. The eccrine gland consists of a secretory coil and a duct. The secretory coil has a layer of serous and mucous cells which produce the precursor of sweat[1,3]. It also contains a cholinergic responsive myoepithelial cell that provides support for the coil and assists in the secretion of water and sodium chloride into the duct. The basal cell

Clinical Uses of Botulinum Toxins, eds. Anthony B. Ward and Michael P. Barnes. Published by Cambridge University Press. © Cambridge University Press 2007.

within the duct is responsible for the majority of sodium chloride reabsorption thereby producing a hypotonic solution on the skin. Although the eccrine sweat glands continually produce secretions, they are further stimulated by heat, exercise, anxiety, or stress[3,4]. Up to 10 liter of sweat can be produced in a day under severe heat stress, but the normal rate is 0.5–1.0 ml / min[1,5]. The sweating rate within individuals depends on the local concentration of acetylcholine and the number of active sweat glands in the area[1]. Males sweat more than females, and it is thought that males either have more active glands or their response is greater to autonomic or endocrine stimuli[6].

The apo-eccrine gland was discovered in a patient with axillary hyperhidrosis and is known to develop in puberty from eccrine-like precursor glands. It is larger than the eccrine gland, has a long duct, and opens directly onto the skin. It responds to acetylcholine and produces a clear fluid secretion; it may secrete up to ten times more fluid than the eccrine gland. Its function is unknown, but patients with hyperhidrosis tend to have more of these glands than those without the condition[1].

Apocrine sweat glands open into the hair follicle, are concentrated in the axillae and perineum, and become functional around puberty. The glands have three layers of cells that are rich in protein and deficient in lipid. They lack myoepithelial cells in the duct. The glands respond to adrenergic stimuli, epinephrine more than norepinephrine, and their pulsatile secretions produce an odor when combined with bacteria on the skin. They do not function in thermoregulation but are thought to function as chemical attractants, signals, or markers[1,3,7].

9.2 Hyperhidrosis

Dysfunction of sweating may occur within any portion of the system. Problems may occur in the hypothalamic nuclei, with pre- and post-ganglionic fibers, with secretion of the neurotransmitter, or secretion by the sweat gland or the sweat duct[2]. Hyperhidrosis is the condition of excessive sweating beyond that required to maintain physiologic homeostasis. The amount of sweating necessary to be considered excessive is not clearly defined, is variable between individuals, and has not been standardized.

Hyperhidrosis may be generalized or focal, bilateral and symmetric or unilateral, primary or secondary in origin. Generalized hyperhidrosis affects the entire body while focal hyperhidrosis occurs in discrete sections of the skin. Generalized hyperhidrosis is usually secondary in nature and the differential diagnosis is extensive (Table 9.1). Infections such as tuberculosis or malaria, and myeloproliferative disorders such as leukemia and lymphoma can result in significant sweating. The use of medications has also been implicated and drugs

Table 9.1. Forms of hyperhidrosis. Hyperhidrosis can be primary or secondary, generalized or focal[5,8,9]

Generalized	Focal/Regional
Fever	Primary focal hyperhidrosis
Infections	Intrathoracic tumors
Malignancy and tumors	Atrioventricular fistula
Thyrotoxicosis	Rheumatoid arthritis
Pheochromocytoma	Spinal cord disease or injury
Hypoglycemia	Stroke
Diabetes mellitus	Syringomelia
Diabetes insipidus	Ross syndrome
Hypopituitarism	Localized unilateral hyperhidrosis[a]
Prinzmetal angina	Gustatory sweating/Frey's syndrome
Endocarditis	Cold-induced hyperhidrosis
Gout	Eccrine nevus
Medications	
Menopause	
Anxiety	
Drug withdrawl	

[a]Also referred to as unilateral circumscribed idiopathic hyperhidrosis.

include propranolol, physostigmine, tricyclic antidepressants, opioids, serotonin reuptake inhibitors, naproxen, acyclovir, gluoxetine, and venlafaxine[2,5,8,9].

Focal or localized hyperhidrosis may result from a secondary process, such as tumors or lesions of the central or peripheral nervous system (Table 9.1). Very rare causes include eccrine nevus, pachyonychia congenita, and nail–patella syndrome (POEMS). Ross' Syndrome, caused by the deterioration of the sympathetic system, produces classic symptoms of anhidrosis, tonic pupils, hyporeflexia, and localized hyperhidrosis of the trunk[2,9–11].

This chapter will focus on idiopathic hyperhidrosis. Primary localized hyperhidrosis, most commonly referred to simply as 'hyperhidrosis,' is characterized by excessive sweating of small regions of the skin, such as the axilla, palms, soles, or face. The onset is usually in adolescence (usually under 25 years of age), although it can begin early in childhood, especially the palmar-plantar variants[9]. The disease manifests as bilateral and relatively symmetric sweating, often with cessation during sleep (Table 9.2). The differential diagnosis for hyperhidrosis is large and secondary causes must be considered, especially when the hyperhidrosis is generalized, asymmetrically distributed or has a late onset[9,12]. A detailed history and examination is the first step with careful detail to the review of symptoms.

Table 9.2. Diagonis of primary focal hyperhidrosis

Criteria for establishing the diagnosis of primary focal hyperhidrosis
Focal, visible excessive sweating of at least 6 months duration
No apparent secondary cause
At least two of the following characteristics
• Bilateral and relatively symmetric
• Impairs daily activities
• Frequency of at least one episode per week
• Age of onset less than 25 years
• Positive family history
• Cessation of focal sweating during sleep

The type and extent of further testing is based on the findings from the history and physical examination.

The incidence of hyperhidrosis was thought to be 0.6−1 per cent, but recent studies found that hyperhidrosis is common with a prevalence of 2.8 per cent[13]. It most commonly presents within the second or third decades, and the prevalence is similar in men and women. A family history is discovered in up to 30−50 per cent of family members[16]. Although many patients sweat on a continuous basis throughout the day, most report that they suffer from the sudden onset of profuse sweating. There can be trigger factors such as emotional stress; stress at work or in the public; higher environmental temperatures; or stimulants such as caffeine; it can also occur without any explanation when patients are cool, comfortable, and calm[15]. Less than half of those afflicted seek care and guidance from physicians with only 38 per cent discussing their condition with a health care provider[13].

Hyperhidrosis has a negative impact on many aspects of patients' daily living − physically, psychologically, and occupationally. Skin that is continuously exposed to moisture can become irritated and macerated, allowing for secondary infections but this plays no role in making the diagnosis of primary hyperhidrosis, nor is it necessary for treatment initiation[14].

The greatest impact of hyperhidrosis is the significant reduction in the quality of life and the alterations it has on daily functioning. Many patients lack confidence, feel depressed, and refrain from meeting new people. Others avoid intimate activities. Often people with hyperhidrosis will not maintain public service positions due to embarrassment and the frequent need to change clothing. Many will not shake hands with others because of the excessive amount of sweat on their hands. Some work from home so their peers do not see their disorder. Patients report limitation at work due to their symptoms and some will spend more than

60 min daily to treat their disease[16]. Using the Dermatology Life Quality Index (DLQI) as a measure of disease burden, patients with hyperhidrosis rate 8.8–18 as compared to patients with psoriasis who average 4.51–13.9 on the DLQI scale[13,17–22].

9.3 Measuring hyperhidrosis

The Minor starch iodine test is a simple way to detect the presence of sweat. After the area to be studied is dried thoroughly, iodine solution is painted over the affected area, and a starch powder such as corn starch is applied. With the interaction of sweat, the area turns a purple–black color (decolorized iodine solutions do not perform the colorimetric change properly and should not be used). While the Minor iodine starch test is useful in the clinic to localize areas of sweat production, it is not a quantitative test. For iodine-sensitive patients, Alizarin or Ponceau red dye and starch can be used. The pink powder turns to a bright red color when wet[23,24]. The Ninhydrin sweat test is another variant that can be used[25], but regardless of which test is performed, they all achieve a colorimetric outline of the sweating area.

Gravimetric assessment identifies the amount of sweat produced during a given time. The technique involves applying pre-weighed filter paper to the affected area (typically 5 min) and then measuring the production of sweat by reweighing the filter paper. Evaporation must be prevented from occurring[26]. There is no standard or validated quantity that separates hyperhidrosis from euhidrosis, although it can exceed 30 times that of normal non-hyperhidrotic individuals. Hund suggests a minimum of 100 mg/5 min for men and 50 mg/5 min for women to identify axillary hyperhidrosis. A study of 60 patients demonstrated that the mean axillary sweat production was 346 mg/5 min for men and 186 mg/5 min for women (healthy control subjects had values of 72 and 46 respectively[6]). Likewise the mean palmar gravimetric measurement was approximately 300 mg/5 min[27].

A third method used to measure disease severity is the use of quality of life scales and questionnaires. Several tools are available, but two of the more commonly used scales are the DLQI and the HyperHidrosis Impact Questionnaire (HHIQ), which help to quantify the impact, burden and disease severity[22]. A newer tool, the hyperhidrosis disease severity scale (HDSS) is based on one question that the patient can answer in the office (Table 9.3). Moderate to strong correlations with the HHIQ, DLQI, and gravimetric sweat production make this a valuable and simple tool to use in the clinical setting. The HDSS is responsive to treatment with a one-point HDSS improvement being associated with approximately

Table 9.3. Hyperhidrosis disease severity scale

'Which best describes the impact of sweating on
your daily activity?'

1	Never noticeable, never interferes
2	Tolerable, sometimes interferes
3	Barely tolerable, frequently interferes
4	Intolerable, always interferes

a 50 per cent reduction in sweat production. This validated scale can aid in selecting patients appropriate for therapy and for assessing effectiveness of the treatment[28].

9.4 Therapy

Many treatments are available for hyperhidrosis, but none are effective in everyone. Therapy should be tailored to the needs of the individual based on factors such as age and health status of the patient, location of disease, occupation and lifestyle.

Antiperspirants are used as first line medical treatment and are thought to function by decreasing eccrine sweat secretion through blockage of the distal secretory ducts[20]. Over-the-counter (OTC) antiperspirants contain 1–2 per cent salt concentrations and do not routinely provide relief from true hyperhidrosis. Prescription strength antiperspirants containing increasing salt concentrations up to 20–30 per cent can be more effective than OTC products. Aluminum salts are typically used, particularly aluminum chloride solutions, like Drysol® and Xerac®[18]. The higher salt concentrations improve the efficacy of the antiperspirant and the likelihood of side effects. The antiperspirant should be applied to the affected area, which has been completely dried. Nightly application is recommended since decreased sweating occurs at night. Continuous use is required as the beneficial effect is sustained for a limited time[20,29]. Some patients will find relief with this treatment but most will not due to lack of efficacy or intolerability. Common side effects of high strength antiperspirants are skin irritation, erythema, dryness, pruritus, and even fissures[9,18].

Systemic anticholinergic drugs such as glycopyrronium bromide, glycopyrrolate, atropine, or oxybutynin provide the patient with a generalized acetylcholine blockade[30]. Their use can result in many adverse effects, and patients frequently experience dry eyes, dry mouth, and urinary retention at the doses required to achieve euhidrosis. Few patients are able to tolerate the systemic treatments well or are willing to live with these effects and the drugs have very limited clinical usefulness. However, this class of therapy is most applicable for patients with hyperhidrosis affecting several areas of the body.

Iontophoresis is the second line treatment for palmar and plantar hyperhidrosis. The procedure is easily performed on the hands and feet but is technically challenging and impractical for the axilla, face and other areas of the body. The hands or feet are placed in a tap water solution, charged with an electrical current. It is thought that either the electrical current changes the ability of the pores to secrete sweat or ions enter the pores and physically block the secretion of sweat[18,31,32]. Initially, iontophoresis requires treatment every 48 hours but, once euhidrosis is achieved, therapy can be tapered to 1–2 treatments per week to maintain clinical benefit. Treatments will take approximately 20 min to treat the hands or feet and 40 min to treat all four extremities. Side effects are relatively minimal but include mild discomfort during the treatment, and erythema and vesicle formation[32]. Sometimes anticholinergic medications are placed into the solution for added benefit, but systemic anticholinergic side effects may then be seen.

En bloc excision of the axillary vault is rarely performed today due to the resulting scarring, contractures, and decreased range of motion[18]. Liposuction and curettage can be used alone or in combination to treat axillary hyperhidrosis. The eccrine units are suctioned or scraped away, although ensuing fibrosis may also play a role. The surgery is 'blinded' and the outcome is technique dependent[33,34]. Side effects include bruising, pain, and tenderness and only partial reduction in sweating.

Endoscopic thoracic sympathectomy (ETS) offers a more permanent answer but is not universally accepted. The sympathetic chain is interrupted using cautery, excision or clipping the T2, T3, and sometimes the T4 ganglion. This provides immediate anhidrosis and the success rate for palmar disease is 95 per cent. The recurrence rate is approximately 6.6 per cent, although the percentage of relapse increases with time[19,35]. The benefit is much less when treating axillary hyperhidrosis with up to 65 per cent of these patients experiencing a recurrence of their hyperhidrosis[35]. ETS is not performed for plantar hyperhidrosis due to the increased likelihood of inducing sexual dysfunction with a lumbar sympathectomy[9].

The major issue surrounding ETS is the potential for patients to develop compensatory sweating, especially of the trunk, abdomen, back and thighs. It can develop within 6 months after surgery and the occurrence or severity is unpredictable. Many patients report that this adverse effect is actually worse and more devastating than the original symptoms[36]. The incidence varies depending on series but approximately 60–70 per cent of patients seem to develop compensatory hyperhidrosis after ETS[35,37,38]. Other complications of ETS include Horner's Syndrome, gustatory sweating, ptosis, pneumothorax, hemothorax, excessive dryness, and those related to any surgical procedure[19,39].

9.5   Botulinum toxin

Since excessive sweating is mediated by acetylcholine and botulinum toxin modulates the release of acetylcholine, it is the logical choice to alter the amount of sweat secreted by the body's sweat glands. The chemodenervation with botulinum toxin is localized, reversible, and can be long-lasting. Botulinum toxin A (BoNT-A) has been most extensively studied and used clinically for the treatment of hyperhidrosis, but there are a few publications related to the use of botulinum toxin B (BoNT-B) as well. Previous chapters have reviewed these toxins in detail.

The basic principle for using botulinum toxins to treat excessive sweating is to first identify the area involved with a test such as the Minor's Starch Iodine test. Since the sweat glands are located at the junction of the dermis and subcutaneous tissue, botulinum toxin is most effective when placed there in a deep intradermal injection. It is important to avoid injecting deeper structures such as muscle to prevent unwanted affects on the underlying muscles and for optimal interaction at the neuro-eccrine interface. The injections are generally placed 1–2 cm apart to allow for diffusion of the toxin to the entire area. This technique decreases the total number of injections needed while maximizing coverage of the drug and preventing 'skipped' areas. Although the technique is similar to treat all areas of the body, the more commonly treated sites will be covered in more detail.

9.6   Axillary hyperhidrosis

Perhaps no area has been as extensively studied as the axilla. Numerous studies have shown the beneficial effect of BoNT-A, including large multicenter randomized, placebo-controlled trials in Europe and the USA[20,26,40–45]. Naumann et al. reported on 320 patients entering the European double-blind, randomized study evaluating BOTOX® in the treatment of axillary hyperhidrosis[40]. Either 50 U of BoNT-A or placebo were injected into each axilla. Three hundred and seven patients completed the study. At 4 weeks, 94 per cent of the BoNT-A group had responded compared with 36 per cent of the placebo group (measured as ≥50 per cent reduction from baseline of spontaneous sweat production). By 16 weeks the response rates were 82 per cent and 21 per cent respectively. Long-term data collected over 16 months in an extension study confirmed that repeated injections of BoNT-A produced similar outcomes with significant reductions in the mean sweat production. The mean duration between

BoNT-A treatments was approximately 7 months[44]. Patient satisfaction after treatment was consistently high and their quality of life improved.

Similar results were recorded in a large phase III multicenter, double-blind, placebo-controlled North American trial of 322 patients. In this study, subjects were randomized to receive either 50 U BoNT-A, 75 U BoNT-A or placebo in each axilla. The hyperhidrosis disease severity scale was the primary efficacy measure with gravimetric measurements being secondary[41]. Success was seen in 75 per cent of patients in both treatment groups compared with 25 per cent in the placebo group (defined as ≥ 2 point reduction in HDSS), while 80–85 per cent of the treated patients had >75 per cent reduction in their baseline sweat production. Patients requiring more than one treatment in the 12-month period had similar results with their repeated injections. Like the European trial, the durability of the treatment with BoNT-A was excellent with the median duration in the treatment groups being approximately 7 months. Treatment satisfaction was very high (85%) and there were no significant differences in any of the parameters between the two treatment groups.

The efficacy of Dysport® has been shown in a multicenter trial of 145 patients[26]. One axilla was treated with 200 U and placebo was used for the contra-lateral axilla. After two weeks, the placebo arm was revealed and those axillae received 100 U BoNT-A. Axillary sweating decreased immediately in all axillae, and the result was maintained for 6 months. Of the patients involved, 98 per cent said they would recommend this therapy for others.

Although studies have consistently shown that 50 U of BOTOX® per axilla provides safe and durable results over an average of 7 months, there is some debate whether higher doses of BoNT-A can provide prolonged duration. One small open-label study utilizing 200 U BoNT-A in each axilla of 47 patients achieved improvement for 29 months in one patient and 19 months for 22 patients. The first relapse in this series occurred at 7 months. Likewise, 250 U of Dysport® in each axilla resulted in prolonged benefit in a small study of 12 patients. Seven remained symptom-free for 12 months, and 9 months for three patients[29]. Currently, the standard dose in the USA and that listed in the package insert for BOTOX® is 50 U per axilla, which achieves excellent results, high patient satisfaction, and helps to keep costs at a minimum.

To optimize treatment, the area of axillary involvement should be identified so that the BoNT-A can be concentrated into the affected region. A starch iodine test is easy to perform using simple povidine–iodine swabs. The key is to thoroughly dry the region before beginning the procedure. The axilla does not need to be shaved prior to performing a starch iodine test or injecting BoNT-A. The BoNT-A is injected into the deep dermis at the dermal-subcutaneous level and is placed 1.5–2 cm apart. Because of the thin skin in the axilla, a wheal may be seen with each injection. An average of 10–15 injections is required but may vary depending on the size of the hyperhidrotic area[46]. Pain is minimal and the procedure is very well tolerated. In the event that a starch iodine test cannot be performed, or is equivocal, the physician should treat the hair-bearing skin in the manner described above. Should symptoms not be alleviated within two weeks, the patient can return to the office and a starch iodine test may help to locate any active areas. Patients should be retreated when the sweating returns at a level of concern for the patient or when the HDSS score is 3 or 4. Some clinicians have patients use a topical therapy twice a week when the sweating starts to return to extend the time interval between injections and help to keep costs down[47]. Side effects noted in the studies include painful injection, hematoma, headache, muscle soreness, increased facial sweating, some compensatory sweating, and axillary pruritus[4,26,40,42–44,48].

9.7 Palmar hyperhidrosis

Botulinum toxin injections are useful in the treatment of palmar hyperhidrosis. No large-scale studies have been published but multiple small studies have demonstrated its ability to establish anhidrosis and clinical improvement in patients' symptoms (Table 9.4). There are several challenges with palmar BoNT-A treatment, including that of optimal dosing, control of pain during injection and potential side effects, especially muscle weakness.

The optimal dose is not known and the issue is complicated by large variations in hand size. Published data is present on doses as low as 50 U per hand[49] and as high as 200 U[50]. Some authors have suggested using a defined dose per injection with Swartling's group using 0.8 U cm^{-2} and Naumann's group using 2 U injected every 1.5 cm on the palm but three injections per fingertip pad and two injections

Table 9.4. Anesthesia techniques used for palmar injections

Topical anesthesia

Nerve blocks	
Intravenous regional anesthesia (Bier's block)	
Cryoanalgesia	Dichlorotetrafluoroethane
	CryAc liquid nitrogen
	Cold packs or ice bath
	Machine-assisted cold air
General anesthesia or sedation anesthesia	
Vibration	

into each of the middle and proximal phalanx using 1–2 U per injection[51]. It is unclear whether or not larger doses add to the duration of symptom relief or increase the risk of muscle weakness. When Wollina used 200 U per hand in 10 patients, his relapse time varied from 3 to 22 months[50]. Saadia studied 24 patients; 11 received 50 U BoNT-A per hand and 13 received 100 U per hand. There was higher patient satisfaction reported in the high-dose group, but he found no difference in the duration (measured as a percentage of the palm area sweating) between the two doses. There were more patients with hand and finger weakness in the high-dose treatment group[49]. Until larger studies help to address this issue, a good starting point is 75–100 U BOTOX® per hand with adjustments being made as needed based on the size of the hand and past responses.

Another challenge with palmar therapy is the shorter duration of response when compared with axillary or facial injections. Responses range from 3–12 months. The reason is unknown but may be related to a smaller diffusion radius in thicker palm skin and compartmentalized areas of the phalanges, the higher number of cholinergic nerve endings or a differential recovery rate between the nerves of the palm and those in the axilla. Backflow of the drug upon injection may also play a role[52].

Injection of the hand can be painful due to the density of nerve receptors and the large numbers of injections that are required. Pain during injection of the palms is much greater with patients reporting an average pain of 68.1 ± 31.8 for palms vs. 29.9 ± 24.5 for axillary treatment (visual analogue scale 1–100)[21]. Several methods of pain control have been tried (Table 9.5), although a few patients will not require any anesthesia. Topical anesthetics and ice packs do not tend to provide adequate control[53,54]. The use of more intensive cold exposure can be used; submersion of the hand in an ice bath, the use of dichlorotetrafluoroethane or liquid nitrogen and machines to emit chilled air may have benefit[55,56]. The use of a dermojet to inject BoNT-A was found to be less painful than standard needle injections, but was much less effective in controlling the hyperhidrosis and not recommended as a useful tool to treat palms[57].

Nerve blocks are one of the more common methods of anesthesia used for injecting the palms and, since special equipment is not required, they can be performed in the office[51,54,58]. The palm is innervated by three nerves that can be anesthetized at the level of the wrist. The median nerve is blocked by injecting between the palmaris longus and flexor carpi radialis tendons at the proximal crease of the volar wrist. The ulnar nerve is located beneath the flexor carpi ulnaris tendon. The needle should be inserted on the radial side of the tendon toward the ulnar styloid process. The superficial branch of the radial nerve can be blocked by injecting in the 'anatomic snuff box' or at the base of the thumb. The landmarks

Table 9.5. Studies of botulinum toxins in palmar hyperhidrosis

Author	Year	Design/Controls	No.	Preparation BoNT-A and dose/hand	Weakness
Naver[90]	1999	One palm treated Other palm, no Rx	94	BoNT 0.8 U cm^{-2} (mean 170 U)	66% lasting 2 days–2 months
Vadoud-Seyedi[63]	2001	Both palms treated	23	BoNT 50 U	0%
Saadia[49]	2001	High dose vs. low dose	24	BoNT 100 U $N=13$ BoNT 50 U $N=11$	77% high dose 45% low dose
Wollina[50]	2001	Both palms treated	10	BoNT 200 U	0%
Glaser[62]	2001	Three groups: different dilution, injection pattern	43	BoNT 60 U all groups	23% mean <3 weeks
Solomon[91]	2002	Both palms treated	20	BoNT 165 U	21% ≤ 6 weeks
Lowe[27]	2002	One palm treated Other palm placebo	19	BoNT 100 U	5% lasted <2 weeks
Schnider[25]	1997	One palm treated Other palm, placebo	11	Dys 120 U	27% lasting 2–5 weeks
Schnider	2001	Both palms treated	21	Dys 230 U	43% lasting 4–8 weeks
Moreau[92]	2003	One palm BoNT Other palm Dys	8	BoNT mean 69 U Dys mean 283 U	25% BoNT (15–21 days) 50% Dys (8–30 days)

are accentuated by having the patient gently flex the wrist and approximating the thumb and index finger. The use of a short, beveled, small-gauge needle such as a 30-gauge, is important to minimize trauma to the underlying nerves and vessels[58]. If the patient feels pain during a nerve block, it must be assumed that the needle has entered the nerve, and should be withdrawn several millimeters. The author prefers to use 1 per cent lidocaine without epinephrine and inject $2-4\,cm^3$ of solution around each nerve. Risks of a nerve block include infiltration of the nerve with subsequent neural injury and vascular puncture.

Intravenous regional anesthesia (IVRA), also known as a Bier's block is effective[53]. An anesthetic such as prilocaine is injected intravenously following the application of a tourniquet cuff on the forearm. First ex-sanguination of the extremity is achieved with an Esmarch bandage and then an electronic double cuff is used. Complete anesthesia can be obtained in 20 min using 40–60 ml of 0.5 per cent prilocaine for most patients. The total tourniquet time for IVRA ranges from 50–80 min and is well tolerated. Due to the risk of toxic cardiovascular and central nervous system reactions, blood pressure and electrocardiograms are monitored during the IVRA and for about 30 min after the procedure[59].

A growing number of physicians are using vibratory anesthesia for palmar injections. The theory is that the nervous system is unable to perceive fully two different types of sensory inputs simultaneously[60]. A hand-held vibrator is applied to the volar and dorsal surface of the hand near the site of BoNT-A injection. This requires an assistant and there is some 'movement' of the patients' hand with the vibration. One vibrator can be used on the volar aspect but does not diminish the pain as much as the use of two (personal experience). Neither technique results in a pain-free injection, but rather a diminishment of perceived pain. A study by Sherer found that pain threshold is significantly higher during vibration compared to pre- or post-vibration, and that vibration applied distal to the site of pain provided better analgesia than vibration applied proximal to the site of pain[61].

Weakness of both the hand and fingers is possible, but is usually minor and of limited duration. The incidence varies upon the series but ranges from 0–77 per cent of patients. The most common area of weakness is the thenar eminence and can be measured in the thumb-index pinch whereas gross strength or grip strength is not affected[49,62]. Rarely, patients report numbness, tingling, or decreased dexterity. Injections of BoNT-A should be administered in the dermal layer, especially over the thenar eminence to limit the chance that the toxin will come in contact with the muscle layer. Subepidermal injections may however, increase the incidence of hematoma[63].

In an attempt to prevent muscle weakness, Zaiac advocates the use of the ADG needle, a device designed for the injection of collagen[64]. He found that the average depth of the eccrine glands in 10 consecutive palmar biopsies was 2.6 mm. By adjusting the needle to a length of 2.6 mm, and using a total of 60–70 U BoNT-A per palm, he had no weakness in 10 consecutive patients[64]. Likewise, Almeida uses an adapter to shorten her 7 mm 30-guage needle to measure 2.5–3.0 mm for palmar injections[54,65].

9.8   Plantar hyperhidrosis

Very little has been published on botulinum toxin treatment for plantar hyperhidrosis. Like the palms, there is no consensus on the optimal dose; the injections are painful, and the duration of response is variable. Naumann used 42 and 48 U of BOTOX® to treat two soles by injecting 3 U (0.15 ml) into each 2 × 2 cm squares[66]. Blaheta's group used 100 U per sole (100 U/5 ml sterile saline) in a study of eight patients with severe plantar hyperhidrosis[67].

A starch iodine test will delineate the hyperhidrotic area, which can extend up the sides and even the dorsum of the foot. BoNT-A should be evenly distributed every 1–2 cm using a small gauge needle and injecting into the deep dermis at the level of the dermal–adipose junction. Technically injections of the plantar surface can be more challenging due to the thickness of the stratum corneum in some areas, especially if calloused. The physician will have to adjust for the variations in depth to accurately place BoNT-A into the appropriate cutaneous level.

The need for pain control has to be addressed similar to palmar injections. IVRA can provide sufficient anesthesia of the sole and has been reported to be effective when administering BoNT-A to the foot. In a small series of eight patients, IVRA was found to be more effective than a peripheral nerve block in reducing the pain of BoNT-A injections[67].

Adequate plantar anesthesia can also be obtained with nerve blocks, generally performed at the level of the ankle. The tibial nerve is blocked by injecting at the level of the medial malleolus posterior to the posterior tibial artery (between the Achilles tendon and the medial malleolus). A second injection is performed at the lateral ankle between the Achilles tendon and the superior border of the lateral malleolus to provide blockade of the sural nerve[52]. Rarely, the dorsum of the foot may need to be treated for some patients and the superficial peroneal nerve can be blocked. A dose of 3–5 ml 1 per cent lidocaine without epinephrine is injected at each site.

Vadoud-Seyedi reported on the role of the Dermojet in plantar hyperhidrosis, treating 10 patients with 50 U BoNT-A in 5 ml saline per foot. Fifteen to twenty sites were injected per foot and no analgesia was utilized. The injections were tolerated well by all patients. One developed a localized hematoma but no weakness or other complications were noted. The duration of benefit lasted 3–6 months, although 20 per cent of patients reported that the treatment had no effect on their condition. The starch iodine test revealed absence of plantar sweating in both of these patients for approximately 3 months[68].

9.9 Facial hyperhidrosis

Facial hyperhidrosis has two distinct clinical pictures. The first presents as excessive sweating of the forehead with or without involvement of the scalp. Some patients with craniofacial hyperhidrosis also have excessive sweating of the nose, chin, cheeks or upper lip. Gustatory sweating or Frey's syndrome is a common complication after surgery or injury in the region of the parotid gland. It most likely stems from aberrant regeneration of the secreto-motor para-sympathetic neurons that normally innervate the parotid and salivary glands[69]. Gustatory sweating can also occur in diabetics with nephropathy or neuropathy[70]. All respond to BoNT-A, with gustatory sweating responding for very long periods of time.

There is a paucity of literature published on craniofacial hyperhidrosis. Kinkelin et al. injected a mean of 86 U of BOTOX® (3 units per injection site) over the forehead at equidistant locations (1–1.5 cm) in 10 men with frontal hyper-hidrosis[71]. To prevent drooping of the eyelids, the injections were kept 1 cm above the eyebrow and injections were performed intracutaneously. Five patients had partial disability in frowning of the forehead, limited to a maximum of 8 weeks. There were no cases of ptosis. Satisfaction was excellent or good in 90 per cent of the subjects. This effect was maintained for 5 months in nine patients[71]. Tan and Solish report that symptoms return in an average of 4½ months after treatment of the forehead[21].

Böger treated 12 men suffering from bilateral craniofacial hyperhidrosis with Dysport injections of 0.1 ng per injection[72]. Half of the forehead was treated using a total of 2.5–4 ng injected equidistantly over one-half. A total of 25–40 injections were administered intradermally to the treatment area. At 4 weeks the patients were re-evaluated and the other side of the face was injected in the same fashion. Decreased sweating was seen within 1 to 7 days after injection and lasted a minimum of 3 months. One patient experienced anhidrosis for 27 months. Side effects were limited to temporary weakness of the frontalis muscle (100%), with 17 per cent experiencing slight brow asymmetry that lasted 1–12 months. There was no relationship between the dose and the strength of the side effect. One patient did not respond initially to 3 ng but had a partial response upon re-treatment with a higher dose.

Table 9.6. The use of BoNT-A in the treatment of gustatory sweating (Frey's syndrome)

Author	Year	Drug and Dose	N	Duration	Side effects
Naumann[93]	1997	BoNT 1–2 U/2.25 cm^2 Mean 21 U	45	>6 months	Small hematomata 11%
Bjerkhoel[94]	1997	BoNT 17.5–62.5 U Mean 37 U	15	>13 months	Mimic muscle corner of mouth 6%
Laskawi[75]	1998	BoNT 2.5 U/4 cm Average 31 U	19	17.3 months mean	None
Laccourrege[76]	1998	BoNT 2.5 U/2 cm 25–88 U	14	>3–9 months	Weakness upper lip 14%
Eckardt[95]	2003	BoNT 16–80 U	33	>12 months	None
Kyrmizakis[69]	2004	BoNT 2.5 U/3–4 cm^2 15–52 U	11	>16–23 months	None
Guntinas-Lichius[73]	2002	Dysport® 148 U mean ($N=20$) 248 U mean ($N=20$)	40	8 months 16 months	None
Beerens[96]	2002	Dys 67.5–150 U Mean 100 U	13	3–24 months	Paresis at corner of mouth 15%

BoNT = BOTOX®; Dys = Dysport®.

The treatment of Frey's syndrome requires small doses of BoNT-A and provides long lasting relief. It is crucial that the affected area be mapped out and the sweating may need to be stimulated by having the patient eat something; sour candy can be very useful. Typical doses used are 1–2 U injected every 2 cm (Table 9.6). Therapy is well-tolerated although some patients will have weakness of the mimic muscles when injections are placed too close to the corner of the mouth.

Treatment of gustatory sweating complicating diabetes with BoNT-A provides symptomatic relief up to 6 months. Restivo used Dysport® 5 U/2.25 cm^2 (mean of 8.3 injections per patient) in 14 patients with diabetes related gustatory sweating. No adverse effects were noted except an occasional cutaneous hematoma at the site of injection[70].

It is unclear why the duration of benefit is so long when treating gustatory sweating. There is some evidence that higher doses of BoNT-A may provide longer durations of symptom relief[73], but even with relatively small doses, the duration of effect is outstanding and can be longer than 3 years[74]. The varying lengths of time seen may be related to different susceptibilities of sweat glands or the specific etiology of the condition[14,69]. Laskawi describes three potential mechanisms[75]:

1. the sweat gland function may be partially or completely abolished in the long time during which they were denervated;

2. once chemically denervated, autonomic nerve fibers are regenerated feebly or not at all;

3. post-surgical and post-traumatic changes locally in the tissue may compromise the regeneration of axon terminals.

There is one report of a patient with Frey's syndrome that developed clinical resistance to Dysport®. Her first treatment in 1999 with 620 U Dysport® lasted only 4 months and a frontalis muscle test to the drug was negative. 13 500 U BoNT-B was injected with recurrence of symptoms at 9 months[76]. Also, there is a report of a patient with torticollis that was immunoresistant to BoNT-A after 2 years. This Frey's syndrome patient was successfully treated with BoNT-F, although the benefit lasted only 3½ months[24].

9.10   Other indications

Inguinal hyperhidrosis affects 2−10 per cent of individuals with primary hyperhidrosis. It usually develops in adolescence and may be associated with excessive sweating of other body sites. It can be debilitating for patients. Intradermal injections of BoNT-A can control the symptoms for 6 months or more[77]. Before treatment can begin, the affected area must be identified with a starch iodine test. BoNT-A is injected in a typical fashion, using 2−3 U BOTOX® every 1−2 cm. The total recommended dose is 100 U but 60−80 U may be used for less severe cases.

Compensatory hyperhidrosis is the most common complication of endoscopic transthoracic sympathectomy, ranging from 44 per cent to 91 per cent of patients reported to develop the problem following surgery. Its development is unpredictable, irreversible, and can be even more severe than the original hyperhidrosis. Treatment has been particularly difficult but two reports note success treating compensatory hyperhidrosis with BoNT-A. Huh used 300 U Dysport® to treat the chest and abdomen area after localizing the disease with a starch iodine test. He diluted each 100 U with 10 cm^3 of saline and injected 0.1 ml into each square centimeter. The effects gradually reduced but remained for 8 months[78]. Belin and Polo treated a patient with severe compensatory hyperhidrosis of the upper abdomen with good results in the treated areas[36]. Unfortunately this man's compensatory sweating was from the nipple line down to his knees and the entire area was not treated due to the extensive surface area.

Chromhidrosis is a rare disorder characterized by the excretion of colored or pigmented sweat. It is most commonly confined to the face or axilla but has been noted on the chest, abdomen, thighs, and groin areas. The colored sweat may be black, blue, green, or yellow. Several etiologies have been implicated. In true eccrine chromhidrosis water soluble pigments are thought to be excreted by the eccrine glands. In pseudo-eccrine chromhidrosis, compounds on the skin surface mix with normally colorless eccrine sweat. Suspected chromogens include dyes, colored chemicals or microorganisms such as *Corynebacterium*. Apocrine chromhidrosis results from lipofuscin granules.

This disorder has been successfully treated with BoNT-A. Matarosso used 15 U of BOTOX® into the affected area of each cheek which measured 3 cm in diameter for a total of 30 U. He injected 3 U of toxin intradermally at 1 cm intervals. Within 48 hours his patient had a marked reduction in the amount of discharged black sweat[79].

Botulinum toxin can be used to treat almost any localized or focal area of hyperhidrosis. Several case reports describe success with various rare forms of hyperhidrosis[11,80]. The key is to follow the basic principles of localizing the area affected, injecting in the correct dermal plane and avoiding the underlying musculature. The dosing will need to be adjusted based on the surface area. A good starting point is to use 2–3 U of BOTOX® every 1–2 cm. Repeating the starch iodine test 2–3 weeks after treatment can help to localize untreated areas that may require additional injections.

9.11 Botulinum toxin type B

Botulinum toxin type B use has been primarily limited to the treatment of cervical dystonia and there are only a few reports of its use for treating hyperhidrosis[81]. Injection of BoNT-B can induce focal anhidrosis; the response being dose-dependent. Birklein found that a threshold dose of 8 U lead to anhidrotic skin spots >4 cm after 3 weeks. The duration was prolonged for 3 months when 15 U were injected, and for 6 months when 125 U BoNT-B were injected[82].

Despite its ability to induce anhidrosis, the use of BoNT-B is limited by the occurrence of systemic adverse events[81]. Dressler reported that 100 U BOTOX®, 2000 U Neurobloc® and 4000 U Neurobloc® are equally effective in blocking axillary hyperhidrosis based on a study of 19 patients. The extent of improvement was similar, approximately 16 weeks. The onset of action was earlier in the BoNT-B treated side, but there was greater discomfort in the BoNT-B treated side compared to the BoNT-A treated axilla. In addition, one patient developed severe dryness of the mouth starting 1 week after the injection and which lasted for 5 weeks. The subject also developed accommodation difficulties and conjunctival irritation that lasted for 3 weeks. Likewise, when patients were treated with

5000 U Neurobloc® in each axilla for primary focal hyperhidrosis, excellent reduction in sweating was achieved but the incidence of side effects was high and included dry mouth (52%), headache (10%) and sensory motor symptoms of the hand (10%)[83,84].

A patient with palmar hyperhidrosis was treated with 2500 U Neurobloc® (Elan Pharmaceuticals, San Francisco, CA) in each palm for a total dose of 5000 U. The hyperhidrosis stopped within 24 hours but 2 days after the injection he developed bilateral blurred vision, indigestion, dry sore throat and dysphagia[85]. The largest study to date using BoNT-B to treat palmar hyperhidrosis included 20 subjects[86]. Three quarters of the patients were treated with 5000 U Neurobloc® per palm and one quarter of the subjects received placebo but were allowed to cross over into treatment at one month. The duration of action ranged from 2.3–4.9 months. Adverse events were common with 90 per cent of treated patients experiencing dry mouth or throat. Other complications reported were indigestion (60%), excessively dry hands (60%), muscle weakness (60%), and decreased grip strength (50%).

Lower dosing may be the key to reducing the high incidence of side effects. A small pilot study of four patients with axillary hyperhidrosis were safely injected with 2500 U Neurobloc® subcutaneously into each axilla. Excellent results were seen in 75 per cent of the subjects and fair results in 25 per cent. No motor or distant autonomic side effects were seen but after 3 months the axillary sweating recurred[87]. BoNT-B is effective in reducing sweat and may be used to treat focal areas of hyperhidrosis. However, because of the incidence of systemic side effects using BoNT-B and the high safety profile using BoNT-A to treat focal hyperhidrosis, to date, BoNT-A is the neurotoxin of choice.

9.12 Complications

Complications unique to a given body site has already been covered. Two more global complications to be addressed are that of compensatory sweating secondary to the treatment with botulinum toxin, and the development of resistance to therapy during the treatment of hyperhidrosis. Since primary focal hyperhidrosis is a disease of long duration, both deserve consideration.

Compensatory sweating is a common sequela of ETS. Following treatment with other modalities, including botulinum toxins, some patients do report a perceived increase in sweating from other body parts. This may be attributed only to a new or heightened awareness of the problem once the focus of attention has been removed from the primary treated area. One study specifically addresses the issue of compensatory hyperhidrosis following BoNT-A therapy[88].

Seventeen patients were treated with BoNT-A and followed for 6 months. Eight different body sites were monitored bilaterally to record any evidence of compensatory sweating. There was no significant increase of sweating in any nontreated area.

The possibility of antibody production with resulting immunoresistance has been a concern with the use of BoNT-A. There have to date been no published reports of resistance developing secondary to treatment of hyperhidrosis, but data from three large clinical studies of patients treated with BoNT-A for axillary hyperhidrosis are awaited. Serum samples were obtained at baseline, prior to each treatment, and at the study exit. The subjects had received 1–4 different treatments; maximum BoNT-A exposure being 600 U. Of the 931 post-treatment samples that were sufficient to analyze, one (0.1%) had neutralizing antibodies present and fourteen (1.4%) were inconclusive. The one patient who tested positive for toxin neutralizing antibodies demonstrated a clinical response to treatment at the time of testing and subsequent testing did not indicate the presence of antibodies. With the new batches of BoNT-A, there does not appear to be any real risk of immunoresistance developing. Treatment of hyperhidrosis requires relatively small doses and long intervals between treatment sessions.

9.13   Future directions

The use of botulinum toxins has revolutionized the treatment of hyperhidrosis. Compared with other treatments, it is unmatched in its efficacy, ease of administration, and patient satisfaction. Further work is needed to optimize the dose, dilution, and injection pattern. Development of quick, safe, and effective pain control is needed for the treatment of more tender areas such as the palms and soles. Plantar hyperhidrosis has been successfully treated using a dermojet to deliver BoNT-A without the use of analgesia[63]. New delivery devices are already being researched to help provide the most comfortable and efficient therapy. Kavanagh and colleagues have successfully used a small iontophoresis machine to deliver BoNT-A to two patients with severe palmar hyperhidrosis, sparing them the injections[89]. Research is ongoing looking at the clinical applications of different botulinum serotypes. Perhaps combination therapy will prove useful. New research is underway to identify the genetic pattern of the disease, which may give further clues to possible therapies.

For the present, botulinum toxin treatment is a valuable, well-tolerated therapy for hyperhidrosis. Hyperhidrosis is socially disabling, occupationally disruptive, and emotionally debilitating. Botulinum toxin injections can be delivered safely in the office and provide the much needed relief for the many who suffer with hyperhidrosis.

REFERENCE

1. Goldsmith, L. (1999). Biology of eccrine and apocrine sweat glands. In I. Freedberg, A. Eisen, K. Wolff, L. Goldsmith, S. I. Katz and T. Fitzpatrick, eds., *Fitzpatrick's Dermatology in General Medicine*. New York: McGraw-Hill, pp. 157–64.

2. Goldsmith, L. (1999). Goldsmith disorders of the eccrine sweat gland. In I. Freedberg, A. Eisen, K. Wolff, L. Goldsmith, S. I. Katz and T. Fitzpatrick, eds., *Fitzpatrick's Dermatology in General Medicine*. New York: McGraw-Hill, pp. 800–9.

3. Stenn, K. and Bhawan, J. (2000). The normal histology of the skin. In E. Farmer and A. Hood, eds., *Pathology of the Skin*. New York: McGraw-Hill.

4. Glogau, R. (1998). Botulinum A neurotoxin for axillary hyperhidrosis: no sweat BOTOX. *Dermatologic Surgery*, **24**, 817–19.

5. Kreyden, O. and Scheidegger, P. (2004). Anatomy of the sweat glands, pharmacology of botulinum toxin, and distinctive syndromes associated with hyperhidrosis. *Clinics in Dermatology*, **22**, 40–4.

6. Hund, M., Kinkelin, I., Naumann, M. and Hamm, H. (2002). Definition of axillary hyperhidrosis by gravimetric assessment. *Archives of Dermatology*, **138**, 539–41.

7. Odderson, I. (1998). Hyperhidrosis treated by botulinum A exotoxin. *Dermatological Surgery*, **24**, 1237–41.

8. Cheshire, W. and Freeman, R. (2003). Disorders of sweating. *Seminars in Neurology*, **23**(4), 399–407.

9. Hornberger, J., Grimes, K., Naumann, M., Glaser, D., Lowe, N. J., Naver, H. *et al.* (2004). Recognition, diagnosis, and treatment of primary focal hyperhidrosis. *Journal of American Academy of Dermatology*, **51**, 274–86.

10. Dangoisse, C. and Song, M. (2000). Hyperhidrosis. In J. Arper, A. Oranje and N. Prose, eds., *Textbook of Pediatric Dermatology*. London: Blackwell Science Ltd.

11. Kreyden, O., Schmid-Grendelmeier, P. and Burg, G. (2001). Idiopathic localized unilateral hyperhidrosis: case report of successful treatment with botulinum toxin type A and review of the literature. *Archives of Dermatology*, **137**(12), 1622–5.

12. Seline, P. and Jaskierny, D. (1999). Cutaneous metastases from a chondroblastoma initially presenting as unilateral palmar hyperhidrosis. *Journal of American Academy of Dermatology*, **40**, 325–7.

13. Strutton, D., Kowalski, J., Glaser, D. and Stang, P. (2004). US prevalence of hyperhidrosis and impact on individuals with axillary hyperhidrosis: results from a national survey. *Journal of American Academy of Dermatology*, **51**, 241–8.

14. Naumann, M. (2001). Evidence-based medicine: botulinum toxin in focal hyperhidrosis. *Journal of Neurology*, **248**(Suppl. 1), S31–S33.

15. Glagau, R. (2004). Hyperhidrosis and botulinum toxin A: patient selection and techniques. *Clinics in Dermatology*, **22**, 45–52.

16. Kowalski, J., Ravelo, A., Glaser, D. and Lowe, N. J. (2003). *Quality-of-Life Effect of Botulinum Toxin Type A on Patients with Primary Axillary Hyperhidrosis: Results from a North American Clinical Study Population*, p. 196. American Academy of Dermatology Annual Meeting.

17. Kowalski, J., Glaser, D., Lowe, N. and Ravelo, A. (2003). Quality-of-Life and Economic Impact of Primary Axillary Hyperhidrosis: Results from a North American Clinical Study Population, p. 198. American Academy of Dermatology Annual Meeting.

18. Hornberger, J., Grimes, K., Naumann, M., Glaser, D. A., Lowe, N. J., Naver, H., Ahn, S. and Stolman, L. P. (2004). Multi-Specialty Working Group on the recognition, diagnosis, and treatment of primary focal hyperhidrosis. Recognition, diagnosis, and treatment of primary focal hyperhidrosis. *Journal of the American Academy of Dermatology*, **51**(2), 274−86.

19. Adar, R. (1977). Palmar hyperhidrosis and its surgical treatment: a report of 100 cases. *Annals of Surgery*, **186**(1), 34−41.

20. Naumann, M., Hamm, H. and Lowe, N. J. (2002). Effect of botulinum toxin type A on quality of life measures in patients with excessive axillary sweating: a randomized controlled trial. *British Journal of Dermatology*, **147**, 1218−26.

21. Tan, S. and Solish, N. (2002). Long-term efficacy and quality of life in the treatment of focal hyperhidrosis with botulinum toxin A. *Dermatological Surgery*, **28**, 495−9.

22. Swartling, C., Naver, H. and Lindberg, M. (2001). Botulinum A toxin improves life quality in severe primary focal hyperhidrosis. *European Journal of Neurology*, **8**(3), 247−52.

23. Bushara, K. and Park, D. (1994). Botulinum toxin and sweating. *Journal of Neurology, Neurosurgery and Psychiatry*, **57**(11), 1437−8.

24. Tugnoli, A., Ragona, R., Eleopra, R., De Grandis, D. and Montecucco, C. (2001). Treatment of Frey syndrome with botulinum toxin type A. *Archives of Otolaryngology − Head and Neck Surgery*, **127**, 339−40.

25. Schnider, P., Binder, M., Auff, E., Kittler, H., Berger, T. and Wolff, K. (1997). Double-blind trial of botulinum A toxin for the treatment of focal hyperhidrosis of the palms. *British Journal of Dermatology*, **136**, 548−52.

26. Heckmann, M., Ceballos-Baumann, A. and Plewig, G. (2001). Botulinum toxin A for axillary hyperhidrosis (excessive sweating). *New England Journal of Medicine*, **344**(7), 488−93.

27. Lowe, N., Yamauchi, P., Lask, G., Patnaik, R. and Iyer, S. (2002). Efficacy and safety of botulinum toxin type A in the treatment of palmar hyperhidrosis: a double-blind, randomized, placebo-controlled study. *Dermatological Surgery*, **28**, 822−7.

28. Glaser, D., Kowalski, J., Eadie, N., Solish, N., Ravelo, A., Weng, Y. *et al.* (2004). Hyperhidrosis disease severity scale (HDSS): validity and reliability results from three studies. *Journal of the American Academy of Dermatology*, **51**(2), 241−8.

29. Heckmann, M., Breit, S., Ceballos-Baumann, A., Schaller, M. and Plewig, G. (1999). Side-controlled intradermal injection of botulinum toxin A in recalcitrant axillary hyperhidrosis. *Journal of the American Academy of Dermatology*, **41**, 987−90.

30. Klaber, M. and Catterall, M. (2002). Treating hyperhidrosis: anticholinergic drugs were not mentioned. *British Journal of Dermatology*, **321**(7262), 703.

31. Stolman, L. (1987). Treatment of excess sweating of the palms by iontophoresis. *Archives of Dermatology*, **123**, 893–6.

32. Stolman, L. (1998). Treatment of hyperhidrosis. *Dermatologic Clinics*, **16**, 863–7.

33. Swinehart, J. (2000). Treatment of axillary hyperhidrosis: combination of the starch-iodine test with the tumescent liposuction technique. *Dermatological Surgery*, **26**, 392–6.

34. Luh, J. and Blackwell, T. (2002). Craniofacial hyperhidrosis successfully treated with topical glycopyrrolate. *Southern Medical Journal*, **95**(7), 756–8.

35. Gossot, D., Galetta, D., Pascal, A. and Debrosse, D. (2003). Long-term results of endoscopic thoracic sympathectomy for upper limb hyperhidrosis. *Annals of Thoracic Surgery*, **75**, 1075–9.

36. Belin, E. and Polo, J. (2003). Treatment of compensatory hyperhidrosis with botulinum toxin type A. *Cutis*, **71**, 68–70.

37. Kim, B., Oh, B. and Park, Y. (2001). Microinvasive video-assisted thoracoscopic sympathectomy for primary palmar hyperhidrosis. *American Journal of Surgery*, **181**(6), 540–2.

38. Andrews, B. and Rennie, J. (1997). Predicting changes in the distribution of sweating following thoracoscopic sympathectomy. *British Journal of Surgery*, **84**(12), 1702–4.

39. Kao, M., Chen, Y., Lin, J., Hsieh, C. and Tsai, J. (1996). Endoscopic sympathetic treatment for craniofacial hyperhidrosis. *Archives of Surgery*, **131**(10), 1091–4.

40. Naumann, M. and Lowe, N. J. (2001). Botulinum toxin type A in treatment of bilateral primary axillary hyperhidrosis: randomised, parallel group, double blind placebo-controlled trial. *British Medical Journal*, **323**, 596–9.

41. Glaser, D., Lowe, N. J., Eadie, N., Daggett, S., Mordaunt, J. and Kowalski, J. (2004). 52-Week prospective randomized double-blind placebo-controlled safety and efficacy study of two dosages of botulinum toxin type A treatment for primary axillary hyperhidrosis. *56th Annual Meeting American Academy Neurology*, **P158**, 4–29.

42. Odderson, I. (2002). Long-term quantitative benefits of botulinum toxin type A in the treatment of axillary hyperhidrosis. *Dermatological Surgery*, **28**, 480–3.

43. Wollina, U., Karamfilov, T. and Konrad, H. (2002). High-dose botulinum toxin type A therapy for axillary hyperhidrosis markedly prolongs the relapse-free interval. *Journal of American Academy of Dermatology*, **46**, 536–40.

44. Naumann, M., Lowe, N., Kumar, C. and Hamm, H. (2003). Botulinum toxin type A is a safe and effective treatment for axillary hyperhidrosis over 16 months: a prospective study. *Archives of Dermatology*, **139**(6), 731–6.

45. Galadari, I. and Alkaabi, J. (2003). Botulinum toxin in the treatment of axillary hyperhidrosis. *Skinmed*, **2**(4), 209–11.

46. Glaser, D. (2004). Treatment of axillary hyperhidrosis by chemodenervation of sweat glands using botulinum toxin type A. *Journal of Drugs in Dermatology*, **3**(6), 627–31.

47. Lowe, N. J., Campanati, A., Bodokh, I., Cliff, S., Jaen, P., Kreyden, O. *et al.* (2004). The place of botulinum toxin type A in the treatment of focal hyperhidrosis. *British Journal of Dermatology*, **151**, 1115–22.

48. Schnider, P., Binder, M., Kittler, P., Birner, D., Starkel, K., Wolff, K. *et al.* (1999). A randomized, double-blind, placebo-controlled trial of botulinum A toxin for severe axillary hyperhidrosis. *British Journal of Dermatology*, **140**, 677—80.

49. Saadia, D., Voustianiouk, A., Wang, A. and Kaufmann, H. (2001). Botulinum toxin type A in primary palmar hyperhidrosis: randomized, single-blind, two-dose study. *Neurology*, **57**, 2095—9.

50. Wollina, U. and Karamfilov, T. (2001). Botulinum toxin A for palmar hyperhidrosis. *J. European Academy of Dermatology and Venereology*, **15**, 555—8.

51. Hund, M., Rickert, S., Kinkelin, I., Naumann, M. and Hamm, H. (2004). Does wrist nerve block influence the result of botulinum toxin A treatment in palmar hyperhidrosis? *Journal of American Academy of Dermatology*, **50**, 61—2.

52. Glogau, R. (2004). Treatment of hyperhidrosis with botulinum toxin. *Dermatologic Clinics*, **22**, 177—85.

53. Vollert, B., Blaheta, H., Moehrle, E., Juenger, M. and Rassner, G. (2001). Intravenous regional anaesthesia for treatment of palmar hyperhidrosis with botulinum toxin type A. *British Journal of Dermatology*, **144**, 632—3.

54. Trindade de Almeida, A., Kadunc, B. and Martins de Oliveira, E. (2001). Improving botulinum toxin therapy for palmar hyperhidrosis: wrist block and technical considerations. *Dermatological Surgery*, **27**, 34—6.

55. Baumann, L., Frankel, S., Esperanza, W. and Halem, M. (2003). Communications and brief reports: cryoanalgesia with dichlorotetrafluoroethane lessens the pain of botulinum toxin injections for the treatment of palmar hyperhidrosis. *Archives of Dermatology*, **29**(10), 1057—62.

56. André, P. (2003). An easy and effective local anaesthesia for treating palmar hyperhidrosis. *Journal of European Academy of Dermatology and Venereology*, **17**, 227—9.

57. Naumann, M., Bergmann, I., Hofmann, U., Hamm, H. and Reiners, K. (1998). Botulinum toxin for focal hyperhidrosis: technical considerations and improvements in application. *British Journal of Dermatology*, **139**, 1123—4.

58. Hayton, M., Stanley, J. and Lowe, N. J. (2003). A review of peripheral nerve blockade as local anaesthesia in the treatment of palmar hyperhidrosis. *British Journal of Dermatology*, **149**, 447—51.

59. Blaheta, H., Vollert, B., Zuder, D. and Rassner, G. (2002). Intravenous regional anesthesia (Bier's block) for botulinum toxin therapy of palmar hyperhidrosis is safe and effective. *Dermatologic Surgery*, **28**, 666—72.

60. Reed, M. (2001). Surgical pearl: mechanoanesthesia to reduce the pain of local injections. *Journal of the American Academy of Dermatology*, **44**, 671—2.

61. Scherer, C., Clelland, J., O'Sullivan, P., Doleys, D. and Canan, B. (1986). The effect of two sites of high frequency vibration on cutaneous pain threshold. *Pain*, **25**(1), 133—8.

62. Glaser, D., Kokoska, M. and Kardesch, C. (2001). *Botulinum Toxin Type A in the Treatment of Palmar Hyperhidrosis: the Effect of Dilution and Number of Injection Sites.* American Academy of Dermatology Annual Meeting, Poster Presentation.

63. Vadoud-Seyedi, J., Heenen, M. and Simonart, T. (2001). Treatment of idiopathic palmar hyperhidrosis with botulinum toxin. *Dermatology*, **203**, 318—21.

64. Zaiac, M., Weiss, E. and Elgart, G. (2000). Botulinum toxin therapy for palmar hyperhidrosis with ADG needle. *Dermatological Surgery*, **26**, 230.

65. Doris, H. (2002). *Cosmetic Use of Botulinum Toxin*. São Paulo: AGE Editora, p. 120.

66. Naumann, M., Hofmann, U., Bergmann, I., Hamm, H., Toyka, K. and Reiners, K. (1998). Focal hyperhidrosis: effective treatment with intracutaneous botulinum toxin. *Archives of Dermatology*, **134**(3), 301−4.

67. Blaheta, H., Deusch, H., Rassner, G. and Vollert, B. (2003). Intravenous regional anesthesia (Bier's block) is superior to a peripheral nerve block for painless treatment of plantar hyperhidrosis. *Journal of American Academy of Dermatology*, **48**(2), 301−3.

68. Vadoud-Seyedi, J. (2004). Treatment of plantar hyperhidrosis with botulinum toxin type A. *International Journal of Dermatology*, **43**, 969−71.

69. Kyrmizakis, D., Pangalos, A., Papadakis, C., Logothetis, J., Maroudias, N. and Helidonis, E. (2004). The use of botulinum toxin type A in the treatment of Frey and crocodile tears syndromes. *Journal of Oral and Maxillofacial Surgery*, **62**(7), 840−4.

70. Restivo, D., Lanza, S., Patti, F., Giuffrida, S., Marchese-Ragona, R. and Bramanti, P. (2002). Improvement of diabetic autonomic gustatory sweating by botulinum toxin type A. *Neurology*, **59**(12), 1971−3.

71. Kinkelin, I., Hund, M., Naumann, M. and Hamm, H. (2000). Effective treatment of frontal hyperhidrosis with botulinum toxin A. *British Journal of Dermatology*, **143**, 824−7.

72. Böger, A., Herath, H., Rompel, R. and Ferbert, A. (2000). Botulinum toxin for treatment of craniofacial hyperhidrosis. *Journal of Neurology*, **414**, 857−61.

73. Guntinas-Lichius, O. (2002). Increased botulinum toxin type A dosage is more effective in patients with Frey's syndrome. *Laryngoscope*, **112**, 746−9.

74. Laccourreye, O., Muscatelo, L., Bonan, B., Naude, C. and Bransu, D. (1998). Botulinum toxin type A for Frey's syndrome: a preliminary prospective study. *Annals of Otorhinolaryngology*, **107**(1), 52−5.

75. Laskawi, R., Drobik, C. and Schonebeck, C. (1998). Up-to-date report of botulinum toxin type A treatment in patients with gustatory sweating (Frey's Syndrome). *Laryngoscope*, **108**, 381−4.

76. Guntinas-Lichius, O. (2003). Injection of botulinum toxin type B for the treatment of otolaryngology patients with secondary treatment failure of botulinum toxin type A. *Laryngoscope*, **113**, 743−5.

77. Hexsel, D. M., Dal'forno, T. and Hexsel, C. L. (2004). Inquinal or Hexsel's hyperhidrosis. *Clinical Dermatology*, **22**(1), 53−9.

78. Huh, C., Han, K., Deo, K. and Eun, H. (2002). Botulinum toxin treatment for compensatory hyperhidrosis subsequent to an upper thoracic sympathectomy. *Journal of Dermatologic Treatment*, **13**, 91−3.

79. Matarasso, S. (2005). Treatment of facial chromhidrosis with botulinum toxin type A. *Journal of American Academy of Dermatology*, **52**(1), 89−91.

80. Sanli, H., Ekmekci, P. and Akbostanci, M. (2004). Idiopathic localized crossed (left side of the upper part of the body, right side of the lower part of the body) hyperhidrosis: successful treatment of facial area with botulinum A toxin injection. *Dermatologic Surgery*, **30**, 552−4.

81. Schlereth, T., Mouka, I., Eisenbarth, G., Winterholler, M. and Birklein, F. (2005). Botulinum toxin A (BOTOX) and sweating-dose efficacy and comparison to other BoNT preparations. *Autonomic Neuroscience: Basic and Clinical*, **117**, 120−6.

82. Birklein, F., Eisenbarth, G., Erbguth, F. and Winterholler, M. (2003). Botulinum toxin type B blocks sudomotor function effectively: a six month follow up. *Journal of Investigative Dermatology*, **121**(6), 1312−16.

83. Dressler, D., Adib Saberi, F. and Benecke, R. (2002). Botulinum toxin type B for treatment of axillar hyperhidrosis. *Journal of Neurology*, **249**(12), 1729−32.

84. Nelson, L., Bachoo, P. and Holmes, J. (2005). Botulinum toxin type B: a new therapy for axillary hyperhidrosis. *British Journal of Plastic Surgery*, **58**, 228−32.

85. Baumann, L. and Halem, M. (2003). Systemic adverse effects after botulinum toxin type B (Myobloc®) injections for the treatment of palmar hyperhidrosis. *Archives of Dermatology*, **139**, 226−7.

86. Baumann, L., Slezinger, A., Halem, M., Vujevich, J., Mallin, K. and Charles, C. (2005). Double-blind, randomized placebo controlled pilot study of the safety and efficacy of Myobloc (botulinum toxin type B) for the treatment of palmar hyperhidrosis. *Dermatologic Surgery*, **31**, 263−70.

87. Hecht, M., Birklein, F. and Winterholler, M. (2004). Successful treatment of axillary hyperhidrosis with very low doses of botulinum toxin B: a pilot study. *Archives of Dermatology Research*, **295**, 318−19.

88. Krogstad, A., Skymne, A., Pegenius, G., Elam, M. and Wallin, B. (2005). No compensatory sweating after botulinum toxin treatment of palmar hyperhidrosis. *British Journal of Dermatology*, **152**, 329−33.

89. Kavanagh, G., Oh, C. and Shams, K. (2004). BOTOX® delivery by iontophoresis. *British Journal of Dermatology*, **151**, 1093−5.

90. Naver, H., Swartling, C. and Aquilonius, S. (1999). Treatment of focal hyperhidrosis with botulinum toxin type A; a brief overview of methodology and two years' experience. *European Journal of Neurology*, **6**(4), S117−S120.

91. Solomon, B. and Hayman, R. (2000). Botulinum toxin type A therapy for palmar and digital hyperhidrosis. *Journal of American Academy of Dermatology*, **42**, 1026−9.

92. Moreau, M., Cauhepe, C., Magues, J. and Senard, J. (2003). Therapeutics: a double-blind, randomized, comparative study of Dysport® vs. BOTOX® in primary palmar hyperhidrosis. *British Journal of Dermatology*, **149**, 1041−5.

93. Naumann, M., Zellner, M., Toyka, K. and Reiners, K. (1997). Treatment of gustatory sweating with botulinum toxin. *Annals of Neurology*, **42**(6), 973−5.

94. Bjerkhoel, A. and Trobbe, O. (1997). Frey's syndrome: treatment with botulinum toxin. *Journal of Laryngology and Otology*, **111**(9), 839−44.

95. Eckardt, A. and Kuettner, C. (2003). Treatment of gustatory sweating (Frey's Syndrome) with botulinum toxin A. *Head and Neck*, **25**, 624−8.

96. Beerens, A. and Snow, G. (2002). Botulinum toxin A in the treatment of patients with Frey Syndrome. *British Journal of Surgery*, **89**, 116−19.

Hypersalivation

M. Fiorella Contarino[1] and Alberto Albanese[2]

[1]Academic Medical Centre, Amsterdam, The Netherlands
[2]Istituto Nazionale Neurologico Carlo Besta, Università Cattolica del Sacro Cuore, Milano, Italy

10.1 Introduction

The terms drooling, hypersalivation and sialorrhoea have been used inter-changeably in scientific jargon. Drooling and sialorrhoea can be considered as synonymous, both indicating 'unintentional loss of saliva from the mouth', perhaps being more profuse in drooling. They usually refer to difficulty in swallowing, either because of pharyngeal muscle weakness, or of reduced spontaneous swallowing or incoordination, leading to excessive pooling of saliva in the anterior mouth and consequent spillage. Hypersalivation (or absolute hypersalivation) is an 'abnormally increased production of saliva', and does not necessarily lead to drooling, if swallowing is efficient. Drooling is sometimes simply referred to as 'relative hypersalivation'.

10.2 Background and clinical description

Saliva performs a number of functions: it facilitates swallowing, keeps the mouth moist and teeth clean, conveys molecules to stimulate the taste, and has digestive and antibacterial functions. Normal daily salivary production is about $1-2 \mathrm{l}$ ($0.5-1.5 \mathrm{ml/min}$). The majority of daily salivary production is secreted by the parotid and submandibular glands; the parotids account for about 20 per cent of all saliva production, whilst the submandibular glands produce about 70 per cent (Table 10.1). Sympathetic impulses modulate the output of preformed components, including amylase and lysozyme, from salivary cells.

The swallowing reflex normally prevents drooling. Swallowing is a complex task requiring intact neuromuscular coordination: the mean number of swallowing actions per hour is 25.

Clinical Uses of Botulinum Toxins, eds. Anthony B. Ward and Michael P. Barnes. Published by Cambridge University Press. © Cambridge University Press 2007.

Table 10.1. Role of the salivary glands in the production of saliva

Salivary glands	Relative contribution	Quality
Parotid	~20–25%	Watery, containing ptyalin; stimulus-induced
Submandibular and sublingual	~60–70%	Submandibular: mixed (watery and viscous); sublingual: viscous; basal
Minor glands: lingual, labial, buccal and palatal	~5–10%	Mixed (watery and viscous); basal

10.2.1 The salivary glands

The parotid gland is located dorsally and laterally to the mandible. Most of the gland lies superficially and can be easily detected using ultrasound anterior to the tragus, inferiorly to the zygomatic arc and behind the posterior margin of masseter muscle. Posteriorly, the gland overlaps the sternocleidomastoid muscle and anteriorly the masseter muscle. The inferior tip of the gland extends into the neck. The facial nerve enters the deep surface of the parotid gland and thereafter divides into the temporal and cervicofacial branches. Both further subdivide into five terminal branches within the gland parenchyma (Figure 10.1). The parotid duct opens into the oral cavity opposite to the upper second molar tooth. The parotid glands are made of serous cells, and therefore secrete a watery saliva containing ptyalin, particularly as a response to specific stimuli (e.g. smell or sight of food).

The submandibular glands lie behind the descendent branch of the mandible (Figure 10.2). They are rather superficial and can be easily found with ultrasound, when approached from the neck. The submandibular glands encompass mixed cell types (serous and mucinous). They are responsible for most of the basal secretion rate and, because of the anterior position of Wharton's duct, for the production of most of the spilled saliva.

The sublingual glands lie under the floor of the mouth. They are predominately mucinous, and rather secrete viscous saliva, acting as a lubricant for the oral cavity.

The salivary glands are controlled by the autonomic nervous system. Parasympathetic or sympathetic stimulations produce saliva, but acetylcholine-mediated muscarinic parasympathetic stimulation predominates, leading to the production of a watery saliva. Sympathetic impulses modulate the output of preformed components, including amylase and lysozyme, from salivary cells[1]. Absence of both nerve impulses causes atrophy of the salivary gland parenchyma.

In the parotid gland, parasympathetic stimulation originates in the inferior salivatory nucleus, and enters the gland on the auriculotemporal nerve, whereas

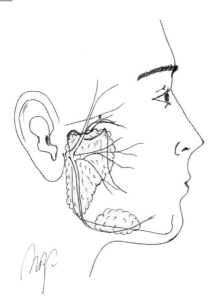

Figure 10.1 Anatomicalillustration of the position of parotid and submandibular gland, with surface reperi, lateral view. Branches of the facial nerve are also shown. Modified from Ref. 59.

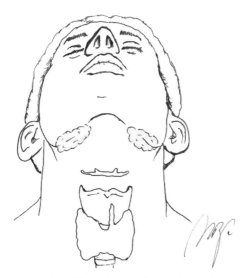

Figure 10.2 Anatomical illustration of the position of parotid and submandibular gland, with surface reperi, neck view. Modified from Ref. 59.

sympathetic innervation lies around the carotid artery. In the submandibular gland, parasympathetic innervation originates at the superior salivatory nucleus, and enters the gland via the corda tympani and lingual nerves; instead, the sympathetic plexus innervating the gland lies around the facial artery.

10.2.2 Drooling

Drooling is normal in young infants; it usually subsides by 18 months as result of physiologic maturity of the orolingual motor function. Drooling beyond 4 years of age is considered abnormal, although otherwise normal children may occasionally achieve complete saliva control only in the early teens[2]. Children who drool in the early stages may improve as dental age and oral musculature mature.

Absolute hypersalivation is quite rare. Transient hypersalivation follows physiological stimuli (i.e. smell or sight of food). Hypersalivation can be due to lesions or foreign bodies placed into the mouth, to rabies infections or mercurial poisoning. It can also be a pharmacological side effect of some antiepileptic drugs, or of atypical neuroleptics (such as clozapine). In the case of clozapine, it has been suggested that hypersalivation occurs in as many as 74 per cent of patients; however, the pathophysiology of clozapine-induced sialorrhoea remains unclear, as no differences in average saliva flow have been demonstrated. Hypersalivation is also observed in a rare autosomal-recessive disorder known as familial dysautonomia that exclusively affects children of Jewish Ashkenazi origin. In this case it may be the result of a combination of impaired swallowing and progressive autonomic neuropathy, leading to denervation supersensitivity and salivary hyperfunction[1]. Similarly, in familial amyloid polineuropathy, which also affects the autonomic nerves, an increased secretion after gum chewing has been found and also attributed to denervation supersensitivity. Finally, a common cause of transient hypersalivation is gastro-oesophageal reflux.

Relative hypersalivation (or drooling) primarily results from infrequent or improper swallowing, dysfunctional voluntary oral motor activity, inadequate lip closure, or forward head posture. It can be seen in association with a wide number of neurological disorders in which swallowing and motility of the lower face musculature are variably affected.

Sialorrhoea occurs in about 50 per cent of patients with amyotrophic lateral sclerosis (ALS); 20 per cent of them have continuous and troublesome drooling[3-5].

From 40 to 80 per cent of patients with parkinsonism may have difficulties with sialorrhoea at some point in their disease course[6,7]. It has been hypothesized that hypersalivation in Parkinson's disease (PD) may occur as a consequence of the involvement of autonomic ganglia, as Lewy bodies have been found therein. Most probably, however, drooling in these patients is not caused by increased salivation, but rather by disturbed swallowing mainly resulting from akinesia; indeed, it has been demonstrated that PD patients have normal and often reduced salivation when compared to age-matched controls[8]. Moreover, the forward flexion of head and trunk are likely to contribute to sialorrhoea.

Other neurological disorders that can be associated with drooling are myopathies, myasthenia gravis, multiple sclerosis, post-stroke, and post-traumatic encephalopathy with involvement of bulbar muscles.

Children with neurological disorders such as cerebral palsy (CP), neuromuscular diseases, autism, language disorders or mental retardation may drool. It has been reported that 10–37.5 per cent of children with CP have significant enough drooling problems as to interfere with their daily life. In a prevalence study conducted on children with CP afferent to special schools, it has been reported that 58 per cent of them had drooling, which was severe in 33 per cent, moderate in 9 per cent and mild in 6 per cent[9]. Studies in children with CP showed normal pharyngeal and oesophageal phases of deglutition, with a marked dysfunction in the oral phase, specifically in the initial suction stage, which hampered initial swallowing[10]. Lack of adequate strength in lip closure is also correlated to dribbling in children. Oral and pharyngeal sensory disturbances or central interruption of normal swallowing reflexes may play a role too. Absolute hypersalivation does not occur in children with CP[10].

Sialorrhoea may also be secondary to sensory dysfunctions in the larynx or to surgical procedures in the upper aerodigestive tract, all resulting in dysphagia. Following oropharingeal surgery, sialorrhoea, albeit transitory, may interfere with wound healing by leading to fistula forming.

Frey's syndrome consists in sweating from the face skin after an appropriate gustative stimulus; it is consequent to abnormal cholinergic reinnervation of denervated cutaneous sweat glands. It can occur as a complication of parotid gland surgery or after sympathetic denervation due to autonomic neuropathies (such as diabetes)[11].

Persistent drooling is socially stigmatizing and may affect interpersonal relationship and self-esteem, because of unpleasant smells and unhygienic appearance. Drooling leads to problems with articulation, feeding, swallowing, and work activities. In addition to irritation and ulceration of perioral skin, in some cases associated with infections, excessive drooling can cause aspiration, choking and *ab-ingestis* pulmonitis. Children and intellectually disabled patients often experience a sizeable improvement in their social behaviour and mood after reduction of drooling after a specific treatment of sialorrhoea.

Evaluation of drooling

Saliva production is influenced by a number of factors, such as the time elapsed from or required to complete feeding, time of the day, concomitant medication, talking, and stressful circumstances. Some different methods have been proposed to measure drooling and evaluate treatment efficacy.

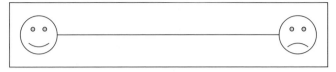

Figure 10.3 This visual analogic scale (VAS) scores the evaluation performed by the patient himself or the caregiver; one extreme indicates the best possible condition and the other is the worst possible condition. The scale line is 10-cm long.

Subjective methods to evaluate drooling are provided by the Visual Analogic Scale (VAS) (Figure 10.3), the Drooling Frequency Scale (DFS), the Drooling Severity Scale (DSS) and the Drool Rating Scale (DRS)[12], which are based on observations performed by the patients or by their caregiver. These subjective evaluations largely rely on the patient's expectations, mood, and general conditions.

Semi-quantitative methods, aimed at measuring the daily production of saliva, include counting the number of paper handkerchiefs or the number of napkins changed in the course of the day, with evaluation of the degree of moistness (i.e. from $1 =$ dry to $3 =$ soaking wet). These methods, too, depend on subjective interpretations and variable behaviour, such as the judgement on cloth wetness or the decision on when to change them[13].

Saliva production at a given time can be measured by inserting dental cotton rolls into the mouth for a short period of time (e.g. from 2 to 5 min). The quantity of saliva produced will result from the difference between the weight of the wet and dry rolls or from the volume of saliva collected after centrifugation of the rolls. These evaluations should be performed at the same time of the day and in standardized conditions. The patient should be in the upright position, having not drunk or eaten since 1 hour before assessment; measurements should be performed after an initial swallow of saliva. In addition, specific collecting systems have been engineered. These rely on cup-like collection devices that can be connected to a system of calibrated test tubes, to measure the total volume of saliva produced[10]. Objective methods account only for the moment of the evaluation, not taking into account daily and weekly fluctuations in saliva production, mechanical and gustatory stimuli, emotional state or body posture. The influence of daily variability can be reduced by performing repeated measurements, possibly on different days.

Finally, ultrasound evaluation of the gland appearance and size or salivary gland scintigraphy (using $[^{99m}Tc]$pertechnetate) could help define changes in gland volume, consistency and activity after treatment[3]. These methods are not fully reliable and standardized and do not give any information on the functional impairment brought about by drooling.

None of the methods described here are truly satisfactory: two or more of these evaluations should be performed in combination to reach an accurate estimate of treatment efficacy, ideally combining at least one subjective and one objective measure. This view is supported by a number of studies that failed to demonstrate a direct correlation between objectively measured saliva reduction and the reported subjective improvement. This discrepancy is explained not only by the inadequate accuracy of the measuring tools, but also by the fact that drooling, and most of the subjective impact of it, is only partially related to the absolute flow of saliva, as it greatly depends on the performance in swallowing and on the efficacy of the oral musculature.

10.3   Alternative treatments

Several treatments have been used over time to treat drooling. Oral treatment as well as local and surgical interventions have been proposed. Benefit is most likely to be achieved in young children, where maturation of oral function may occur, and in adults with relatively mild problems of salivary control.

10.3.1   Anticholinergic drugs

Various anticholinergic drugs have been used to treat sialorrhoea. These drugs act by reducing cholinergic activity that stimulates secretion of saliva, but are usually ineffective at low doses. Higher dosages, instead, often produce unacceptable systemic side effects, such as confusion, memory impairment, hallucinations, insomnia and sedation, blurred vision, exacerbation of acute angle glaucoma, urinary retention, constipation, and cardiac arrhythmia. Moreover, this symptomatic treatment only produces a temporary relief. Anticholinergic drugs can be given orally, sublingually, transdermally, subcutaneously, intramuscularly, or intravenously.

Glycopyrronium bromide (glycopirrolate) is a quaternary anticholinergic that is thought to be less likely to cross the blood—brain barrier, thus producing fewer central effects. The sparse studies performed in adults and children have agreed that the benefit of orally administered glycopirrolate is generally in the range of 70—90 per cent of improvement at doses up to 2 mg daily (or up to 0.4 mg/kg/day in children)[13-15]. However, reported side effects are behavioural problems, urinary retention and constipation. These occurred even at lower doses and were more pronounced in children than in adults and often led to discontinuation of the treatment[16]. Topical application of glycopirrolate has been proposed for the treatment of Frey's syndrome, with infrequent mild adverse events[17].

Studies on benztropine mesylate and trihexyphenidyl, reported inconsistent data on efficacy and side effects. It has been suggested that, at least in children with CP, trihexyphenidyl is more indicated than other oral drugs because of its potential benefit on dystonia associated to CP. This anticholinergic drug can be started at the dose of 0.02–0.04 mg/kg/day, and slowly increased on need.

Transdermal scopolamine has been used to treat drooling, but the results were inconsistent. It is not infrequent to observe allergic reactions to the self-adhering skin patch. Moreover, chronic treatment with scopolamine has been associated with dizziness, blurred vision, psychosis or confusion. A different route of administration has been attempted in three patients with drooling who were treated by local nebulization of 800 µg of scopolamine. Benefit without side effects has been reported, but a short-lived effect and the need for repeated prolonged applications through a mouth mask make this treatment uncomfortable[18].

Significant improvement on subjective evaluation, despite a non-significant objective reduction of saliva flow, has been achieved in seven patients with sialorrhoea secondary to parkinsonism, treated with sublingual atropine twice daily. Two of them, however, experienced worsening of hallucinations[7]. Sublingual atropine was also effective in controlling clozapine-induced sialorrhoea[19].

10.3.2 Surgical treatment

Various reports have suggested that over 80 per cent of patients undergoing a surgical procedure would benefit from surgery. It has been demonstrated that, at least in children, neuromuscular oral impairment and the severity of drooling are inversely related to postoperative improvement[20,21]. Surgical interventions are invasive and irreversible, and are therefore inadequate in young children, elderly patients with poor general conditions or when sialorrhoea is a temporary feature. In children, surgical treatments should be postponed until full dental development has been reached[9]. Those who undergo surgical procedure without additional risks are generally young, otherwise fit, patients. A number of studies have pointed out the complications that can occur during surgery and the potential long-term side effects, such as dental caries, salivary glands calculi or a number of symptoms due to excessive dryness of the mouth (burning sensations, fissuring of commissures, tongue paraesthesias). Finally, it should also be taken into account that few surgeons have adequate experience or are willing to engage themselves in these rather uncommon procedures.

Surgical treatment can be directed to each of the salivary glands or to the excretory ducts in different combinations. Excision of the parotid glands can be complicated by facial nerve palsy or by Frey's syndrome (see above); the latter occurs in up to 96 per cent of patients, as demonstrated by the starch iodine testing (Minor test). Excision of the submandibular gland can be associated with ligation[22] or rerouting of the parotid duct (so-called Wilkie's procedure). Benefits have been reported in up to 80–100 per cent of patients, but side effects are common (up to 30 per cent, including wound dehiscence, duct stenosis or cyst, oral/dental problems, septic parotitis, xerostomia). Furthermore, excision of the submandibular gland can be complicated by permanent (up to 7 per cent) or temporary (up to 36 per cent) damage to the marginal mandibular nerve or by damage to other nerves, such as the lingual or the hypoglossal.

Salivary duct transposition consists in rerouting of the ducts and orifices to the pharynx to bypass the oral phase of deglutition. A reasonably efficient pharyngeal phase is needed in order to avoid the risk of aspiration. Submandibular salivary duct transposition is the most common type of surgery[20,21,23–25]. This procedure is commonly complicated by unwanted events, such as lateral neck cyst or a mucous retention pseudocystis of the sublingual ducts and gland (ranula), which could eventually require additional surgery. Duct obstruction, gland infection or transient airway obstruction have also been reported[21,24]. Transient swelling of the cheek, the mouth floor or of the submandibular region is a common finding after this type of surgery and can last for several weeks. Recently, the transposition of parotid duct orifices using vein grafts has been introduced. This procedure is still anecdotal and requires high surgical competence and a microsurgical approach[26].

Surgical ligation of the parotid excretory ducts involves the danger of gland swelling and abscess formation, because of a congestion of the secretory product. The efficacy of this procedure, when performed alone, is controversial[27]. The four-duct ligation (bilateral parotid and submandibular duct ligation) can be efficacious and less invasive than gland excision[27,28].

Transtympanic neurectomy produces a parasympathetic denervation of the parotid gland. Sialorrhoea control by approximately 75 per cent has been reported in the immediate, while long-term studies show a high failure rate. It is usually performed in association with a division of the corda tympani, inevitably causing loss of taste in the anterior two-thirds of the tongue.

10.3.3 Radiotherapy

Radiation-induced xerostomia is a well-known side effect of radiotherapy delivered to the head and neck region. The serous acinic cells of the salivary tissue are the target of radiation injury. Very few reports in the literature refer to the use of this technique for treating sialorrhoea. In a report on 31 cases of sialorrhoea of different origin, referred to radiotherapy after failure of medical treatment, an initial satisfactory response (complete to partial, but with drooling not interfering any longer with social activities) was achieved in 82 per cent of patients[29]. In 64 per cent of cases, benefit was maintained for a mean follow-up period of 39 months. Response rates were higher with electrons than with orthovoltage, and when larger fields (including both submandibular glands and the whole of parotids) were used. Twenty-six per cent of the patients reported acute side effects (oral candidiasis, skin reactions, mucositis), while 13 per cent reported permanent side effects (troublesome thick secretions and temporo-mandibular joint fusion). In another series, including only patients with sialorrhoea due to ALS, benefit was achieved in all the patients, but symptoms sometimes recurred after a few months. Reported side effects were erythema and burning of the skin, sore throat, nausea, and thicker secretions, all of which receded from a few hours to 4 weeks[5].

The elderly and those in poor general conditions, or with limited life expectancy, can be offered radiation therapy. This treatment, however, should be avoided in children, because of the risk of inducing malignancies or impeding a normal growth, thereby leading to facial asymmetry or osteonecrosis.

10.3.4   Occupational, physical, and speech therapies

It has been suggested that facilitation of mouth closure can effectively decrease drooling. Exercises, stimulation programmes or the intraoral appliance of training devices have been proposed to improve the strength of lip seal and deglutition mechanisms[30,31]. Intraoral appliances are not suitable for children under the age of six, in whom presumably dentition is not fully completed. Vibration and/or icing have been used to improve sensation and movement. Behavioural modification programmes use a conditioning technique with auditory or visual signals as cues to prompt swallowing (biofeedback). The target end-points of these programmes are the child's awareness of drooling and his ability to swallow on command, which correlate with the overall treatment outcome. These techniques are time-consuming and require full cooperation, in addition to the integrity of the neuromuscular system in the facial district. Success largely depends on the intellectual ability and motivation of the patient. Motor rehabilitation should be aimed to enhance head control, improve muscle tone, and stabilize the relation of body position.

10.3.5   Acupuncture

Tongue acupuncture has been proposed as a treatment of alternative medicine for children with drooling. Five of the 40 points thought to correspond somatotopically to specific skills or body regions are usually addressed. Thirty sessions are normally required for a total course of 6 weeks. Good results, according to subjective evaluations, have been obtained in 10 children. Improvement of drooling still persisted over 6-month follow-up[32].

10.4   Botulinum toxin

10.4.1   Introduction

Autonomic symptoms of the cranial district and particularly dry mouth have been observed in the majority of patients with human botulism. In 1822 Justinus Kerner, analysing 155 cases of food-borne botulism, made the first accurate description of botulinum toxin (BoNT)-induced autonomic failure. Kerner also developed the idea of a possible therapeutic use of the substance causing botulism, not only for muscular hypercontractions, but also for units of hyperhidrosis and hypersalivation[33].

Two BoNT serotypes (BoNT-A and BoNT-B) are available in the clinic; their relative potency has not been univocally assessed and therefore direct comparisons have a limited value. The possible use of BoNT for the treatment of sialorrhoea was first considered by Bushara, who proposed to inject BoNT type A into the parotid glands in patients with ALS[34]. However only in the last few years has BoNT type A, and very recently also type B, been used for this purpose.

10.4.2   Efficacy

BoNT inhibits acetylcholine release in nerve terminals not only at the neuromuscular junction, but also in the sympathetic and parasympathetic ganglion cells and in postganglionic parasympathetic nerves. This action is exerted by blocking the fusion of acetylcholine-containing vesicles with the plasma membrane. In animals it has been demonstrated that in the parotid and submandibular glands BoNT-A inhibits the release of acetylcholine from the synaptic vesicles into the synaptic cleft, resulting in reduced function of parasympathetic controlled glands. In rats treated in just one parotid gland the acinar volume is increased in the treated gland, probably as a result of retention of the excretion products in the cell bodies. The increased number of acinar cells observed in the contralateral gland could be due to a reactive enhancement of saliva production. This phenomenon has not been observed after treatment of the submandibular glands[35]. Studies in dogs have demonstrated that BoNT types A and D significantly decrease the production of saliva from the submandibular gland through an anticholinergic, rather than toxic, effect[36]. BoNT-B produces similar effects at the neuromuscular junction and autonomic terminals, acting on a different intracellular target. The blockade of nerve terminals by BoNTs is irreversible; the clinical effects, however, are temporary as new nerve terminals sprout giving rise to new connections.

Anticholinergic side effects seem to be more common with BoNT-B. Trials on patients with cervical dystonia treated with BoNT-B have reported an increased incidence of dysphagia and dryness of the mouth[37,38]. These adverse events increase with increasing dosage[37] and account for up to 44 per cent of the cases treated with 10.000 NeuroBloc[TM38]. The most frequent side effects reported with BoNT-B are dryness of the mouth (76%), impaired accommodation (36%), irritation of the conjunctiva (20%), reduced sweating, swallowing difficulties, heartburn, constipation, difficult bladder voiding, head instability, dryness of nasal mucosa or thrush[39–41]. BoNT-A is from 10 to 50 times more potent than BoNT-B as a treatment of the motor symptoms of dystonia, although it is only 2.5–20 times more potent than BoNT-B when sudomotor blockade is considered[41,42]. It appears that BoNT-B is clearly more potent in blocking sudomotor nerves than motor neurons in humans, probably due to a different affinity for the BoNT serotypes of cholinergic synapses of the autonomic and motor systems. A higher affinity of BoNT-B for the autonomic than somatic motor nerves could account for the higher frequency of autonomic side effects observed in patients treated for dystonia with BoNT-B. It is therefore hypothesized, albeit not yet confirmed, that less unwanted weakness of surrounding muscles could occur following injections of BoNT-B into the salivary glands.

Treatment of salivary drooling with BoNT has proven promising, especially when compared to other available treatments. Parotid was the initially targeted gland, mainly because it is easily reached. This gland, however, accounts for only about 20 per cent of all saliva production. Since the submandibular glands produce most of the saliva, the simultaneous or sequential combined treatment of the parotid and submandibular glands has been attempted. In cases in which only the parotid glands are injected, the remaining viscous secretions of the submandibular and sublingual glands is sufficient to protect against the unwanted effects due to dry mouth[4]. Still, when the parotid and submandibular glands are both injected, dry mouth is uncommon, because the basal secretion of the remaining salivary glands is sufficient. Treatment of submandibular glands alone is far less effective than combined treatments[12]. No detailed reports are available concerning injection of BoNT in the sublingual glands. It has only been mentioned that dysphagia occurred in half of four patients who received direct injections into the sublingual glands without benefiting in any reduction of sialorrhoea[43]. Salivary flow is reduced after BoNT treatment, but the secretion of salivary components is not, because BoNT does not affect adrenergic innervation[44].

The clinical efficacy of the BoNT is appreciable within 7 days and anyway within 2 weeks after treatment. The duration of the effect has not always been accurately measured and seems to vary between 6 and 30 weeks (Tables 10.2 and 10.3). Therefore, the injections must be repeated periodically. An inverse correlation has been reported between the amount of drooling before treatment and the duration and the scale of clinical benefit[12,45]; this may suggest that BoNT doses need to be tailored on each patient. The reported duration of efficacy following BoNT treatment of sialorrhoea is longer than that following treatments for focal dystonia or spasticity and is similar to that of hyperhidrosis. The reason for this difference is unclear at present; one possibility is that this effect may be related to a different rate for the synthesis of the synaptic proteins inhibited by BoNT in the autonomic nerves compared to somatic motor nerves. In addition, re-sprouting in autonomic nerve endings has not been observed to date[46]. It has been hypothesized that autonomic innervation may have a trophic function on glands, that would be lost following BoNT treatment[47], but histological findings on sweat glands after BoNT treatment do not reveal gland atrophy[46].

There are only three published studies on BoNT-B injections for drooling[43,48,59]. The reported magnitude and duration of efficacy and the frequency of side effects are similar to those reported in trials using BoNT-A.

BoNT treatment has been successfully used also to treat clozapine-induced hypersalivation[49] and Frey's syndrome[50,51]. In this latter condition, it has been administered subcutaneously.

Results of BoNT treatment largely depend on the accuracy of injection placement into the glands, on the dose used, on the choice of glands to inject (based on their relative role in salivary secretion), on the patient's condition and on the underlying pathology[59]. Some studies failed to demonstrate objectively a significant saliva reduction, despite subjective improvement. This discrepancy could be explained by a placebo effect, since only three controlled studies have been conducted[43,45,52], or by limitations in the accuracy of the outcome measures. The variety of dosages, of toxin brands, of assessment methods, and of the causes of drooling make it very difficult to compare the available studies. In general terms, most studies reported that the overall benefit was reasonably good and capable of improving the patients' quality of life (Tables 10.2 and 10.3).

10.4.3 Injection techniques

BoNT injections are made percutaneously into the parotid or into the submandibular gland. One pilot study has attempted to deliver BoNT directly through Stenson's duct, but this retrograde approach has produced unacceptable side effects[53].

In most of the studies, the injections have been performed without guidance, but recent evidence suggests that a better outcome can be obtained when ultrasound guidance is used. This allows us to accurately reach the gland parenchyma, compensating for the anatomical variability of gland location observed in different patients. Ultrasound guidance is an essential aid to avoid vascular structures and branches of the facial nerve. It has been suggested that electromyographic guidance could prevent inadvertent injection into the masseter

Table 10.2. Synopsis of studies on botulinum toxin treatments for sialorrhoea in adults including more than 1 patient

Patients	Gland	BoNT dose	US	Efficacy	Outcome measure	Latency	Adverse events	Duration	Notes	Ref.
4 (1 CP, 1 PD, 1 PSP, 1 ALS)	P	20 (D)	N	Good. No effect in ALS	Subjective	7 days	Dysphagia, chewing problems; dry mouth	6–16		54
5 PD	P	10 (B)	N	Moderate to good in four no effect in one	Subjective	?	Masseter and mouth opening weakness	17–30		55
9 PD	P	7.5–7 pts 15–9 pts (B)	N	Good in three, partial in three	DFS, DSS rolls weight	7–10 days	Pain	8	Difference low/high dose not evaluated.	6
5 ALS	P±SM	P: 6–20 SM: 5 (B)	N	Good in four, no effect in one	DLQI, No. handkerchiefs, Scintigraphy	3–5 days	Sialorrhoea increase	?	Progressive additional treatment	3
11 PD	P	5 (B)	N	Good (significant reduction)	UPDRS II, rolls weight	?	No	6	Assessment only at 1 week	58
10 (1 idiopathic, 4 ALS, 2 PD,	P+SM	P: 15–40	Y	Good in two, partial in	VAS	3–8 days	Dry mouth	17–30	Dose adjusted with respect	47

1 CP, 1 post-traumatic, 1 post-encephalitic)		SM: 10–15 (B)		seven, no effect in one	Rolls	7–14 days	No	8–28	to salivation rate and body weight	44
13 (8 post-neoplastic, 4 neurodegenerative, 1 post-stroke)	P+SM	P: 22,5 SM: 10 (B)	Y	Good	Centrifugal, Subjective				Lower dose for two patients	45
10 (7 PD, 3 MSA)	P+SM	P: 146,25 SM: 78,75 (D)	Y	Good (significant reduction)	ADL, DSS, DFS	7 days	Pain at injection site	3–6	RCT	48
9 (6 PD, 2 LBD, 1 MSA)	P	1000 (N)	N	Good. VAS reduction 61%. Weight reduction 42% (NS)	VAS (0–4), Rolls weight	?	Dry mouth, increased sialorrhoea	8–20		
32 (12 ALS, 12 PD, 4 MSA, 4 CBD)	P	a) 18.75 b) 37.5 c) 75 (D)	N	Good for c) (50%), nonsignificant for a) and b)	Rolls weight, Subjective counter. ADL questionnaire	?	No	?	RCT, dose-finding study	52
16 PD	P+SM	P: 1000 SM: 250 (N)	N	Good	DRS, DFS, DSS, VAS, GIS, scintigraphy	5 ± 5 days	Dry mouth, gait worsening,	12–20	RCT. Duration not specifically addressed.	43

Table 10.2. (*Cont.*) Synopsis of studies on botulinum toxin treatments for sialorrhoea in adults including more than 1 patient

Patients	Gland	BoNT dose	US	Efficacy	Outcome measure	Latency	Adverse events	Duration	Notes	Ref.
18 (9 ALS, 9 PD)	P+SM	P: 1000 SM: 250 (N)	Y	Good (significant reduction)	Rolls weight, DSS, DFS, DRS, VAS	2.4 ± 0.9 days	Viscous saliva, pain, dry mouth, parotitis, haematoma, bleeding. diarrhea, neck pain	ALS: 3.4 ± 0.5 PD: 4.8 ± 0.8 months		59

BoNT doses are expressed in Units. Duration is expressed in weeks, unless specified. Abbreviations: ADL = activities of daily living scale; ALS = amyotrophic lateral sclerosis; B = BOTOX®; CBD = cortico-basal degeneration; CP = cerebral palsy; D = Dysport®; DFS = drooling frequency scale; DLQI = dermatology life quality index; DRS = drool rating scale; DSS = drooling severity scale; GIS = global impression scale; LBD = Lewy body dementia; MSA = multiple system atrophy; MU = mouse units; N = NeuroBloc™; NS = not significant; P = parotid; PD = Parkinson's disease; PSP = progressive sopranuclear palsy; pt = patient; RCT = randomized controlled trial; SM = submandibular; UPDRS = unified Parkinson's disease rating scale; US = ultrasound; VAS = visual analogic scale.

Table 10.3. Synopsis of botulinum toxin treatments for sialorrhoea in children

Patients	Gland	BoNT dose (units)	Needle	US	Efficacy	Outcome measure	Latency of effects	Adverse events	Duration	Notes	Ref.
3 CP	SM	(1) 30 (2) 40 (3) 50 (B)	25G	Y	51–63% reduction of salivary flow	DFS, DSS, rolls weight	?	1 thick saliva	>16 weeks (2 pts) 4 weeks (1 pt)	Weight-adjusted dose: 1) <15 Kg 2) 15–25 Kg 3) >25. General anaesthesia.	2
17 CP	(1) SM (2) SM+P	(1) SM: 10, 20, 30 (2) SM/P: 30/20, 30/30, 30/40 (B)	22G	Y	(1) benefit in 33% (2) benefit in 80%	Speech therapist evaluation, radiographic swallowing evaluation DRS, DQ	7–10 days	No	2–26 weeks	Dose escalation. Additive gland treatment. Local anaesthesia.	12
9 (6 CP, 1 congenital CMV infection, 1 chromosomal abnormality, 1 mental retardation)	P	5 (B)	30G	N	Over 75% (3 pts) 27–46% (2 pts) 15% (1 pt) No benefit (3 pts)	Rolls weight, DQ, DFS, DSS	Within 4 weeks	1 increase of saliva production for 8 weeks (mild dysphagia?)	8–16 weeks	Local anaesthesia.	56

Abbreviations: B = BOTOX®; CMV = cytomegalovirus; CP = cerebral palsy; DFS = drooling frequency scale; DQ = drool quotient; DRS = drool rating scale; DSS = drooling severity scale; MU = mouse units; P = parotid; pt = patient; SM = submandibular.

muscle, but this procedure can be difficult, painful and time-consuming, while comparable results can be obtained with ultrasound guidance alone.

The parotid gland can otherwise be targeted considering the surface anatomical reperi (as shown in Figure 10.4). The cholinergic innervation is equally distributed within the gland, and there is no need to target any specific area. The aim of the treatment is to reach the entire gland volume; for this purpose usually 2–3 injections are performed. The preferred injection points are:

(1) in the space between the mandibular ascendent branch, the anterior border of mastoid process and the adjoining upper part of SCM muscle;

(2) preauricularly, between the posterior margin of the masseter muscle, the tragus and the mandibular corner, or

(3) between the mandibular ascendent branch and the posterior margin of the masseter muscle.

If the injections are placed in more than one site, at least one should be in the gland body, while the others could be in the tail or in the region above the masseter muscle.

The submandibular glands are targeted considering, as anatomical reperi, the margin of mandibular descendent branch (as shown in Figure 10.5). BoNT can be injected in a single site per each gland.

Injection depth in parotid glands can vary, according to the site chosen. Studies on BoNT-A diffusion show its ability to disseminate beyond fascial planes.

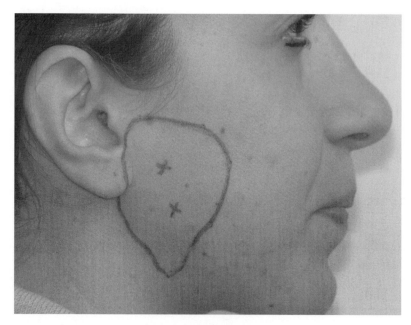

Figure 10.4 Suggested injection points for the parotid gland.

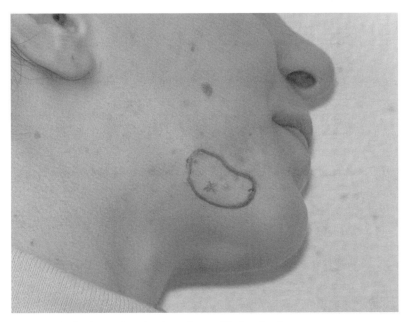

Figure 10.5 Suggested injection points for the submandibular gland.

When ultrasound guidance is used, delivering the toxin in the middle of the gland can minimize the risk of diffusion, yielding a more favourable dose−response relationship. We suggest using a 55 mm 22G needle; a depth of 30 mm can be necessary to reach the centre of the gland. When the injections are made without guidance, the depth should be kept around 10−15 mm, in order to avoid nervous and vascular structures within the gland. Extra-fascial parotid injections have also been proposed[4].

The patient can be placed supine, with the head turned on one side to treat the parotids and with the head in a backward tilt to treat the submandibular glands. It is good usage to provide appropriate antisepsis and to withdraw the syringe plunger, thus ensuring that the needle has not penetrated any vessel. The diluted toxin should be injected slowly within the gland.

10.4.4   Dosage guidelines

For the parotid gland the reported doses of BoNT-A vary between 5 and 40 BOTOX® U, usually diluted in 2 ml of saline, or 20−150 Dysport® U (Table 10.2). The reported doses of BoNT-B were 1000 NeuroBloc™ U in each parotid gland. The total dose was injected in one or up to three sites. In the submandibular glands doses of 5−15 BOTOX® U were used in each gland in three studies, whereas 78.75 Dysport® U were injected in one study and 250 NeuroBloc™ U were used in two study. In all these studies, the injections were placed in a single site (Table 10.2).

In order to prevent the potentially serious side effect of dysphagia in patients with bulbar symptoms it is prudent to initially begin treatment with a lower dosage (i.e. between 5 and 10 BOTOX® U) in each parotid gland, depending on the amount of drooling. If these are ineffective, higher dosages can be used in the parotid gland or the submandibular glands may be additionally injected.

Some authors attempted to determine if any features could predict the outcome of treatment. At least in adults, weight does not influence the efficacy following a fixed dose[48]; some authors have suggested the adjustment of dosage in children in consideration of the low weight and the smaller dimensions of the targeted glands[2]. This does not apply to adults where the efficacy of BoNT depends entirely on its local action without any appreciable weight influence.

10.4.5 Side effects

Side effects are related to injection site, the dosage and dilution of the toxin used, along with the patient's general conditions. Occurrence of side effects is usually higher in patients with poor physical conditions (i.e. patients with ALS in the late stages). Ultrasound guidance greatly increases the safety of the treatment, and helps avoiding vascular and nerve structures, as well as the masseter muscle. The most frequent potential side effect of this treatment is excessive dryness of the mouth; this has been reported only in few patients and has always been mild and short-lasting. In keeping with this, potential aftermaths of this side effect (such as salivary duct calculi or dental caries) have never been reported. A theoretically relevant complication could be dysphagia, due to diffusion to nearby bulbar muscles; this, however, has been reported in just one patient, who experienced mild worsening of a pre-existing dysphagia[54]. Chewing can also be weakened, due to diffusion of BoNT to the masseter muscles; this has been reported in two studies in which the injections were made without guidance[54,55]. Excessive weakness of a masseter muscle can induce dislocation of the temporo-mandibular joint.

Damage to the facial nerve or the facial artery that cross the parotid are theoretically possible complications that have never been reported, even when the injections were performed without guidance. This could be due to the common use of short and thin needles (less than 25 G), that penetrate the parotid only superficially. Infection of the salivary gland or of the salivary duct or local haematomas are also possible, theoretical, complications. Surprisingly, increase of sialorrhoea has been reported twice (in an adult and a child); this is possibly due to the occurrence of mild dysphagia and consequent further reduction of swallowing[3,56]. Pain at the injection site is frequently reported, particularly when larger needles are used. In children, local anaesthesia with anaesthetic cream is useful (Table 10.3); general anaesthesia has also been anecdotally used[57], but is rarely necessary. Other reported side effects following BoNT injection are gait worsening, diarrhoea or neck pain[43]; these are unlikely to be related to the treatment, but rather to the underlying pathology. In our experience, the frequency of side effects is very low when patients are in good general condition and ultrasound guidance is used.

10.5 Conclusion

BoNT is an efficacious treatment of drooling, especially when it is administered in more than just one salivary gland. The safety of this treatment can be increased by using ultrasound guidance. The reduction of saliva flow in a patient with hypersalivation can increase dental caries and requires an adequate dental supervision if the treatment is prolonged in time.

In order to fully appreciate the success of BoNT treatment, the underlying pathology and the diverse individual issues are to be taken into account.

Acknowledgment

The authors thank Dr Mario Rigante for artwork.

REFERENCES

1. Wolff, A., Harell, D., Gadoth, N. and Mass, E. (2002). Submandibular and sublingual salivary gland function in familial dysautonomia. *Oral Surg. Oral Med. Oral Pathol. Oral Radiol. Endod.*, **94**(3), 315–19.

2. Johnson, H., King, J. and Reddihough, D. S. (2001). Children with sialorrhoea in the absence of neurological abnormalities. *Child Care Health Dev.*, **27**(6), 591–602.

3. Giess, R., Naumann, M., Werner, E., Riemann, R., Beck, M., Puls, I., Reiners, C. and Toyka, K. V. (2000). Injections of botulinum toxin A into the salivary glands improve sialorrhoea in amyotrophic lateral sclerosis. *J. Neurol. Neurosurg. Psychiatry*, **69**(1), 121–3.

4. Glickman, S. and Deaney, C. N. (2001). Treatment of relative sialorrhoea with botulinum toxin type A: description and rationale for an injection procedure with case report. *Eur. J. Neurol.*, **8**(6), 567–71.

5. Harriman, M., Morrison, M., Hay, J., Revonta, M., Eisen, A. and Lentle, B. (2001). Use of radiotherapy for control of sialorrhoea in patients with amyotrophic lateral sclerosis. *J. Otolaryngol.*, **30**(4), 242–5.

6. Pal, P. K., Calne, D. B., Calne, S. and Tsui, J. K. (2000). Botulinum toxin A as treatment for drooling saliva in PD. *Neurology*, **54**(1), 244–7.

7. Hyson, H. C., Johnson, A. M. and Jog, M. S. (2002). Sublingual atropine for sialorrhoea secondary to parkinsonism: a pilot study. *Mov. Disord.*, **17**(6), 1318–20.

8. Koike, Y. and Takahashi, A. (1997). Autonomic dysfunction in Parkinson's disease. *Eur. Neurol.*, **38**(Suppl. 2), 8–12.

9. Tahmassebi, J. F. and Curzon, M. E. (2003). Prevalence of drooling in children with cerebral palsy attending special schools. *Dev. Med. Child Neurol.*, **45**(9), 613–17.

10. Tahmassebi, J. F. and Curzon, M. E. (2003). The cause of drooling in children with cerebral palsy: hypersalivation or swallowing defect? *Int. J. Paediatr. Dent.*, **13**(2), 106–11.

11. Restivo, D. A., Lanza, S., Patti, F., Giuffrida, S., Marchese-Ragona, R., Bramanti, P. and Palmeri, A. (2002). Improvement of diabetic autonomic gustatory sweating by botulinum toxin type A. *Neurology*, **59**(12), 1971–3.

12. Suskind, D. L. and Tilton, A. (2002). Clinical study of botulinum-A toxin in the treatment of sialorrhoea in children with cerebral palsy. *Laryngoscope*, **112**(1), 73–81.

13. Neverlien, P. O., Sorumshagen, L., Eriksen, T., Grinna, T., Kvalshaugen, H. and Lind, A. B. (2000). Glycopyrrolate treatment of drooling in an adult male patient with cerebral palsy. *Clin. Exp. Pharmacol. Physiol.*, **27**(4), 320–2.

14. Blasco, P. A. and Stansbury, J. C. (1996). Glycopyrrolate treatment of chronic drooling. *Arch. Pediatr. Adolesc. Med.*, **150**(9), 932–5.

15. Olsen, A. K. and Sjogren, P. (1999). Oral glycopyrrolate alleviates drooling in a patient with tongue cancer. *J. Pain. Symptom. Manage.*, **18**(4), 300–2.

16. Mier, R. J., Bachrach, S. J., Lakin, R. C., Barker, T., Childs, J. and Moran, M. (2000). Treatment of sialorrhoea with glycopyrrolate: a double-blind, dose-ranging study. *Arch. Pediatr. Adolesc. Med.*, **154**(12), 1214–18.

17. Kim, W. O., Kil, H. K., Yoon, D. M. and Cho, M. J. (2003). Treatment of compensatory gustatory hyperhidrosis with topical glycopyrrolate. *Yonsei Med. J.*, **44**(4), 579–82.

18. Zeppetella, G. (1999). Nebulized scopolamine in the management of oral dribbling: three case reports. *J. Pain Symptom. Manage.*, **17**(4), 293–5.

19. Comley, C., Galletly, C. and Ash, D. (2000). Use of atropine eye drops for clozapine induced hypersalivation. *Aust. N. Z. J. Psychiatry*, **34**(6), 1033–4.

20. Crysdale, W. S., Raveh, E., McCann, C., Roske, L. and Kotler, A. (2001). Management of drooling in individuals with neurodisability: a surgical experience. *Dev. Med. Child. Neurol.*, **43**(6), 379–83.

21. Mankarious, L. A., Bottrill, I. D., Huchzermeyer, P. M. and Bailey, C. M. (1999). Long-term follow-up of submandibular duct rerouting for the treatment of sialorrhoea in the pediatric population. *Otolaryngol. Head Neck Surg.*, **120**(3), 303–7.

22. Stern, Y., Feinmesser, R., Collins, M., Shott, S. R. and Cotton, R. T. (2002). Bilateral submandibular gland excision with parotid duct ligation for treatment of sialorrhoea in children: long-term results. *Arch. Otolaryngol. Head Neck Surg.*, **128**(7), 801–3.

23. Panarese, A., Ghosh, S., Hodgson, D., McEwan, J. and Bull, P. D. (2001). Outcomes of submandibular duct re-implantation for sialorrhoea. *Clin. Otolaryngol.*, **26**(2), 143–6.

24. Wilson, S. W. and Henderson, H. P. (1999). The surgical treatment of drooling in Leicester: 12 years experience. *Br. J. Plast. Surg.*, **52**(5), 335–8.

25. Uppal, H. S., De, R., D'Souza, A. R., Pearman, K. and Proops, D. W. (2003). Bilateral submandibular duct relocation for drooling: an evaluation of results for the Birmingham Children's Hospital. *Eur. Arch. Otorhinolaryngol.*, **260**(1), 48–51.

26. Ozgenel, G. Y. and Ozcan, M. (2002). Bilateral parotid-duct diversion using autologous vein grafts for the management of chronic drooling in cerebral palsy. *Br. J. Plast. Surg.*, **55**(6), 490–3.

27. Klem, C. and Mair, E. A. (1999). Four-duct ligation: a simple and effective treatment for chronic aspiration from sialorrhoea. *Arch. Otolaryngol. Head Neck Surg.*, **125**(7), 796–800.

28. Shirley, W. P., Hill, J. S., Woolley, A. L. and Wiatrak, B. J. (2003). Success and complications of four-duct ligation for sialorrhoea. *Int. J. Pediatr. Otorhinolaryngol.*, **67**(1), 1–6. Review.

29. Borg, M. and Hirst, F. (1998). The role of radiation treatment in the management of sialorrhoea. *Int. J. Radiat. Oncol. Biol. Phys.*, **41**, 1113–19.

30. Johnson, H. M., Reid, S. M., Hazard, C. J., Lucas, J. O., Desai, M. and Reddihough, D. S. (2004). Effectiveness of the Innsbruck Sensorimotor Activator and Regulator in improving saliva control in children with cerebral palsy. *Dev. Med. Child. Neurol.*, **46**(1), 39–45.

31. Lloyd Faulconbridge, R. V., Tranter, R. M., Moffat, V. and Green, E. (2001). Review of management of drooling problems in neurologically impaired children: a review of methods and results over 6 years at Chailey Heritage Clinical Services. *Clin. Otolaryngol.*, **26**(2), 76–81.

32. Wong, V., Sun, J. G. and Wong, W. (2001). Traditional Chinese medicine (tongue acupuncture) in children with drooling problems. *Pediatr. Neurol.*, **25**(1), 47–54.

33. Erbguth, F. J. (1998). Botulinum toxin, a historical note. *Lancet*, **351**, 1820.

34. Bushara, K. O. (1997). Sialorrhea in amyotrophic lateral sclerosis: a hypothesis of a new treatment – botulinum toxin A injections of the parotid glands. *Med. Hypotheses*, **48**(4), 337–9.

35. Ellies, M., Laskawi, R., Tormahlen, G. and Gotz, W. (2000). The effect of local injection of botulinum toxin A on the parotid gland of the rat: an immunohistochemical and morphometric study. *J. Oral. Maxillofac. Surg.*, **58**(11), 1251–6.

36. Shaari, C. M., Wu, B., Biller, H. F., Chuang, S. and Sanders, I. (1998). Botulinum toxin decreases salivation from canine submandibular glands. *Otolaryngol. Head Neck Surg.*, **118**, 452–7.

37. Brashear, A., Lew, M. F., Dykstra, D. D., Comella, C. L., Factor, S. A., Rodnitzky, R. L., Trosch, R., Singer, C., Brin, M. F., Murray, J. J., Wallace, J. D., Willmer-Hulme, A. and Koller, M. (1999). Safety and efficacy of NeuroBloc (botulinum toxin type B) in type A-responsive cervical dystonia. *Neurology*, **53**(7), 1439–46.

38. Brin, M. F., Lew, M. F., Adler, C. H., Comella, C. L., Factor, S. A., Jankovic, J., O'Brien, C., Murray, J. J., Wallace, J. D., Willmer-Hulme, A. and Koller, M. (1999). Safety and efficacy of NeuroBloc (botulinum toxin type B) in type A-resistant cervical dystonia. *Neurology*, **53**(7), 1431–8.

39. Dressler, D., Adib Saberi, F. and Benecke, R. (2002). Botulinum toxin type B for treatment of axillar hyperhidrosis. *J. Neurol.*, **249**(12), 1729–32.

40. Racette, B. A., Lopate, G., Good, L., Sagitto, S. and Perlmutter, J. S. (2002). Ptosis as a remote effect of therapeutic botulinum toxin B injection. *Neurology*, **59**(9), 1445–7.

41. Dressler, D. and Benecke, R. (2003). Autonomic side effects of botulinum toxin type B treatment of cervical dystonia and hyperhidrosis. *Eur. Neurol.*, **49**(1), 34–8.

42. Birklein, F., Eisenbarth, G., Erbguth, F. and Winterholler, M. (2003). Botulinum toxin type B blocks sudomotor function effectively: a 6 month follow up. *J. Invest. Dermatol.*, **121**(6), 1312–16.

43. Ondo, W. G., Hunter, C. and Moore, W. (2004). A double-blind placebo-controlled trial of botulinum toxin B for sialorrhoea in Parkinson's disease. *Neurology*, **62**(1), 37–40.

44. Ellies, M., Laskawi, R., Rohrbach-Volland, S. and Arglebe, C. (2003). Up-to-date report of botulinum toxin therapy in patients with drooling caused by different etiologies. *J. Oral. Maxillofac. Surg.*, **61**(4), 454–7.

45. Mancini, F., Zangaglia, R., Cristina, S., Sommaruga, M. G., Martignoni, E., Nappi, G. and Pacchetti, C. (2003). Double-blind, placebo-controlled study to evaluate the efficacy and safety of botulinum toxin type A in the treatment of drooling in parkinsonism. *Mov. Disord.*, **18**(6), 685–8.

46. Naumann, M., Hofmann, U., Bergmann, I., Hamm, H., Toyka, K. V. and Reiners, K. (1998). Focal hyperhidrosis: effective treatment with intracutaneous botulinum toxin. *Arch. Dermatol.*, **134**, 301–4.

47. Porta, M., Gamba, M., Bertacchi, G. and Vaj, P. (2001). Treatment of sialorrhoea with ultrasound guided botulinum toxin type A injection in patients with neurological disorders. *J. Neurol. Neurosurg. Psychiatry*, **70**(4), 538–40.

48. Racette, B. A., Good, L., Sagitto, S. and Perlmutter, J. S. (2003). Botulinum toxin B reduces sialorrhoea in parkinsonism. *Mov. Disord.*, **18**(9), 1059–61.

49. Kahl, K. G., Hagenah, J., Zapf, S., Trillenberg, P., Klein, C. and Lencer, R. (2004). Botulinum toxin as an effective treatment of clozapine-induced hypersalivation. *Psychopharmacology (Berl.)*.

50. Naumann, M., Zellner, M., Toyka, K. V. and Reiners, K. (1997). Treatment of gustatory sweating with botulinum toxin. *Ann. Neurol.*, **42**, 973–5.

51. Teive, H. A., Troiano, A. R., Robert, F., Iwamoto, F. M., Maniglia, J. J., Mocellin, M. and Werneck, L. C. (2003). Botulinum toxin for treatment of Frey's syndrome: report of two cases. *Arq. Neuropsiquiatr.*, **61**(2A), 256–8.

52. Lipp, A., Trottenberg, T., Schink, T., Kupsch, A. and Arnold, G. (2003). A randomized trial of botulinum toxin A for treatment of drooling. *Neurology*, **61**(9), 1279–81.

53. Winterholler, M. G., Erbguth, F. J., Wolf, S. and Kat, S. (2001). Botulinum toxin for the treatment of sialorrhoea in ALS: serious side effects of transductal approach. *J. Neurol. Neurosurg. Psychiatry*, **70**, 417–18.

54. Bhatia, K. P., Munchau, A. and Brown, P. (1999). Botulinum toxin is a useful treatment in excessive drooling in saliva. *J. Neurol. Neurosurg. Psychiatry*, **67**(5), 697.

55. Jost, W. H. (1999). Treatment of drooling in Parkinson's disease with botulinum toxin. *Mov. Disord.*, **14**(6), 1057.

56. Bothwell, J. E., Clarke, K., Dooley, J. M., Gordon, K. E., Anderson, R., Wood, E. P., Camfield, C. S. and Camfield, P. R. (2002). Botulinum toxin A as a treatment for excessive drooling in children. *Pediatr. Neurol.*, **27**(1), 18–22.

57. Jongerius, P. H., Rotteveel, J. J., van den Hoogen, F., Joosten, F., van Hulst, K. and Gabreels, F. J. (2001). Botulinum toxin A: a new option for treatment of drooling in children with cerebral palsy. Presentation of a case series. *Eur. J. Pediatr.*, **160**(8), 509–12.

58. Friedman, A. and Potulska, A. (2001). Quantitative assessment of parkinsonian sialorrhoea and results of treatment with botulinum toxin. *Parkinsonism Relat. Disord.*, **7**(4), 329–32.

59. Contarino, M. F., Pompili, M., Tittoto, P., Vanacore, N., Sabatelli, M., Cedrone, A., Rapaccini, G. L., Gasbarrini, G., Tonali, P. A., Bentivoglio, A. R. (2006). Botulinum toxin B ultrasound-guided injections for sialorrhea in Amyotrophic Lateral sclerosis and Parkinson's disease. *Parkinsonism Relat. Disord.* [Epub ahead of print]

Appendix: Rating scales for drooling

Drooling frequency scale

1	Never drools	
2	Occasional drooling	Not every day
3	Frequent drooling	Every day but not all the day
4	Constant drooling	Every day

Drooling severity scale

1	Dry	Never drools
2	Mild	Only lips wet
3	Moderate	Lips and chin wet
4	Severe	Clothing soiled
5	Profuse	Clothing, hands and tray moist and wet

Drooling rating scale

Pre-injection

Salivation

1 Normal
2 Pooling in mouth
3 Minimal drooling
4 Moderate drooling
5 Constant drooling

Bib or shirt changes in a day as a result of excessive drooling

1 None
2 1 bib or shirt change a day

Drooling rating scale (*Cont.*)

3   2–3 bib/shirt changes a day
4   4–5 bib/shirt changes a day
5   6 or more bib/shirt changes a day

Drooling while eating

1   None
2   Minimal, does not interfere with eating
3   Moderate, slight interference with eating
4   Moderate-severe, obviously interferes with eating
5   Severe, prohibits eating

Drooling at night

1   None
2   Minimal, lips slightly moist
3   Moderate, lips and chin wet, pillow slightly moist
4   Moderate to severe, pillow obviously wet
5   Severe, pillow saturated, clothing wet

Choking or severe coughing episodes

1   Never
2   Has happened only once or twice
3   Happens occasionally
4   Happens often
5   Happens every/almost everyday

Noisy breathing or 'gurgling' caused by excess saliva

1   Never
2   Occasional (1 episode/week to 1 episode/day)
3   Frequent (>2 episodes/day)
4   Constant

Degree of skin irritation (face/neck) from drooling

1   None
2   Slight redness, occasionally
3   Slight redness, always
4   Moderate redness, always
5   Severe redness, occasional breakdown

Halitosis (bad breath)

1   None
2   Slight halitosis
3   Moderate halitosis
4   Moderate-severe halitosis
5   Severe halitosis

Patient self-confidence secondary to drooling

1   Drooling does not affect confidence
2   Drooling causes a slight embarrassment
3   Drooling causes moderate embarrassment
4   Drooling causes severe embarrassment

Public response to patient and drooling (please reflect)

1   Normal, do not shy away
2   Minimal, slightly reluctant to have physical contact with the patient
3   Moderately reluctant to have physical contact with the patient
4   Moderate-severe, seem extremely reluctant to touch the patient
5   Severe, will not even touch the patient

Ease in caring for patient related to drooling

1   No problem
2   Slight inconvenience
3   Moderate inconvenience
4   Severe inconvenience

How limiting is the patient's drooling on doing activities outside the home?

1   None
2   Very mild
3   Mild
4   Moderate
5   Severe

Overall, how much of an inconvenience is for the caregiver the excessive saliva and/or drooling of the patient?

1   Not bothered at all
2   Bothered a little
3   Bothered more than a little, but not a lot
4   Bothered a lot
5   Extremely bothered

Overall, how bothered is the patient as a result of excessive drooling

1   Not bothered at all
2   Bothered a little
3   Bothered more than a little, but not a lot
4   Bothered a lot
5   Extremely bothered

Post-injection

Overall, how has the drooling been since the BOTOX® injection?

1   Markedly worse
2   Moderately worse
3   Slightly worse
4   No change

Drooling rating scale (*Cont.*)

5   Slightly improved
6   Moderately improved
7   Markedly improved

If you have seen an improvement, how has it improved for you?

How would you rate your level of satisfaction with treatment for drooling?

1   Markedly dissatisfied
2   Moderately dissatisfied
3   Mildly dissatisfied
4   Mildly satisfied
5   Moderately satisfied
6   Markedly satisfied

Would you undergo botulinum toxin injections again?

1   Yes
2   No

Botulinum toxin type A for the prophylactic treatment of primary headache disorders

David W. Dodick

Mayo Clinic College of Medicine, Scottsdale, Arizona, USA

11.1 Introduction

Migraine is a chronic neurovascular disorder that afflicts 8–15 per cent of the world's population and is the most common primary headache disorder in clinical practice. In the United States there are an estimated 28 million migraine sufferers, with women being affected three times as often as men[1]. It is characterized by severe headaches and is often associated with nausea, vomiting, heightened sensitivity to sound and light, and focal (paresthesias, visual scintillations) and global (impaired concentration) neurological dysfunction. Migraine is considered to be one of the top 20 causes of disability due to chronic diseases, and severe migraine has been judged by the World Health Organization to be as disabling as quadriplegia, psychosis, and dementia[2].

Most sufferers are in their most socially active and productive years (25–55)[1]. Not only is migraine painful and disabling for the sufferer, but it exerts a significant economic burden on society. It causes 112 million bedridden days each year and costs $14 billion in reduced productivity and missed workdays[3]. The economic burden of migraine is comparable with that of diabetes[4] and higher than that of asthma[5].

Even among migraineurs who consult a physician, many are not satisfied with their therapy and report that prescribed medications are not always optimal. Triptan medications, the most effective acute therapy for migraine attacks, are only effective in improving the pain and associated migraine symptoms, such as photophobia and nausea, in up to two thirds of patients[6]. There is a significant need to develop more effective therapies for migraine prevention because 35 per cent of migraineurs suffer from two to three severe attacks per month, whereas 25 per cent suffer from more than four attacks per month[6].

Clinical Uses of Botulinum Toxins, eds. Anthony B. Ward and Michael P. Barnes. Published by Cambridge University Press. © Cambridge University Press 2007.

Furthermore, up to 14 per cent of patients with migraine develop chronic daily headache (transformed migraine >15 headache days per month), and a high baseline headache frequency (>1 attack per week) appears to be one of the most important risk factors for this progression[7]. Of the more than 4 per cent of the United States population that suffers from chronic daily headache, acute headache medication overuse, and treatment resistance are frequent associated features[8].

Patients with frequent, disabling, or refractory migraine should be considered for prophylactic treatment. Current United States guidelines recommend preventive therapy in one or more of the following situations:
(1) frequent headaches;
(2) recurring migraines that significantly interfere with daily routine;
(3) failure of, a contraindication to, overuse of, or adverse events (AEs) with acute migraine therapies;
(4) cost of acute and preventive therapies;
(5) patient preference; and
(6) the presence of uncommon migraine conditions, including hemiplegic migraine, basilar migraine, migraine with prolonged aura, or migrainous infraction[9].

Although numerous therapies are currently available for the prevention and treatment of migraine, most of these agents have significant side effects.

Commonly used agents for migraine prophylaxis include β-adrenergic blockers, calcium channel blockers, tricyclic antidepressants, and anticonvulsants. Moderate to severe adverse events (AEs) are not uncommon with the available prophylactic medications. β-Blockers are known to produce a wide array of AEs, including drowsiness, fatigue, lethargy, sleep disorders, and depression. AEs typically associated with the calcium channel blockers include constipation, peripheral edema, and weight gain[10], whereas the tricyclic antidepressants commonly are associated with a variety of AEs, including sedation, weight gain, dry mouth, constipation, dizziness, mental confusion, palpitations, blurred vision, and urinary retention. The AEs associated with antiepileptic drugs are unique to each medication, but the most common AEs include nausea, vomiting, and gastrointestinal distress[10]. Because of the AE profile and limited efficacy of currently available preventive therapies, there is a need for novel and improved prophylactic therapies.

The modest efficacy and side effect profile are major reasons why prophylactic therapy is underutilized in migraine sufferers. Data from the American Prevalence and Prevention Study, a large population-based study in the United States, demonstrated that of the more than 40 per cent of migraine patients who should be considered for prophylactic therapy (according to frequency and disability criteria) [less than 5 per cent suggests have ever received] a prophylactic drug[11].

The need therefore for more effective and well tolerated prophylactic medications is a treatment priority in this field over the next decade.

11.2 Botulinum toxin type A for the treatment of headache: mechanism of action

Botulinum toxin type A (BoNT-A) is a focally administered neurotoxin that inhibits the release of acetylcholine at the neuromuscular junction[12]. It is used therapeutically in disorders characterized by muscle hyperactivity, including dystonia and movement disorders, spasticity, cerebral palsy, and gastrointestinal, and urological disorders[13]. Although not currently indicated, BoNT-A also has been safely used for hyperkinetic disorders such as tremor, autonomic disorders such as hyperhidrosis, and cosmetically troublesome hyperfunctional facial lines (crow's feet and forehead lines).

The analgesic effect of BoNT-A has long been observed in the treatment of dystonia and spasticity[14]. This led to further investigation of BoNT-A for other painful conditions, including migraine and tension-type headaches. Although the analgesic mechanism of action is still under investigation, preclinical in vitro and in vivo evidence demonstrates that BoNT-A inhibits the release of nociceptive mediators such as glutamate, substance P, and calcitonin gene-related peptide (CGRP) from nociceptive fibers, suggesting that BoNT-A may have direct antinociceptive action distinct from its neuromuscular activity[14–16]. Presumably, through a peripheral mechanism, BoNT-A has also been shown to inhibit central sensitization of central trigeminovascular neurons[17] which is felt to be integral to the development, progression, and maintenance of the headache associated with migraine[18]. Central sensitization is also considered to be a potential mechanism underlying the development of chronic daily headache in patients with migraine[18]. These findings led to several clinical trials the results of which have suggested that BoNT-A may be an effective and safe prophylactic headache medication in the treatment of migraine[19,20]. The results of three large-scale, uncontrolled, retrospective studies involving 1011 patients with a variety of episodic and chronic headache disorders provided further evidence for a potential role for BoNT-A in the prophylaxis of headaches[21–23].

11.3 Episodic migraine

Episodic migraine is distinguished from transformed migraine by having a frequency of headaches less than 15 days per month. The results from placebo-controlled studies evaluating the efficacy of BoNT-A in patients with episodic migraine are mixed. The first double-blind, placebo-controlled randomized clinical trial was published by Silberstein and colleagues[19]. In this study, 123 patients who had experienced between two and eight moderate-to-severe migraine headaches over a 3-month period were randomized to receive a single injection of either placebo, low dose (25 U), or high dose (75 U) BoNT-A. This single dose was injected into multiple sites of pericranial muscles during the injection visit. Injections were performed anteriorly, in the frontalis, glabellar region and temporalis muscle. At the end of the 3-month follow-up period post injection, the low dose BoNT-A group experienced a mean decrease of 1.88 moderate-to-severe migraines compared to the placebo group ($P=0.042$). Furthermore, patients in the low-dose group had a significant reduction in the incidence of migraine-associated vomiting compared to placebo ($P=0.012$). The high dose BoNT-A group, however, did not have a significant effect on migraine pain and associated symptoms. In fact, at the higher dose, there was an increase in adverse events (AEs). The authors suggest that the lack of BoNT-A activity at this higher concentration may actually be due to a lower number of migraine headaches at baseline compared to the low dose BoNT-A group[19]. In this trial BoNT-A was well tolerated with no AEs observed in the low dose group compared to placebo.

Barrientos and Chana also conducted a randomized, placebo-controlled trial that evaluated the efficacy and tolerability of BoNT-A as prophylaxis for episodic migraine[20]. Thirty patients with a history of two to eight migraine attacks per month were enrolled and randomized to receive placebo or 50 U of BoNT-A injected in 15 pericranial muscle sites. During the 3-month study, when compared to baseline, patients treated with BoNT-A experienced fewer attacks at day 30 (3.7 vs. 5.8, $P<0.02$), day 60 (3.2 vs. 5.8, $P<0.2$), and day 90 (2.5 vs. 5.8, $P<0.01$). In contrast, no significant reduction from baseline was observed in the placebo group. Severity, and duration of migraine attacks were also significantly reduced in the BoNT-A group compared to placebo. At the end of the 3-month study, the BoNT-A treated group reported a significant decrease in the use of NSAIDs and triptan medications compared to placebo for acute headache treatment. This supports the previous clinical data that BoNT-A is effective and well tolerated for preventive migraine treatment.

A small double-blind, placebo-controlled study of BoNT-A conducted by Brin and colleagues further support the efficacy of BoNT-A in migraine[24]. In this trial, 56 subjects having a history of two to six migraines per month were randomized into four groups receiving:
(1) BoNT-A in frontal/temporal regions;
(2) BoNT-A frontal/placebo temporal;
(3) placebo frontal/BoNT-A temporal; and
(4) placebo in frontal/temporal regions.

Migraine frequency was reduced by a median of 1.8 headaches/month in BoNT-A treated groups (Groups 1−3) compared with a median reduction of 0.2 headaches/month in the placebo group (Group 4). This study however is limited by its small population size.

In contrast, Evers and colleagues evaluated the efficacy of BoNT-A in 60 patients who were randomly assigned to receive either placebo in the frontal and neck muscles; 16 U botulinum toxin A in the frontal muscles and placebo in the neck muscles; or 100 U BoNT-A in the frontal and neck muscles[25]. In both treatment groups, 30 per cent of patients showed a reduction of migraine frequency in the third month by at least 50 per cent compared with baseline. In the placebo, group 25 per cent of the patients showed such a reduction ($P=0.921$). There were no significant differences between the three study groups with respect to reduction of migraine frequency, number of days with migraine, and the number of total single doses to treat a migraine attack. In the *post hoc* analysis, the reduction of all accompanying symptoms was significantly higher in the 16 U treatment group compared with the placebo group. In the 100 U treatment group, significantly more adverse events occurred compared with the placebo group. All adverse events were mild and transient. This study did not show any efficacy of BoNT-A in the prophylactic treatment of migraine. Only migraine associated symptoms were significantly reduced in the 16 U but not in the 100 U treatment group. The authors recommended that future studies focus on the efficacy of botulinum toxin A in specific subgroups of patients, on the efficacy of repetitive injections, and on other injection sites.

11.4   Chronic daily headache

Chronic daily headache (CDH) refers to a group of headache disorders that are defined in part by the presence of headache on more than 15 days per month for more than 3 months. Approximately 4 per cent (~12 million) of the population worldwide experience daily or near-daily headaches[26−30]. It has been estimated that approximately 70−80 per cent of patients presenting to headache clinics in the United States are suffering from CDH, of whom the vast majority suffer from transformed migraine[31]. The disability and impact associated with this disorder is substantial and touches almost every aspect of the patient's life. These patients experience significantly diminished health-related quality of life and mental health, as well as impaired physical, social, and occupational functioning[32−34]. In addition, for a significant number of patients with CDH, the clinical course is often complicated and perpetuated by the overuse of acute headache medication[35]. The management of patients with CDH represents one of the major challenges for practicing clinicians. The use of prophylactic medications for CDH is supported mainly by open-label studies. A few controlled studies have been performed; however, these studies do not account for symptomatic medication overuse or concomitant prophylactic medication as major confounders, or do not provide specific diagnoses for patients with CDH[36–40].

A number of studies have recently reported on the efficacy of BoNT-A in the treatment of patients with chronic daily headache. Ondo and colleagues conducted a randomized, double-blind, placebo-controlled, parallel clinical trial that examined the effect of BoNT-A treatment on patients with chronic daily headache including chronic tension headache and transformed migraine[41]. Sixty patients who experienced chronic headache more than 15 days each month were enrolled and randomized to receive, based upon the 'follow the pain' rationale, either 200 U of BoNT-A or matching placebo and at 12 weeks and, if the patient consented, a second open-label BoNT-A injection. Following the first injection, patients treated with BoNT-A had significantly fewer headache days from weeks 8–12 compared with placebo. In addition, 10 per cent of patients treated with BoNT-A reported a dramatic improvement and 24 per cent reported a marked improvement compared with 3 and 7 per cent respectively in the placebo-treated group. At week 24, patients who had received two BoNT-A injections had significantly fewer headache days over the second 12-week period than those receiving one injection (40 vs. 19 days, $P < 0.05$).

The therapeutic value of BoNT-A in the prophylaxis of headaches in migraine patients with chronic daily headache has been further investigated in an exploratory phase 2, randomized, double-blind, placebo-controlled study in 355 patients with CDH[42]. The injection sites and dosage employed in this study are outlined in Figure 11.1. The results of this study demonstrated that BoNT-A, at 105–260 U, was safe and well-tolerated. Furthermore, BoNT-A produced beneficial effects relative to placebo on most efficacy parameters assessed, and statistically significant differences relative to placebo were observed for some parameters. Despite the observation of consistent numerical advantages for BoNT-A over placebo in this study, the prospectively-defined primary efficacy end point was not met; however, the secondary and other prospectively-defined efficacy end points were achieved. This suggested that further analysis of the efficacy data was warranted to determine whether consistent statistically significant advantages were present in specific patient subgroups.

In this exploratory phase 2 study, approximately one third of patients were receiving one or more other headache prophylactic therapies. Yet, these patients still qualified for the study by having 16 or more headache-days per the 30-day baseline period. The discontinuation of concurrent prophylactic therapy was not required by the study protocol. The fact that patients taking a prophylactic treatment in this study still reported 16 or more headache-days may be seen as an

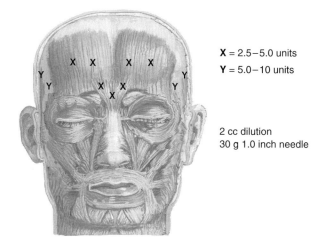

X = 2.5–5.0 units
Y = 5.0–10 units

2 cc dilution
30 g 1.0 inch needle

Figure 11.1 Anterior injection sites.

indication of a distinct refractory subpopulation. Thus, in order to determine the impact of BoNT-A alone, the data were analyzed for the subgroup of patients in this study who were not receiving prophylactic therapy[43].

Of the 355 patients randomized in the study, 228 (64%) were not taking prophylactic medication and were included in this analysis (117 received BoNT-A, 111 received placebo injections)[43]. The mean frequency of headaches per 30 days at baseline was 14.1 for the BoNT-A group and 12.9 for the placebo group ($P=0.205$). After two injection sessions, the maximum change in the mean frequency of headaches per 30 days was −7.8 in the BoNT-A group compared with only −4.5 in the placebo group ($P=0.032$), a statistically significant between-group difference of 3.3 headaches. The between-group difference favoring BoNT-A treatment continued to improve to 4.2 headaches after a third injection session ($P=0.023$). In addition, BoNT-A treatment at least halved the frequency of baseline headaches in over 50 per cent of patients after three injection sessions. Statistically significant differences between BoNT-A and placebo were evident for the change from baseline in headache frequency and headache severity for most time points from day 180 through day 270. Only five patients (four patients receiving BoNT-A treatment; one patient receiving placebo) discontinued the study due to adverse events and most treatment-related events were transient and mild to moderate in severity. The results of this subgroup analysis appeared to indicate that BoNT-A is an effective and well-tolerated, stand-alone prophylactic treatment for migraine patients with CDH.

Thus, the efficacy and safety profile of BoNT-A demonstrated in this analysis suggest that BoNT-A is an effective, well-tolerated prophylactic treatment in patients with CDH who are not using other prophylactic headache treatments.

Furthermore, the results also suggest that assessment of the frequency of headaches is a sensitive measure of efficacy in this patient population and that future studies to confirm these findings are needed.

11.5 Chronic tension-type headache

Given the relief of pain associated with intramuscular injections of BoNT-A for the treatment of dystonia and spasticity, BoNT-A might be expected to effectively treat tension-type headache. When injected into contracted muscle, current data suggests that BoNT-A modifies the sensory feedback loop to the central nervous system by blocking intrafusal fibers, resulting in decreased activation of muscle spindles[45]. This effectively alters the sensory afferent system by reducing the traffic along Ia spindle afferent fibers. Unfortunately, the results from controlled studies does not support the use of BoNT-A in patients with tension-type headache.

In a recent placebo-controlled study, 40 patients were randomized to receive BoNT-A (maximum 100 U) or placebo (saline) in muscles with increased tenderness[46]. After 12 weeks there was no significant difference between the two treatment groups in decrease of headache intensity on VAS (-3.5 mm, 95 per cent confidence interval (CI) -20 to $+13$), mean number of headache days (-7%; 95% CI -20 to $+4$), headache hours per day (-1.4%; 95% CI -3.9 to $+1.1$), days on which symptomatic treatment was taken (-1.9%; 95% CI -11 to $+7$) and number of analgesics taken per day (-0.01%; 95% CI $-0.25-0.22$). There was no significant difference in patient's assessment of improvement after weeks 4, 8, and 12.

In another prospective, multicenter, randomized, double-blind, placebo-controlled trial, 112 patients with chronic tension-type headache were injected with 500 mouse units of botulinum toxin (Dysport®) or placebo into multiple pericranial muscles using a fixed-dose, fixed-site approach[47]. Injections were made following a fixed scheme and not adjusted to the patient's symptoms. There were no significant differences between the two groups when evaluating the area under the headache curve of 6 weeks before and 12 weeks after the treatment as the main effect measure. There were also no differences between the two groups on multiple secondary effect measures such as the number of days with headache, the number of days with intake of analgesics, the duration of the nocturnal sleep, and the Beck Depression Inventory score.

11.6 Tolerability

The clinical dose of BoNT-A commonly used for headache therapy is between 25–260 U, which is 30–120 times below the toxic limit[48]. Most of the trials published have reported mild and transient AEs. In a placebo-controlled double-blind trial, Silberstein and colleagues found that while no serious AEs occurred, some patients receiving BoNT-A injections experienced transient minor AEs including blepharoptosis, diplopia, and injection site weakness[19]. The authors also found that the injection of high doses of BoNT-A (75 U) resulted in a dose-dependent increase in the side effect profile of BoNT-A. Similarly, in the Mathew study, where dosages ranged from 105–265 U, the incidence of adverse events was higher in the BoNT-A group (BoNT-A, 76.1%; placebo, 63.1%; $P = 0.033$)[42]. The incidence of muscular weakness, neck pain, blepharoptosis, and skin tightness was significantly greater in the BoNT-A treatment population, as compared to placebo; however, for most adverse events, the incidence did not differ significantly between treatment groups. Most adverse events were transient and mild to moderate in severity.

11.7 Injection strategy

The most common sites of injections include the glabellar (procerus and corrugator), frontal, temporal, and sometimes the occipital regions (Figures 11.1–11.3). BoNT-A is administered either at fixed injection sites; at sites of pain or tenderness ('follow the pain'); or a combination of both[44]. The total dosage of toxin, the number of units per site of injection, dilution of toxin, and sites of injection varied widely, however, between studies and among investigators. The total dosage ranged from 25 to 300 U over several injection sites.

The fixed-site approach consists of bilateral injections, even if the patient has strictly unilateral headaches. The muscles injected are the procerus, corrugators, frontalis, and temporalis. Follow-the-pain injection sites are identified by history ('Where does it hurt when you have a headache?' and 'Show me with your hands where the pain is') and by examination of the cervical paraspinal, shoulder girdle, and temporomandibular musculature. These sites include the temporalis, occipitalis, trapezius, splenius capitus, suboccipital, and cervical paraspinal muscles.

For patients with migraine or migrainous headache features by history, treatment with a fixed-site approach may be required for successful results. When only a follow-the-pain approach is used in patients with migraine or migrainous headache, two problems arise: first, a poor cosmetic outcome; and second, the headaches may shift to the previously unaffected side. Even in these cases, cosmetic effects in the frontal region need to be obtained, but asymmetric injections can be given in the temporalis, occipitalis, splenius capitus, cervical, and subcervical paraspinal muscles. The doses injected in the cervical-shoulder girdle

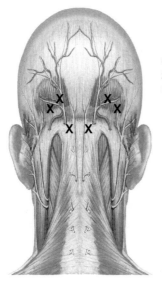

Occipitalis/suboccipital
25–50 units total
(6 injection sites)

Figure 11.2   Posterior injections using a follow-the-pain strategy.

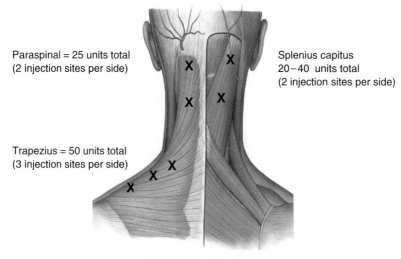

Paraspinal = 25 units total
(2 injection sites per side)

Splenius capitus
20–40 units total
(2 injection sites per side)

Trapezius = 50 units total
(3 injection sites per side)

X = injection sites for
each muscle group

Figure 11.3   Posterior injections using a follow-the-pain strategy.

muscles are low to prevent any possible weakness, which could cause headache. Patients need to be assessed carefully for associated cervical dystonia, which requires injection of the dystonic muscles.

Current available data do not seem to indicate a dose–response benefit. There is a need for further randomized, placebo-controlled clinical trials to identify the optimal dosing regimen and injection sites for BoNT-A. Some data, however, including the recently reported controlled studies in patients with CDH, report greater efficacy with repeated dosing[42,43]. Until results of large, well-conducted trials are available, optimal method of BoNT-A delivery remains unresolved.

11.8 Conclusion

The efficacy and safety profile of BoNT-A suggest that it is an effective, well-tolerated prophylactic treatment in migraine patients with CDH who are not using other prophylactic headache treatments. The data also suggest that assessment of the frequency of headaches is a sensitive measure of efficacy in this patient population and that future studies to confirm these findings are needed. The data at this time do not support the efficacy of BoNT-A for the treatment of episodic migraine or chronic tension-type headache. Further studies are needed to evaluate subgroups of migraine sufferers with frequent headache. Optimal dosing and injection regimens are not yet known. Dosages as low as 25 units are effective, and adverse side effects, which are often mild to moderate and transient, appear to be dose-dependent. A combination of fixed anterior injections with a follow-the-pain approach appears to be optimal, but further controlled studies are necessary to determine the most effective injection regimens.

REFERENCES

1. Lipton, R. B., Stewart, W. F., Diamond, S., Diamond, M. L. and Reed, M. (2001). Prevalence and burden of migraine in the United States: data from the American Migraine Study II. *Headache*, **41**, 646–57.
2. Menken, M., Munsat, T. L. and Toole, J. F. (2000). The global burden of disease study: implications for neurology. *Arch. Neurol.*, **57**, 418–20.
3. Hu, X. H., Markson, L. E., Lipton, R. B., Stewart, W. F. and Berger, M. L. (1999). Burden of migraine in the United States: disability and economic costs. *Arch. Intern. Med.*, **159**, 813–18.
4. Thom, T. J. (1996). Economic costs of neoplasms, arteriosclerosis, and diabetes in the United States. *In Vivo*, **10**, 255–9.
5. Weiss, K. B., Gergen, P. J. and Hodgson, T. A. (1992). An economic evaluation of asthma in the United States. *N. Engl. J. Med.*, **326**, 862–6.
6. Goadsby, P. J., Lipton, R. B. and Ferrari, M. D. (2002). Migraine: current understanding and treatment. *N. Engl. J. Med.*, **346**, 257–70.

7. Scher, A. I., Stewart, W. F., Ricci, J. A. and Lipton, R. B. (2003). Factors associated with the onset and remission of chronic daily headache in a population-based study. *Pain*, **106**, 81–9.

8. Scher, A. I., Stewart, W. F., Liberman, J. and Lipton, R. B. (1998). Prevalence of frequent headache in a population sample. *Headache*, **38**, 497–506.

9. Silberstein, S. D. (2000). Practice parameter: evidence-based guidelines for migraine headache (an evidence-based review). *Neurology*, **55**, 754–62.

10. Silberstein, S. D. and Goadsby, P. J. (2002). Migraine: preventive treatment. *Cephalalgia*, **22**, 491–512.

11. Lipton, R. B., Scher, A. I., Kolodner, K. *et al.* (2002). Migraine in the United States: epidemiology and patterns of health care use. *Neurology*, **58**, 885–94.

12. Dolly, O. (2003). Synaptic transmission: inhibition of neurotransmitter release by botulinum toxins. *Headache*, **43**(Suppl. 1), S16–S24.

13. Zalvan, C., Bentsianov, B., Gonzalez-Yanes, O. and Blitzer, A. (2004). Noncosmetic uses of botulinum toxin. *Dermatol. Clin.*, **22**, 187–95.

14. Aoki, K. R. (2003). Evidence for antinociceptive activity of botulinum toxin type A in pain management. *Headache*, **43**(Suppl. 1), 9–15.

15. Cui, M., Khanijou, S., Rubino, J. and Aoki, K. R. (2004). Subcutaneous administration of botulinum toxin A reduces formalin-induced pain. *Pain*, **107**, 125–33.

16. Durham, P. L. and Cady, R. (2004). Regulation of calcitonin gene-related peptide secretion from trigeminal nerve cells by botulinum toxin type A: implications for migraine therapy. *Headache*, **44**, 35–42; discussion 42–3.

17. Oshinsky, M. L., Pozo-Rosich, P., Luo, J., Hyman, S. and Silberstein, S. (2004). Botulinum toxin type A blocks sensitization of neurons in the trigeminal nucleus caudalis. *Cephalalgia*, **24**, 781.

18. Burstein, R. and Jakubowski, M. (2004). Analgesic triptan action in an animal model of intracranial pain: a race against the development of central sensitization. *Ann. Neurol.*, **55**, 27–36.

19. Silberstein, S., Mathew, N., Saper, J., Jenkins, S. *et al.* (2000). Botulinum toxin type A as a migraine preventive treatment. *Headache*, **40**, 445–50.

20. Barrientos, N. and Chana, P. (2003). Botulinum toxin type A in prophylactic treatment of migraine headaches: a preliminary study. *J. Headache Pain*, **4**, 146–51.

21. Tepper, S., Bigal, M., Sheftell, F. and Rapoport, A. (2004). Botulinum neurotoxin type A in the preventative treatment of refractory headache: a review of 100 consecutive cases. *Headache*, **44**, 794–800.

22. Troost, B. T. (2004). Botulinum toxin type A (BOTOX®) in the treatment of migraine and other headaches. *Expert Rev. Neurotherapeutics*, **41**, 27–31.

23. Blumenfeld, A. (2003). Botulinum toxin type A as an effective prophylactic treatment in primary headache disorders. *Headache*, **43**, 853–60.

24. Brin, M. F., Binder, W. J., Blitzer, A, Schenrock, L. and Pogoda, J. M. (2002). Botulinum toxin type A for pain and headache. In M. F. Brin, M. Hallett and J. Jankovic, eds., *Scientific and Therapeutic Aspects of Botulinum Toxin*. New York: Lippincott Williams & Wilkins, pp. 233–50.

25. Evers, S., Vollmer-Hasse, J., Schwaag, S. *et al.* (2004). Botulinum toxin A in the prophylactic treatment of migraine – a randomized, double-blind, placebo-controlled study. *Cephalalgia*, **24**, 838–43.

26. Scher, A. I., Stewart, W. F., Liberman, J. and Lipton, R. B. (1999). Prevalence of frequent headache in a population sample. *Headache*, **38**(7), 497–506.

27. Castillo, J., Munoz, P., Guitera, V. and Pascual, J. (1999). Epidemiology of chronic daily headache in the general population. *Headache*, **39**(3), 190–6.

28. Wang, S. J., Fuh, J. L., Lu, S. R., Liu, C. Y., Hsu, L. C., Wang, P. N. *et al.* (2000). Chronic daily headache in Chinese elderly: prevalence, risk factors and biannual follow-up. *Neurology*, **54**(2), 314–19.

29. Pascual, J., Colas, R. and Castillo, J. (2001). Epidemiology of chronic daily headache. *Curr. Pain Headache Rep.*, **5**(6), 529–36.

30. Lanteri-Minet, M., Auray, J. P., El Hasnaoui, A., Dartigues, J. F., Duru, G., Henry, P. *et al.* (2003). Prevalence and description of chronic daily headache in the general population in France. *Pain*, **102**(1–2), 143–9.

31. Mathew, N. T., Reuveni, U. and Perez, F. (1987). Transformed or evolutive migraine. *Headache*, **27**, 102–6.

32. D'Amico, D., Usai, S., Grazzi, L., Rigamonti, A., Solari, A. and Leone, M. *et al.* (2003). Quality of life and disability in primary chronic daily headaches. *Neurol. Sci.*, **24**(Suppl. 2), S97–S100.

33. Guitera, V., Munoz, P., Castillo, J. and Pascual, J. (2002). Quality of life in chronic daily headache: a study in a general population. *Neurology*, **58**(7), 1062–5.

34. Wang, S. J., Fuh, J. L., Lu, S. R., Juang, K. D. (2001). Quality of life differs among headache diagnoses: analysis of SF-36 survey in 901 headache patients. *Pain*, **89**(2–3), 285–92.

35. Mathew, N. T., Stubits, E. and Nigam, M. R. (1982). Transformation of episodic migraine into daily headache: analysis of factors. *Headache*, **22**, 66–8.

36. Saper, J. R., Silberstein, S. D., Lake, A. E. and Winters, M. E. (1994). Double-blind trial of fluoxetine: chronic daily headache and migraine. *Headache*, **34**, 497–502.

37. Krymchantowski, A. V., Silva, M. T., Barbosa, J. S. and Alves, L. A. (2002). Amitriptyline versus amitriptyline combined with fluoxetine in the preventative treatment of transformed migraine: a double-blind study. *Headache*, **42**, 510–14.

38. Spira, P. J., Beran, R. G., for the Australian Gabapentin Chronic Daily Headache Group. (2003). *Neurology*, **61**, 1753–9.

39. Saper, J. R., Lake, A. E., Cantrell, D. T., Winner, P. K. and White, J. R. (2002). Chronic daily headache prophylaxis with tizanidine: a double-blind, placebo-controlled, multicenter outcome study. *Headache*, **42**, 470–82.

40. Silvestrini, M., Bartolini, M., Coccia, M., Baruffaldi, R., Taffi, R. and Provinciali, L. (2003). Topiramate in the treatment of chronic migraine. *Cephalalgia*, **23**, 820–4.

41. Ondo, W. G., Vuong, K. D. and Derman, H. S. (2004). Botulinum toxin A for chronic daily headache: a randomized, placebo-controlled, parallel design study. *Cephalalgia*, **24**, 60–5.

42. Mathew, N. T., Frishberg, B. M., Gawel, M., Dimitrova, R., Gibson, J., Turkel, C., for the BOTOX CDH Study Group. (2005). *Headache*, **45**, 293–307.

43. Dodick, D. W., Mauskop, A., Elkind, A. H., DeGryse, R., Brin, M. F. and Silberstein, S. D., for the BOTOX CDH Study Group. (2005). *Headache*, **45**, 315–24.

44. Dodick, D. W. (2003). Botulinum neurotoxin for the treatment of migraine and other primary headache disorders: from bench to bedside. *Headache*, **43**, 25–9.

45. Rosales, R., Arimura, K., Takenaga, S. and Osame, M. (1996). Extrafusal and intrafusal muscle effects in experimental botulinum toxin-A injection. *Muscle Nerve*, **19**, 488–95.

46. Padberg, M., de Bruijn, S. F. T. M., de Haan, R. J. *et al.* (2004). Treatment of chronic tension-type headache with botulinum toxin: a double-blind, placebo-controlled clinical trial. *Cephalalgia*, **24**, 675–80.

47. Schulte-Mattler, W. J. and Krack, P., BoNTTH Study Group. (2004). Treatment of chronic tension-type headache with botulinum toxin A: a randomized, double-blind, placebo-controlled multicenter study. *Pain*, **109**, 110–14.

48. Brin, M. F. (1997). Botulinum toxin: chemistry, pharmacology, toxicity, and immunology. *Muscle Nerve*, **20** (Suppl. 6), S146–S168.

Botulinum toxin in the management of back and neck pain

Áine Carroll

The National Rehabilitation Hospital, Dun Laoghaire, Co. Dublin, Ireland

12.1 Introduction

Musculoskeletal problems are the most common cause of disability in the UK[1].

Most literature regarding spinal pain concentrates on acute or chronic low back pain rather than neck and thoracic spine pain. Pain from the spinal region, e.g. neck and the low back, is a major health problem in the industrialized world[2-5]. Although spinal pain is common, its aetiology remains obscure. The association between symptoms, imaging results and anatomical or physiological changes, is weak. Despite often exhaustive investigations, up to 85 per cent of patients with low back pain, will find no definite causal diagnosis[5]. Similar findings apply to neck and shoulder pain[6].

The most common site of spinal pain is the lower back. Neck pain appears to be almost as frequent, while thoracic pain is less prevalent[3,4]. Neck symptoms are often poorly differentiated from pain in the shoulder region and the two are therefore often combined[3]. Low back pain and neck pain frequently occur together.

In developed countries, in excess of 70 per cent of the population can expect to experience back pain at some time in their lives [2,3]. Each year, 15–45 per cent of adults suffer from back pain, and one in 20 people present to a hospital with a new episode. Low back pain presents most commonly between the ages of 35 and 55 years[3]. The vast majority of patients suffer from pain, which is usually moderate or severe and is generally benign. In most, the episode of back pain is acute and resolves spontaneously within 6 weeks. However, in approximately 20 per cent, the pain may persist or relapse over the following year[7].

The Clinical Standards Advisory Group (CSAG) was set up in 1991 as an independent source of expert advice to the UK Health Ministers and to the NHS on standards of clinical care for, and access to and availability of services to

Clinical Uses of Botulinum Toxins, eds. Anthony B. Ward and Michael P. Barnes. Published by Cambridge University Press. © Cambridge University Press 2007.

NHS patients. In October 1992 CSAG was asked by the Health Ministers to 'advise on the standards of clinical care for, and access to and availability of services to, NHS patients with back pain'. Its recommendations were published in 1994, together with the government's response[8]. The CSAG found that at the time of the survey, 6 per cent of employed people with back pain lost at least one working day secondary to the back pain in the previous four weeks[9]. This is equivalent to 1.9 per cent of all employed people losing at least one day in 4 weeks, and includes 0.3 per cent who were on sick leave for the entire 4 weeks. The estimate of total working days lost in Britain is 52 million days (with 95% confidence intervals of 35–69 million days).

They also found that half the total days lost due to back pain are due to the 85 per cent of people who are off work for short periods (less than seven days), and half by the 15 per cent of people who are off work for longer than one month. The longer a person is off work with back pain, the lower their chance of returning to work. After six months there is about a 50 per cent chance of returning to work; this has fallen to about 25 per cent at 1 year and 10 per cent by 2 years.

12.2 Costs

The CSAG estimated that the annual cost of managing back pain to the National Health Service (NHS) is £481 million a year (range £356–£649 million). Non-NHS costs (such as private consultations and prescriptions) add an additional £197 million to the bill. The costs of social security benefits is estimated at approaching £1.4 billion with the price of lost production as a result of sick leave being estimated at £3.8 billion[9]. This breaks down to an annual NHS cost to a purchasing authority of 250 000 people of £2.2 million (range £1.6–£2.9 million). Thus, in a typical general practice (GP) with five GPs and 10 000 patients, the cost of such patients is approximately £88 000 per annum (range £65 000–£118 000).

12.3 Clinical management

It is clear therefore that it is in the interest of the individual and society as a whole that back and neck pain are treated efficiently and effectively to reduce the socio-economic burden of such conditions. There are guidelines available from the UK Royal College of General Practitioners and also the UK Department of Health to assist in the management of patients with back and neck pain, covering history, examination, radiographic investigations and treatment[10]. Koes et al. in 2001 compared national clinical guidelines for the management of low back pain in primary care from 11 different countries. They concluded that the comparison of the clinical guidelines showed that diagnostic and therapeutic recommendations were generally similar. They found that updates of the guidelines were planned in most countries, although so far produced only in the UK. They felt that new evidence might lead to stronger conclusions and enable future guidelines to become more concordant[12].

12.4 Treatment

The aim of treatment is to relieve pain and return patients to their normal activities as soon as possible. It is clear from the CSAG that the time scale of management is important. There is clear evidence that the longer the duration of back pain and of time off work, the less successful the outcome of treatment and the lower the chance of getting back to work. Therefore, the first six weeks are crucial in reducing the development of chronic pain and disability.

Any treatment strategy depends on establishing a working diagnosis. Back pain can be divided into those patients with pain associated with serious spinal pathology (around 1 per cent), nerve root compression (up to 4 per cent), and those with mechanical or 'simple' low back pain (around 95 per cent).

Laboratory and imaging studies, performed as indicated, provide information that can be useful in establishing a diagnosis and developing a treatment plan in a patient with acute back pain. If no significant improvement in symptoms is noted after 4–6 weeks of treatment, the physician should reassess the patient. To avoid misdiagnosis and unnecessary or inappropriate treatments, the physician may then want to refer the patient to a spine specialist.

There is an abundance of research to guide in the management of acute low back pain and to a lesser extent neck pain. Research, however, is lacking to advise in the management of chronic spinal pain.

12.5 General guidance

12.5.1 Reassurance

People with acute simple low back pain should be reassured that the condition is not serious and should resolve quickly[13].

12.5.2 Bed rest

This was once a mainstay of management but has been found in recent times to not be of benefit or indeed to be detrimental.

Bed rest for 2–7 days is worse than placebo or ordinary activity[12]. It is less effective than alternative treatments for pain relief, rate of recovery, return to daily activities, or days lost from work[14]. Prolonged bed rest may lead to debilitation, chronic disability, and increasing difficulty in rehabilitation. There is insufficient evidence to recommend bed rest in people with chronic low back pain[15].

12.5.3 Activity modification

Patients should be advised to remain active. Current evidence suggests that staying active accelerates recovery from the acute attack and leads to reduced chronic disability and less time off work[16,17]. There is currently insufficient evidence on the effect of this advice in people with chronic low back pain. Additional advice on improving posture, taking exercise, lifting, bending, sitting, driving, and choice of mattress may be helpful[18]. Patient education about low back pain is recommended if the treatment programme is to succeed[19].

12.5.4 Medication

Simple analgesia

Simple analgesics such as paracetamol are first line in the management of acute spinal pain. They provide symptomatic relief during the days or weeks in which natural recovery is expected. Paracetamol is more effective when used regularly than as required for reducing low back pain. Long-term use is not well established in chronic pain[11].

Nonsteroidal anti-inflammatory drugs (NSAIDs)

These tend to be the pharmacological mainstay of treatment in acute spinal pain[20], they are appropriate for second-line use in the absence of contraindications and when simple analgesia alone is inadequate. The efficacy of NSAIDs in chronic low back pain has been assessed by only a few trials and the methodology was too different for the data to be pooled. The evidence to support their use is therefore limited[11].

Compound analgesics

Combinations of paracetamol and weak opioids may be effective alternatives when paracetamol or NSAIDs alone do not provide adequate pain control, although no quality studies compare their relative efficacy in acute spinal pain. Codeine is the agent of choice to be taken with paracetamol, as there is more established risk: benefit data available to support its use over other weak opioids[22]. Compound analgesics are often associated with an increased incidence of adverse effects. Separate prescriptions of paracetamol and codeine are preferred, to facilitate titration of the most effective and safe analgesic dose to match the individual's requirements[21].

Strong opioids

Strong opioids, e.g. morphine, appear to be no more effective in relieving acute spinal pain than other analgesics such as paracetamol and NSAID. Strong opioids have many adverse effects, including drowsiness, decreased reaction times, and potential physical dependence. The use of strong opioid analgesics in the management of chronic, nonmalignant, low back pain is controversial because of the risk of addiction. It is therefore not endorsed[23].

Muscle relaxants

Muscle relaxants have been shown to effectively reduce acute low back pain and muscle tension, and improve mobility[24]. There is limited evidence from the literature to support use of muscle relaxants in neck pain[25]. Their efficacy in reducing acute low back pain is fairly well established[26] and they may provide relief in acute episodes[16]. Diazepam is the most widely prescribed. Muscle relaxants have significant adverse effects, including drowsiness and potential physical dependence, even after relatively short courses. For these reasons they should only be used in people who have significant spasm. The optimal course length is 3−7 days, and for a maximum of 2 weeks. Comparisons of effectiveness with NSAIDs have been inconclusive.

Antidepressants

Antidepressants as analgesics are not licensed for this purpose in the UK although they are widely prescribed for this purpose. There are currently no randomized controlled trials of their use in acute spinal pain and therefore insufficient evidence of their relative efficacy is available[11,16]. A recent systematic review of the effect of antidepressants (from different classes) on chronic low back pain filtered out nine randomized placebo-controlled trials that included 504 people[27]. The systematic review found that people treated with antidepressants demonstrated a small but significant improvement in pain severity (standardized mean difference 0.41; 95% CI +0.22 to +0.61) but there was no statistically significant improvement in the ability to perform activities of daily living (standardized mean difference 0.24; 95% CI −0.21 to +0.69). The benefit of tricyclic antidepressants (TCAs) in chronic low back pain remains controversial, but an initial 1-month trial of therapy may be worth considering[26,28,29].

Anticonvulsants

Anticonvulsants such as carbamazepine and gabapentin are sometimes used in the management of chronic pain but no trial data is available to support their use in chronic low back pain.

12.5.5 Physical therapy modalities

Superficial heat (hydrocolloid packs), ultrasound (deep heat), cold packs, and massage are useful for relieving symptoms in the acute phase after the onset of low back pain. These modalities provide analgesia and muscle relaxation. However, their use should be limited to the first 2–4 weeks after the injury. The use of deep heat may be subject to a number of restrictions[30].

No convincing evidence has demonstrated the long-term effectiveness of lumbar traction[31] and transcutaneous electrical stimulation[32] in relieving symptoms or improving functional outcome in patients with acute low back pain. Therapy should emphasize the patient's responsibility for spine care and injury prevention.

Lumbar corsets and supports

Lumbar corsets and supports are used in the prevention and treatment of non-specific low back pain. There is limited evidence that lumbar supports are more effective than no treatment. However, a recent systematic review found the methodological quality of comparative studies to be poor and consequently the effect of lumbar supports remains unclear[33].

Back schools

Back schools, where groups of people with back pain receive education and skills (e.g. exercises), supervised by a specialist. There is conflicting evidence on the effects of back schools in people with acute or chronic low back pain. However, in occupational settings back schools have been found to be more effective than no treatment in people with chronic low back pain[34].

Behavioural therapy

There is limited evidence that cognitive, operant, and respondent behavioural therapy improved pain relief compared with certain other interventions in acute low back pain[35]. In people with chronic low back pain, evidence has found that behavioural therapy has a moderate effect on pain and a mild effect on disability compared with no treatment[35]. There is conflicting evidence on the effectiveness of behavioural therapy compared to other treatments.

Multidisciplinary programmes

These intensive physical and psychosocial programmes involve a variety of different health professionals and aim to improve function and help people to cope with their symptoms. Limited evidence has found that multidisciplinary rehabilitation led to a faster return to work[36]. In people with severe chronic low back pain, multidisciplinary intervention improved pain relief, functional status, and return to work moderately more than traditional inpatient rehabilitation or usual care, up to 1 year.

Evidence for the benefit of other osteopathic or chiropractic treatments is inconclusive. Only registered members of a recognized professional association should carry out these treatments.

12.5.6 Epidural, facet joint, and local injections with anaesthetics and/or steroids

These interventions have been evaluated in chronic low back pain. Because of a lack of well-designed trials, there is insufficient evidence to demonstrate whether they are effective. The evidence to support the use of facet joint injections appears to be particularly limited[37,38,39].

12.5.7 Percutaneous radiofrequency neurotomy

Chronic pain following whiplash injury has been treated with percutaneous radiofrequency neurotomy to denature the nerves innervating the painful joint. One small open trial found complete relief from pain in 71 per cent of patients[40] but the procedure has been unsuccessful in treating low back pain.

12.5.8 Indications for surgical evaluation

Research comparing the outcomes of conservative and surgical management of back pain have revealed no clear advantage for surgery[41]. Patients with acute low back pain that have 'red flags' on history and examination should undergo immediate surgical evaluation. Patients with suspected cauda equina lesions require immediate surgical investigation. Surgical evaluation is also indicated in patients with deteriorating neurological deficits or intractable pain that is resistant to conservative treatment.

12.5.9 Surgical interventions

Intervertebral disc herniation causing nerve root impingement is one of the more common indications for surgical intervention, although most patients respond to conservative therapy without surgery[42]. Therefore, a trial of conservative noninvasive treatment, followed by surgical intervention in nonresponders, is recommended. Many patients continue to experience some degree of pain postoperatively. Patients with spinal stenosis may require decompressive laminectomy to decrease direct pressure on neural elements. Finally, spinal fusion is performed on some patients with medically refractory mechanical low back pain, without obvious structural cause, to immobilize segments of the spinal column and to alleviate pain presumably caused by movements of these segments[43].

However, this procedure cannot be considered the definitive treatment for mechanical low back pain; in some patients, back pain becomes even more severe after surgery[44].

12.5.10   Other Recognized Modalities

Other therapies for chronic low back pain include facet joint anaesthetic and steroid injections, radiofrequency, and thermocoagulation of the intervertebral disc[45,46]. More rigorous study is needed to identify the subsets of patients who might benefit from such procedures, as well as the efficacy of the various modalities.

Botulinum toxin

Recently, botulinum toxin has emerged as a treatment option in the management of various musculoskeletal disorders and should be considered as a treatment option in those patients who have not responded to a more conventional approach[46–64].

Botulinum toxin is a neurotoxin produced by the anaerobic bacillus *Clostridium botulinum*. The bacteria produces seven serologically distinct toxins that are potent neuroparalytic agents. Although the seven neurotoxins are antigenically distinct, they possess similar molecular weights and have a common subunit structure consisting of a heavy chain and a light chain joined by a disulphide bond[65]. All serotypes interfere with neural transmission by blocking the release of acetylcholine (ACH), which is the principal neurotransmitter at the neuromuscular junction. After synaptic transmission is blocked by botulinum toxin, the muscles become clinically weak and atrophic.

Botulinum toxin appears to have a beneficial effect in various pain conditions, and this effect seems to be separate from the effects caused by neuromuscular transmission blockade. There are several hypotheses as to how botulinum toxin might exert its analgesic effect, including direct effects on muscle nociceptors, influence on sensitizing mediators, alteration of afferents derived from muscle spindles, physiological changes in reflex and synergistic movements, direct and secondary autonomic effects, and induced neuroplasticity in the central nervous system (CNS)[66]. Whether these mechanisms work in isolation or in combination is a matter for conjecture and may be related to the specific condition generating the pain, in addition to the behaviour and possibly the genetics of the patient.

Botulinum toxin in low back pain

To date, there is only one published randomized, placebo-controlled study of botulinum toxin type A for treatment of back pain[46,47]. Other data have been presented showing variable results for the use of type A for treatment of back pain, some failing to show statistical significance of efficacy[48,49]. However, it is difficult to extrapolate results across studies due to small sample sizes, differing methodologies, and varying back pain pathologies. As yet, there have been no randomized, placebo-controlled studies investigating the use of botulinum toxin type B in back pain. Current research suggests a positive role for botulinum toxin in the management of back pain but larger, more rigorously designed studies using similar methodologies and outcome measures are required to better clarify its efficacy.

Foster *et al.* in 2001 conducted a randomized, double-blind study investigating the effect of administration of type A into the paravertebral muscles of patients with chronic low back pain[46]. Thirty-one adults with low back pain of more than 6 months' duration and no acute lesions on magnetic resonance imaging (MRI) were enrolled in the study. They were randomized to receive type A ($n=15$) or normal saline ($n=16$). A physiatrist performed physical examinations and rated pain levels, and a neurologist performed all injections, which were administered at the site of the predominant pain at five paravertebral levels. Injections of 40 U of type A (0.4 ml of 100 U ml^{-1}) or 0.4 ml of saline was given at each level. Each patient was assessed before treatment and again at 3 and 8 weeks after treatment.

Of those who had received type A, 73 per cent reported significant pain relief at 3 weeks ($P=0.012$) and 60 per cent reported sustained relief at 2 months ($P=0.009$). Using the Oswestry Low Back Pain Questionnaire (OLBPQ), 66 per cent of type A recipients displayed a significant response at 8 weeks ($P=0.011$). In a follow-up interview at 6 months, responders indicated dissipation of the analgesic effect 3–4 months after treatment. There were no reported side effects. This double-blind study clearly demonstrated the efficacy of botulinum toxin type A in patients with unilateral low back pain although the sample size was small.

The use of botulinum toxin type B for the management of pain syndromes is now emerging in pain management circles. As with type A, initial data for type B suggest a possible role in treating back pain. In a recent prospective open label study, type B was evaluated for safety and efficacy as a treatment for chronic low back pain[48]. In Opida's study, participants ($n=35$) had chronic back spasms and back pain without radiating leg pain. They also had a reduced lumbar range of motion. Symptom severity was assessed using a numeric rating scale (NRS) before treatment and again at 4 and 12 weeks. The mean pretreatment NRS score was 9.4. Patients received 10 000 U of botulinum toxin type B divided equally among lumbar muscles (L2–L3, L3–L4, L4–L5, and L5–S1). After treatment, 23 patients (66%) reported a reduction in lumbar pain and improved lumbar range of motion. At 4 weeks and 12 weeks after injection, the mean NRS scores were significantly improved with scores of 3.6 ($P<0.001$) and 4.8 ($P<0.001$) respectively. The study limitations included its open-label design and the large number of patients lost to follow-up, which make any conclusions questionable.

Botulinum toxin in the management of myofascial pain syndrome (MPS)

There have been several reports of the beneficial effect of botulinum toxin in the management of refractory MPS[50–52]. More recently there have been more robust studies reported.

Lalli et al. studied 20 patients with MPS in a double-blind randomized trial of 50 U of botulinum toxin type A (BOTOX®; Allergan Pharmaceuticals, Irvine, CA) or 1% lidocaine[53]. Those that received toxin showed a statistically significant improvement in pain score and muscle spasm at weeks 2 and 4. Adding steroid did not appear to provide additional efficacy. Porta evaluated lidocaine/methylpred-nisolone versus type A (BOTOX®) in 40 patients with MPS in the psoas, piriformis, and scalenus anterior muscles in a single-blind randomized trial[54]. Patients received 80–150 U of type A or a similar volume of a steroid combined with a local anaesthetic. The reduction in pain scores was better in the toxin group at 30 days ($P=0.0598$) but did not reach significance until 60 days ($P=0.0001$). These studies support earlier findings of efficacy in treating refractory cases of MPS with type A[23–26]. Similar efficacy has been shown in studies of type B used to treat MPS[55–57].

De Andrés et al. performed an open-label interventional prospective trial in 77 patients with refractory MPS[58]. The outcome measures used were visual analogue scale (VAS) applied before enrollment, 15, 30, and 90 days and upon completion of the study; the Lattinen test to establish relationship between pain intensity and its corresponding impact on daily living; the hospital anxiety and depression scale (HAD) to assess psychologic stress, performed both before treatment and at the end of the study; and the Oswestry Questionnaire was used to evaluate patients' ability to carry out daily life activities according to their degree of physical impairment and disability scores. The global analysis revealed a positive correlation between the VAS score prior to treatment and the scoring at 15, 30, and 90 days. This correlation was maintained when analysing independently for superficial or deep muscles. The correlation coefficients for HAD scores and the Lattinen test values showed a significant association between pre- and post-treatment findings.

Some of the studies involving the use of botulinum toxin have been methodologically flawed. There have been studies that have included a mixed population of both MPS and fibromyalgia patients[59]. Questionable injection technique and suboptimal dosing may have affected response rates in some studies[49,60].

Botulinum toxin in the management of whiplash associated disorder

Intervention with botulinum toxin has been utilized in the management of chronic-whiplash patients in a pilot study in Canada, with encouraging results[61].

The pilot study was a randomized, double-blind, placebo-controlled study comparing outcome measures in 26 patients with chronic whiplash-associated disorder. Fourteen subjects received botulinum toxin and 12 received saline. The patients that received the toxin had a significant ($P < 0.01$) improvement in range of movement and subjective pain compared with the placebo group, but there was a trend to improvement only in subjective functioning.

Opida also demonstrated that type B may be of benefit in such patients in a prospective trial of 31 patients with whiplash-type neck pain and headaches[62]. In this study, 71 per cent of patients had significant reductions in pain and headache frequency and severity.

Taqi *et al.* also demonstrated significant positive results using type A in a prospective randomized trial in a more generic group of patients with cervicothoracic MPS[63]. He also found similar results in a retrospective study of type B in 40 patients. The results indicated that patients with cervicothoracic MPS appeared to respond better than those with lower back or gluteal pain[64].

12.6 Treatment protocol

12.6.1 Identification and injection of trigger points

There is currently no consensus on optimal injection technique and it would appear, on reviewing the current evidence, that the results of treatment seem positive regardless of the technique employed. It would appear that as long as the botulinum toxin is delivered to the targeted muscle, technique is of secondary importance. Targeting and technique will obviously be of more significance in smaller and less accessible muscles, e.g. the anterior muscles of the neck, when ultrasound guidance or EMG techniques will have to be employed.

The techniques involved usually involve the identification and injection of trigger points or the point of maximal pain on a muscle (Table 12.1).

Table 12.1. Equipment needed for trigger-point injection

Rubber gloves

Gauze

Alcohol wipes for skin cleansing

2.5/5 ml syringe

Botulinum toxin

Various gauge needles

Adhesive dressing

Most patients with back or neck pain exhibit tender areas in the larger muscles, often in conjunction with tight bands or knots. These tender areas do not always meet the definition of classic trigger points but it would seem reasonable to target treatment to the most tender areas or to trigger points if present.

Trigger points are discrete, focal, hyperirritable-table points located in a taut band of skeletal muscle. These points are painful on compression and can produce referred pain, referred tenderness, motor dysfunction, and autonomic phenomena[67].

The palpation of a hypersensitive bundle or nodule of muscle fibre of harder than normal consistency is the physical finding most often associated with a trigger point.

There are two techniques that can be used to palpate the trigger point (Figure 12.1):
1. Flat palpation
2. Pincer palpation

Flat palpation involves simply moving the fingertip(s) transversely across the muscles fibres, exerting a slight degree of pressure until a 'taut band' is located. Having found this tight section of the muscle, explore along its length to locate the spot of maximum tenderness with minimum pressure: that is the trigger point.

Pincer palpation involves grasping the belly of the muscle between the thumb and finger and squeezing the fibres between them with a back and forth rolling

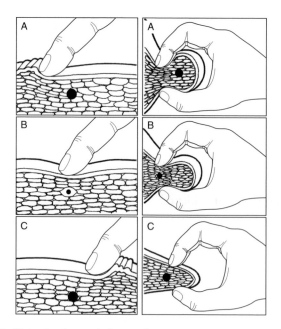

Figure 12.1   Flat palpation and pincer grip.

motion to locate taut bands. When a taut band is identified, it is then explored along its length to locate the point of maximal tenderness in response to minimal pressure; that is the trigger point.

12.7 Preinjection assessment

Botulinum toxin should be used only under close supervision in patients with disturbed neuromuscular transmission — for example, in myasthenia gravis or Lambert—Eaton myasthenic syndrome or during treatment with aminoglycosides. A history of coagulopathy should be checked and an enquiry made about anti-platelet or anticoagulant therapy. Botulinum toxin is contraindicated in preg-nancy and while breast-feeding.

The patient should have given written informed consent prior to the procedure.

The patient should be placed in a comfortable position to promote muscle relaxation. This is usually achieved by positioning the patient in the prone or supine position. This positioning may also help the patient to avoid injury where there is a vasovagal syncopal reaction.

12.8 Needle selection

The choice of needle size depends on the location of the muscle being injected. The needle must be sufficiently long to reach the most tender point or contraction knot in the trigger point to disrupt it. A 22-gauge, 1.5-inch needle is usually sufficient to reach most superficial muscles. For thick subcutaneous muscles such as the gluteus maximus or paraspinal muscles in persons who are not obese, a 21-gauge, 2.0-inch needle is usually necessary.

12.9 Injection solution

The amount of toxin used depends on the size of the muscle being injected and the number of trigger points. Table 12.2 shows suggested dosage regimens for par-ticular muscles based on current evidence.

12.10 Injection technique

Once the most tender area or trigger point has been identified and the overlying skin has been cleansed with alcohol, the clinician should immobilize the area either using a pinch between the thumb and index finger or between the index and middle finger (Figure 12.2).

Table 12.2. Suggested doses of botulinum toxin

Muscle	Suggested doses of botulinum toxin (units)		
	Allergan	Dysport	Myobloc
Trapezius	50–100	200–400	1000–5000
Sternocleidomastoid	20–50	80–200	1000–3000
Rhomboids	50–100	200–400	1000–5000
Supraspinatus	20–50	80–200	1000–3000
Scalaneus anterior or medius	20–50	80–200	1000–3000
Iliopsoas	20–50	80–200	1000–3000
Quadratus lumborum	20–50	80–200	1000–3000

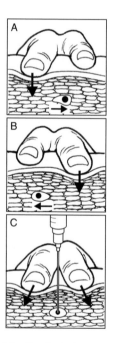

Figure 12.2 Injection technique.

Using an aseptic technique, the needle should be inserted 1–2 cm distant from the trigger point so that the needle can be advanced into the tender point/trigger point at an acute angle of 30 degrees to the skin. The stabilizing fingers should apply pressure on either side of the injection site, ensuring adequate tension of the muscle fibres to allow accurate penetration of the trigger point. As with all injection techniques, the plunger should be withdrawn before injection to ensure that the needle is not within a blood vessel. The injectant should then be introduced once the needle is in position.

12.11   Post-injection management

After injection, pressure should be applied to the injected area for a couple of minutes to promote haemostasis. A simple adhesive bandage may be applied if required, ensuring to check that the patient is not sensitive to such dressings.

12.12   Possible complications

The complications associated with treatment with botulinum toxin are rare – 1.1 per cent in >350 procedures. Transient swelling around the site of injection has been reported. Clinical weakness in the treated muscle and in adjacent musculature is thought to be dose related. Some people treated with botulinum toxin have reported a flu-like syndrome and a feeling of general fatigue[68].

There is as yet little evidence about how frequently these injections should be repeated and for how long. The follow-up in the published studies is relatively short. Experience in the management of dystonia and spasticity would suggest that treatment can be repeated every 3–4 months long-term without any adverse effects.

The use of botulinum toxin in spinal pain is usually well localized and the doses will therefore be insufficient to cause excessive weakness of paravertebral muscles. However, patients should be warned of this as a potential side effect.

12.13   Conclusion

Botulinum toxin is emerging as a useful adjunct therapy in the arsenal of weaponry against spinal pain. As long as patients have had serious spinal pathology excluded, botulinum toxin can be used to successfully treat pain in conjunction with simple analgesics and exercise programmes.

REFERENCES

1. Health Survey for England 2001 – Disability: A survey carried out on behalf of the Department of Health, Edited by Madhavi Bajekal, Paola Primatesta and Gillian Prior, Joint Health Surveys Unit National Centre for Social Research, Department of Epidemiology and Public Health at the Royal Free and University College Medical School. Published by The Stationery Office (ISBN 0-11-322601-2).
2. Waddell, G. (1996). Low back pain: a twentieth century health care enigma. *Spine*, **21**, 2820–5.
3. Andersson, G. B. J. (1997). The epidemiology of spinal disorders. In J. W. Frymoyer, ed., *The Adult Spine: Principles and Practice*, 2nd edn. Philadelphia: Lippincott-Raven Publishers, pp. 93–141.

4. Linton, S., Hellsing, A.-L. and Hallden, K. (1998). A population-based study of spinal pain among 35−45-year-old individuals: prevalence, sick leave and health care use. *Spine*, **23**, 1457−63.

5. Deyo, R. A. and Weinstein, J. N. (2001). Low-back pain. *New England Journal of Medicine*, **344**, 363−70.

6. Mäkelä, M., Heliövaara, M., Sievers, K., Impivaara, O., Knekt, P. and Aromaa, A. (1991). Prevalence, determinants, and consequences of chronic neck pain in Finland. *American Journal of Epidemiology*, **134**, 1356−67.

7. Webb, R., Brammah, T., Lunt, M., Urwin, M., Allison, T. and Symmons, D. (2003). Prevalence and predictors of intense, chronic and disabling neck and back pain in the UK general population. *Spine*, **28**(11), 1195−202.

8. Back Pain. Report of a CSAG Committee on Back Pain, 1994, HMSO.

9. Epidemiology Review: The Epidemiology and Cost of Back Pain. Clinical Standards Advisory Group, 1994, HMSO.

10. RCGP Clinical Guidelines for the Management of Acute Low Back Pain Review Date: December 2001.

11. Koes, B. W., van Tulder, M. W., Ostelo, R., Burton, K. and Waddell, G. (2001). Clinical guidelines for the management of low pain in primary care: an international comparison. *Spine*, **26**(22), 2504−14.

12. Deyo, R. A., Diehl, A. K. and Rosenthal, M. (1986). How many days of bed rest for acute low back pain? *New England Journal of Medicine*, **315**, 1064−70.

13. Van der Hoogen, H. J. M., Koes, B. W., van Eijk, K. T. M. *et al.* (1998). On the course of low back pain in general practice: a one year follow up study. *Annals of the Rheumatic Diseases*, **57**, 13−19.

14. Vroomen, P., de Krom, M., Wilmink, J. T. *et al.* (1999). Lack of effectiveness of bed rest for sciatica. *New England Journal of Medicine*, **340**, 418−23.

15. Hagen, K. B. (2001). *Bed Rest for Acute Low Back Pain and Sciatica* (Cochrane Review). The Cochrane Library (Issue 2), Oxford.

16. Waddell, G., Feder, G., McIntosh, A. *et al.* (1999). *Low Back Pain Evidence Review*. London: Royal College of General Practitioners.

17. Waddell, G., Feder, G. and Lewis, M. (1997). Systematic reviews of bed rest and advice to stay active for acute low back pain. *Br. J. Gen. Pract.*, **47**(423), 647−52.

18. Waddell, G. (1999). Chiropractic for low back pain. Evidence for manipulation is stronger than that for most orthodox medical treatments. *BMJ*, **318**(7178), 262.

19. Gilbert, J. R., Taylor, D. W., Hildebrand, A., *et al.* (1985). Clinical trial of common treatment for low back pain in family practice. *BMJ* (*Clin. Res. Ed*)., **66**, 791−4.

20. Porter, R. W. and Ralston, S. H. (1994). Pharmacological management of back pain syndromes. *Drugs*, **48**, 189−98.

21. de Craen, A. J., Di Giulio, G., Lampe-Schoenmaeckers, J. E., Kessels, A. G. and Kleijnen, J. (1996). Analgesic efficacy and safety of paracetamol−codeine combinations versus paracetamol alone: a systematic review. *BMJ*, **313**(7053), 321−5.

22. Moore, A., Collins, S., Carroll, D. and McQuay, H. (1997). Paracetamol with and without codeine in acute pain: a quantitative systematic review. *Pain*, **70**(2−3), 193−201.

23. Medicines Resource (1997). Management of chronic pain in the community. *Medicines Resource*, **41**, 159–60.

24. van Tulder, M. W., Touray, T., Furlan, A. D., Solway, S. and Bouter, L. M. (2003). Muscle relaxants for nonspecific low back pain: a systematic review within the framework of the Cochrane collaboration. *Spine*, **28**, 1978–92.

25. Aker, P. D., Gross, A. R., Goldsmith, C. H. and Peloso, P. (1996). Conservative management of mechanical neck pain: systematic overview and meta-analysis. *BMJ*, **313**, 1291–6.

26. Van Tulder, M. W., Koes, B. W. and Bouter, L. M. (1997). Conservative treatment of acute and chronic non-specific low back pain: a systematic review of randomized controlled trials of the most common interventions. *Spine*, **22**, 2128–56.

27. Salerno, S. M., Browning, R. and Jackson, J. L. (2002). The effect of antidepressant treatment on chronic back pain: a meta-analysis. *Archives of Internal Medicine*, **162**, 19–24.

28. Turner, J. A. and Denny, M. C. (1993). Do antidepressant medications relieve chronic low back pain? *Journal of Family Practice*, **37**, 545–53.

29. Fishbain, D. (2000). Evidence-based data on pain relief with antidepressants. *Annals of Medicine*, **32**, 305–16.

30. Lehmann, J. F. (1982). *Therapeutic Heat and Cold.* 3rd edn. Baltimore: Williams & Wilkins.

31. Beurskens, A. J., De Vet, M. C., Koke, A. J., Regtop, W., van der Heijden, G. J., Lindeman E. *et al.* (1997). Efficacy of traction for nonspecific low back pain. 12-week and 6-month results of a randomized clinical trial. *Spine*, **22**, 2756–62.

32. Herman, E., Williams, R., Stratford, P., Fargas-Babjak, A. and Trott, M. (1994). A randomized controlled trial of transcutaneous electrical nerve stimulation (CODETRON) to determine its benefits in a rehabilitation program for acute occupational low back pain. *Spine*, **19**, 561–8.

33. Van Tulder, M. W., Jellema, P., van Poppel, M. N. *et al.* (2000). Lumbar supports for prevention and treatment of low back pain (Cochrane Review). The Cochrane Library (Issue 2). Oxford

34. Van Tulder, M. W., Esmail, R., Bombardier, C. and Koes, B. W. (2000). Back schools for non-specific low back pain (Cochrane Review). The Cochrane Library (Issue 2). Oxford

35. Van Tulder, M. W., Ostelo, R., Vlaeyen, J. W. *et al.* (2001). Behavioral treatment for chronic low back pain: a systematic review within the framework of the Cochrane Back Review Group. *Spine*, **26**, 270–81.

36. Effective Health Care Bulletin (2000). Acute and chronic low back pain. *Effective Health Care*, **6**, 1–8.

37. Mathews, J. A., Mills, S. B., Jenkins, V. M. *et al.* (1987). Back pain and sciatica: controlled trials of manipulation, traction, sclerosant and epidural injections. *British Journal of Rheumatology*, **26**, 416–23.

38. Koes, B. W., Scholten, R. J., Mens, J. M. and Bouter, L. M. (1995). Efficacy of epidural steroid injections for low-back pain and sciatica: a systematic review of randomized clinical trials. *Pain*, **63**, 279–88.

39. Nelemans, P. J., Bie, R. A.D., Vet, H. C. W. D. and Sturmans, F. (2001). Injection therapy for subacute and chronic benign low back pain (Cochrane Review). The Cochrane Library (Issue 2). Oxford

40. McDonald, G. J., Lord, S. M. and Bogduk, N. (1999). Long-term follow-up of patients treated with cervical radiofrequency neurotomy for chronic neck pain. *Neurosurgery*, **45**, 61–8.

41. Nancy J. O. and Birkmeyer, J. N. (1999). Weinstein medical versus surgical treatment for low back pain. *Evidence and Clinical Practice, Effective Clinical Practice*, September/October.

42. Weber, H. (1983). Lumbar disc herniation. A controlled, prospective study with ten years of observation. *Spine*, **8**, 131–40.

43. Jens, I. B., Sorensen, R., Friis, A., Nygaard, O., Indahl, A., Keller, A., Ingebrigtsen, T., Eriksen, H., Holm, I., Koller, A. K., Riise, R. and Reikeras, O. (2003). Randomized clinical trial of lumbar instrumented fusion and cognitive intervention and exercises in patients with chronic low back pain and disc degeneration. *Spine*, **28**(17), 1913–21.

44. Indahl, A., Velund, L. and Reikeraas (1995). Good prognosis for low back pain when left untampered. A randomized clinical trial. *Spine*, **20**, 473–7.

45. Philip, S. K. (2002). Role of injection therapy: review of indications for trigger point injections, regional blocks, facet joint injections, and intra-articular injections. *Curr. Opin. Rheumatol.*, **14**, 52–7.

46. Foster, L., Clapp, L., Erickson, M. and Jabbari, B. (2001). Botulinum toxin A and chronic back pain: a randomized, double-blinded study. *Pain Practice*, **1**(4), 379–80.

47. Foster, L., Clapp, L., Erickson, M. and Jabbari, B. (2001). Botulinum toxin A and chronic low back pain: a randomized, double-blind study. *Neurology*, **56**(10), 1290–3.

48. Opida, C. L. (2002). Open-label study of MyoblocTM/Neurobloc (botulinum toxin type B) in the treatment of patients with chronic low back pain. Poster 202 presented at the *International Conference 2002: Basic and Therapeutic Aspect of Botulinum and Tetanus Toxins* : June 9, 2002. Hannover, Germany.

49. Knusel, B., DeGryse, R., Grant, M. *et al.* (1998). Intramuscular injection of botulinum toxin type A (BOTOX) in chronic low back pain associated with muscle spasm. Presented at *17th Annual Scientific Meeting, American Pain Society*, November 5–8, San Diego, California.

50. Acquadro, M. A. and Borodic, G. E. (1994). Treatment of myofascial pain with botulinum A toxin. *Anesthesiology*, **80**, 705–6 (Letter).

51. Alo, K. M., Yland, M. J., Kramer, D. L. *et al.* (1997). Botulinum toxin in the treatment of myofascial pain. *Pain Clinics*, **10**, 107–16.

52. Grana, E. A. (1998). Treatment of chronic cervical myofascial pain with botulinum toxin. *Arch. Phys. Med. Rehab.*, **79**, 1172. Royal, M. A., Gordin, V., Huebert, J. D. *et al.* (1999). Botulinum toxin type A botox in the treatment of refractory myofascial pain. Abstract presented at the *International Conference 1999: Basic and Therapeutic Aspects of Botulinum and Tetanus Toxins*, Orlando, FL, November 16–18, p. 73.

53. Lalli, F., Gallai, V., Tambasco, N. *et al.* (1999). Botulinum A toxin versus lidocaine in the treatment of myofascial pain: a double-blind randomized study. Presented at the *International Conference 1999: Basic and Therapeutic Aspects of Botulinum and Tetanus Toxins*, Orlando, FL, November 16–18.

54. Porta, M. (2000). A comparative trial of botulinum toxin type A and methylprednisolone for the treatment of myofascial pain syndrome and pain from chronic muscle spasm. *Pain*, **85**, 101–5.

55. Nalamachu, S. (2002). Treatment with botulinum toxin type B (Myobloc™) injections in three patients with myofascial pain. Abstract presented at the *AAPM 18th Annual Meeting*, San Francisco, CA, February 26–March 3.

56. Smith, H., Audette, J., Dey, R. *et al.* (2002). Botulinum toxin type B for a patient with myofascial pain. Abstract presented at the *AAPM 18th Annual Meeting*, San Francisco, CA, February 26–March 3.

57. Dubin, A., Smith, H. and Tang, J. (2002). Evaluation of botulinum toxin type B (Myobloc™) injections in a patient with painful muscle spasms. *Pain*, **3**(Suppl. 1), 11 (abstract).

58. De Andres, J., Cerda-Olmedo, G., Valia, J. C., Monsalve, V., Lopez-Alarcon and Minguez, A. (2003). Use of botulinum toxin in the treatment of chronic myofascial pain. *Clinical Journal of Pain*, **19**(4), 269–75.

59. Porta, M., Perretti, A., Gamba, M., Luccarelli, G. and Fornari, M. (1998). The rationale and results of treating muscle spasm and myofascial syndromes with botulinum toxin type A. *Pain Digest*, **8**, 346–52.

60. Wheeler, A. H., Goolkasian, P. and Gretz, S. S. (1998). A randomized, double-blind, prospective pilot study of botulinum toxin injection for refractory, unilateral cervicothoracic, paraspinal, myofascial pain syndrome. *Spine*, **23**, 1662–7.

61. Freund, B. J. and Schwartz, M. (2000). Treatment of whiplash-associated neck pain with botulinum toxin A: a pilot study. *Headache*, **40**, 231–6 and *J. Rheum.*, **27**, 481–4.

62. Opida, C. L. (2002). Evaluation of Myobloc™ (botulinum toxin type B) in patients with post-whiplash headaches. Abstract presented at the *AAPM 18th Annual Meeting*, San Francisco, CA, February 26–March 3.

63. Taqi, D., Gunyea, I., Bhakta, B. *et al.* (2002). Botulinum toxin type A in the treatment of refractory cervicothoracic myofascial pain. *Pain*, **3**(Suppl. 1), 16 (abstract).

64. Taqi, D., Royal, M., Gunyea, I. *et al.* (2002). Botulinum toxin type B (Myobloc™) in the treatment of refractory myofascial pain. *Pain*, **3**(Suppl. 1), 16 (abstract).

65. Schiavo, G., Rossetto, O., Santucci, A., DasGupta, B. R. and Montecucco, C. (1992). Botulinum neurotoxins are zinc proteins. *Journal of Biological Chemistry*, **267**, 23479–83.

66. Arezzo, J. C. (2002). Possible mechanisms for the effects of botulinum toxin on pain. *The Clinical Journal of Pain*, **18**(6), S125–S32.

67. Simons, D. G., Travell, J. G. and Simons, L. S. (1999). In Travell and Simons' *Myofascial Pain and Dysfunction: the Trigger Point Manual*. 2nd edn. Baltimore: Williams & Wilkins.

68. Lange, D. J., Brin, M. F., Warner, C. L., Fahn, S. and Lovelace, R. E. (1987). Distant effects of local injection of botulinum toxin. *Muscle and Nerve*, **10**, 552–5.

Clinical uses of botulinum toxin

John Elston

Oxford Eye Infirmary, Radcliffe Infirmary, Oxford, UK

13.1 Ophthalmological uses

13.1.1 Introduction

Botulinum toxin targets the cholinergic neuromuscular complex with exquisite precision producing dose dependent muscle weakness. The concept of using this property therapeutically was an ingenious and bold one, and it came from a thoughtful and innovative ophthalmologist over 30 years ago. Working at the time on extraocular muscle electromyography (EMG) Alan Scott of the Smith Kettlewell Eye Research Foundation was exploring the treatment potential of the ability to locate a needle tip at or near the motor point of extraocular muscles. Using an EMG guided injection technique could enable focal delivery of a drug — for example local anaesthetic — to modify muscle function. The ideal drug would need to remain localized at the injection point and have an effect on muscle function only, without inducing inflammation or scarring, either temporarily enhancing or more probably reducing function, over a predictable time frame. Full recovery of extraocular muscle function would be necessary to restore normal eye movement. During the period of induced muscle underactivity it was hypothesized that the balance between two opposing extraocular muscles (agonist:antagonist balance) would be altered in such a way that a permanent change in the relative position of the two eyes would be achieved after the effect of the drug had worn off. This created the possibility of treating misalignment of the eyes (strabismus or squint) by non-surgical means.

Scott investigated candidate drugs using EMG guided injections into the medial rectus of binocular primates under ketamine anaesthesia using, as well as botulinum toxin A, alpha-bungarotoxin (snake venom), DFP (di-isopropyl-fluoro-phosphate) and absolute alcohol.

Clinical Uses of Botulinum Toxins, eds. Anthony B. Ward and Michael P. Barnes. Published by Cambridge University Press. © Cambridge University Press 2007.

Scott's first publication on the subject was in 1973[1]. He successfully demonstrated that with proper dose control ocular malalignment (the creation of strabismus) could be achieved with a botulinum toxin injection into the medial rectus. A period of muscle paresis was followed by recovery of eye movement but a persistent divergent strabismus. The other substances used had considerable drawbacks; absolute alcohol was unpredictable in effect and caused intense local inflammation. Alpha-bungarotoxin's action was diffuse in the orbit and short-lived: DFP caused systemic toxicity. Work then began on using the method to treat strabismus in human subjects.

It is notable that Scott also speculated that the technique could be adapted to the treatment of unwanted muscle spasms (for example in blepharospasm) thereby anticipating the extraordinary expansion in the clinical use of botulinum toxin that has taken place since.

The two principle ophthalmological indications for botulinum toxin treatment remain the management of some categories of strabismus, and the treatment of blepharospasm and hemifacial spasm. Botulinum toxin has been used in clinical ophthalmology for longer than in any other discipline, giving the opportunity to fully explore and fine tune potential indications. As well as benefiting patients, the development of the treatment potential of botulinum in ophthalmology has given the opportunity to study and understand disorders, such as blepharospasm and extraocular muscle contracture, more fully. This review will detail the ophthalmological indications and highlight areas of clinical development that have been facilitated.

13.2   Strabismus

The injection technique utilizes 37 mm × 27 gauge EMG needles (insulated except at the tip) plus standard ground and reference electrodes. The signal from the muscle to be treated may be recorded with standard EMG equipment, or using a portable auditory signal generator. The lateral, medial and inferior rectus muscles are suitable for treatment. In adults, treatment is under topical anaesthesia, the retrobulbar portion of the muscle to be treated being approached transconjunctivally and activated (to give an EMG signal) by the subject by looking into the field of action of that muscle. In children ketamine anaesthesia (which retains spontaneous eye movements) plus local anaesthetic should be used (Table 13.1).

The extent of the muscle paresis after injection is dose dependent. The onset of paresis is within 24—48 hours, maximal at approximately one week, with a slow recovery over 8—12 weeks. The rationale for the treatment is that the resulting alteration in agonist : antagonist muscle dynamics will achieve some degree of permanent realignment of the visual axes once the full range of movement of the treated muscle returns.

The original hypothesis was that a period of 6–8 weeks botulinum-induced palsy of an extraocular muscle (with associated structural denervation changes in the muscle) would result in long term effective muscle 'lengthening' and contracture or shortening in the ipsilateral antagonist muscle. For example, in an individual with a convergent squint (esotropia), paralysing the medial rectus would lengthen that muscle and cause simultaneous contracture in the lateral rectus of the same eye. When medial rectus function recovered the balance of forces between these two muscles would have been altered so that the alignment of the treated eye would have been permanently changed in respect of the untreated eye.

Unfortunately (with the exception of infants, see below) in the absence of binocular function (i.e. motor and sensory stereopsis) to maintain a normal alignment of the eyes after a single treatment, the strabismus tends to recur to nearly the same angle as pre-treatment[2]. Lasting effects on alignment of the eyes are greatest in esotropia and consecutive exotropia and average 12 prism dioptres or 6 degrees. There is a tendency for a larger change in angle with the treatment of a larger squint. The relatively small change in permanent strabismus angle determines the most suitable cases for treatment as indicated below.

There are a number of preconditions; an adult must be able to understand the proposed treatment and cooperate – a sudden head movement could lead to a penetrating eye injury. High myopia is a contraindication because of the unpredictable thinning and expansion of the posterior segment of the eye (posterior staphyloma) increasing the risk of penetration. Multiple previous strabismus operations is a relative contraindication because of the excessive scar tissue complicating the technique. On the other hand, previous seriously traumatized eyes with low intraocular pressure (pre-phthisical) are unsuitable for eye muscle surgery, but good candidates for botulinum toxin treatment.

The commonest side effect is spread of the toxin to other (untreated) extra-ocular muscles. The lateral rectus and medial rectus are the usual muscles treated, and spread to the inferior rectus (possibly partly determined by gravity) may occur. It almost invariably resolves completely over 4–6 weeks. Partial upper lid ptosis may occur but is also self-limiting[2]. Side effects are commoner in children than in adults, even when using smaller total doses.

Trivial haemorrhage from trauma to the conjunctival vasculature is occasionally encountered; patients on anticoagulants, including aspirin, are at particular risk from this side effect so these drugs are a relative contraindication to the treatment. Anterior ciliary artery puncture can lead to extensive subconjunctival haemorrhage and a few cases of potentially vision damaging orbital haemorrhage have been described, at least one requiring surgical decompression.

13.3　Informed consent

It is important to obtain signed informed consent before treating strabismus with botulinum toxin injections. This imposes on the practitioner the duty to explain the concept of this intervention, the perceived benefits and any advantages it may have in the individual as against standard surgical treatment. Patients need to understand that the purpose of the treatment is to paralyse an eye muscle for a period of time, and that this in itself may produce other symptoms such as double vision as well as a temporary undesirable effect on appearance.

Single use disposable EMG injection electrodes should be used.

13.4　Indications

13.4.1　Childhood

Infantile esotropia

Infantile esotropia denotes a moderate to large angle convergent squint, evident either at birth or within the first few months of life. Each eye is healthy and moves normally. Amblyopia is unusual as the infant 'cross fixates', i.e. uses the left eye to look to the right and vice versa. The cause is not known and in most infants neurological development is otherwise completely normal. Theoretically if the eyes are realigned to normal early enough in the process of visual maturation there may be potential for binocular visual development, but in practice this is almost never achieved. Either standard surgical correction or realignment of the eyes with botulinum toxin carries the potential to create amblyopia, as cross fixation is no longer observed.

There is good evidence that this condition responds at least as well in terms of sensory and motor outcomes to simultaneous treatment of both medial rectus muscles with botulinum toxin in the first year of life as it does to standard surgery[3]. A period of over correction (exotropia) is anticipated after toxin treatment, resolving to leave a small stable residual esotropia. Repeat treatment may be required. This treatment is best given under ketamine and local anaesthetic but has been described under general anaesthetic with the conjunctiva opened to directly inject the muscles.

Unlike the situation in non-binocular adults when strabismus is almost invariably recurrent following botulinum toxin injections, in infants a long term

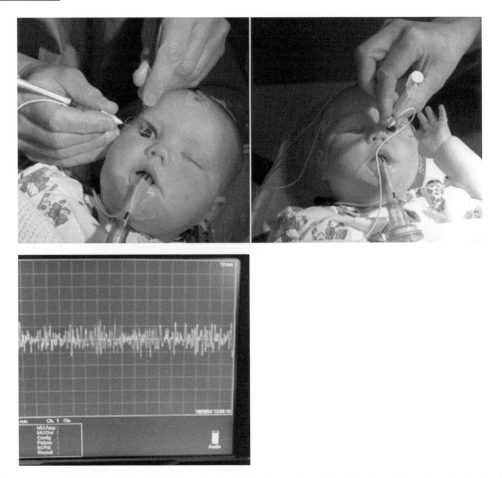

Figure 13.1 Injection of the medial rectus muscles in a 6-month-old using ketamine plus topical anaesthesia (pre-treatment with inhalational anaesthesia to intubate). Inset, the EMG signal from the muscle.

realignment of the visual axes by one simultaneous treatment of both medial rectus muscles may be achieved (Figure 13.1). The age at treatment appears to be critical and in one series a significantly better outcome in terms of alignment was achieved with treatment before or around the age of 6 months rather than from 7 months onwards[4]. As extraocular muscle function recovers a small (approximately 10 prism dioptres) residual esotropia remains with evidence of stability for 5 years and more. Sensory and motor binocular stereoscopic outcomes are as good with this treatment as with incisional surgery.

Children, who have been under-corrected by surgical treatment of infantile esotropia, have a good outcome from botulinum toxin treatment of the residual esotropia without the need for further surgery[5].

A major advantage of botulinum toxin versus surgery is the absence of scarring. Any eye muscle surgery needed later in life should be more predictable. Botulinum toxin treatment can be carried out at an age (4–6 months) when surgical treatment is technically challenging because of the small size of the orbit relative to the eye. Theoretically, the earlier the age of ocular alignment the better the chance of binocular function developing.

Many infantile esotropes will in later childhood develop anomalies of vertical alignment of the eyes, including oblique muscle dysfunction and the phenomenon of dissociated vertical deviation. If some degree of motor and sensory stereopsis can be established by early botulinum toxin treatment, the incidence and extent of these vertical alignment anomalies may be reduced.

Because of the size of the orbit in infants, the side effects of spread of paralytic effect to the levator and vertically acting muscles are more common. This is one reason why small doses of toxin to both medial rectus muscles are used – asymmetric partial ptosis is less likely to lead to amblyopia than a more profound unilateral ptosis.

Parents of children with infantile esotropia are entitled to be offered this effective non-surgical treatment of their child. Failure of toxin treatment does not prejudice future standard strabismus surgery. A detailed explanation of the relative efficacy of injection versus surgical treatment will be required, together with the risks and benefits of the two treatment alternatives.

Other Childhood strabismus

Specific syndromes

1. *Paediatric VIth nerve palsy* (occurring during visual maturation) of any aetiology may cause amblyopia and loss of developing binocular functions. Botulinum treatment of the ipsilateral medial rectus should be considered to prevent this. Low dose treatment is required as the side effects of either ptosis or vertical deviation will nullify the potential benefit of aligning the eyes in the straight ahead position. This treatment may therefore have to be repeated for the required beneficial effect to be achieved. It is obviously of most benefit when spontaneous resolution of the VIth nerve palsy is anticipated (e.g. benign post viral VIth)[6].

2. *Acute onset (normosensorial) esotropia* tends to occur towards the end of the first decade after visual maturity has been achieved. The esotropia may be initially intermittent, most often seen in the morning on waking but tending to become constant. It responds well to botulinum toxin treatment of one medial rectus muscle, which should restore good alignment and binocularity in the majority of cases[7].

Botulinum can also be used to treat small angle primary eso and exotropias, surgical over and under corrections, and for the investigation of binocularity (see below).

Table 13.1. Indications for treatment in strabismus

(a) *Childhood*
    Infantile esotropia
    VIth nerve palsy
    Normosensorial esotropia
    Surgical under and over corrections
(b) *Adults*
    Small angle eso/exotropia with binocular potential
    Investigation of binocularity
    Thyroid ophthalmopathy
    VIth nerve palsy

13.4.2 Adult

Large angle primary or consecutive eso or exotropias (Figure 13.2) without binocularity may respond well in the short term to botulinum treatment, but the strabismus is almost invariably recurrent to the same or similar angle within about 4 months. Maintenance of a good alignment of the eyes in these circumstances can only be achieved by repeated injections. Botulinum toxin treatment of adult strabismus is therefore most useful in situations where:

• Each eye has good vision (no amblyopia or major damage from other ocular pathology, e.g. retinal detachment).
• Normal binocular vision has developed in terms of both sensory stereopsis (ability to see three-dimensional presentations) and motor fusion, that is central ocular motor control mechanisms which maintain the alignment of the eyes against prismatic or other deviation.

The following conditions should be considered suitable for treatment.

1. Small angle, primary or consecutive eso or exotropia without binocularity, or following surgical over- or under-correction of large angle deviations. Botulinum toxin treatment in the absence of binocularity leads to only a small shift of the angle of the strabismus towards zero. If the pre-treatment angle is sufficiently small this shift will have a beneficial effect.

2. Small or moderate angle horizontal strabismus secondary to retinal detachment or other ocular surgery, such as glaucoma drainage surgery with explant

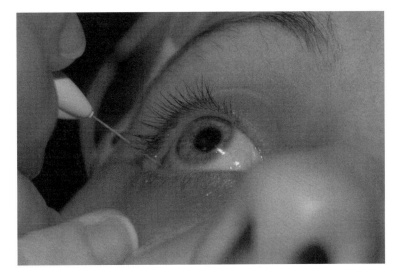

Figure 13.2 Injection of the lateral rectus under topical anaesthesia; an adult with exotropia.

(e.g. Molteno tube). These patients should have good pre-existing motor and sensory stereopsis. Note that the treatment potential may be limited if there is excessive fibrosis around the eye involving the extraocular muscles and limiting movement. Also that (particularly in post-retinal detachment patients) additional barriers to the re-establishment of binocularity other than misalignment of the visual axes may be present, such as differences in image size and quality, macular ectopia and ocular torsion[8].

3. Pre-operative investigation of potential binocularity or risk of post-operative diplopia. In some patients orthoptic testing with prisms suggest that realigning the visual axes surgically will lead to intractable double vision. Patients may be unwilling to trade the improved alignment for a potentially disruptive symptom. Correcting the strabismus with botulinum toxin does not mimic the effect of an operation since an element of extraocular muscle palsy is introduced, so that for at least some of the period following the treatment the deviation of the visual axes is incomitant, i.e. it varies according to the direction in which the patient looks. Nevertheless, this intervention will provide useful information for the patient as to the likely effect of corrective surgery. In some cases it is possible to demonstrate unexpected restoration of binocular function when the eyes are aligned, thus indicating a better prognosis for definitive surgical treatment.

4. Small angle vertical strabismus when the treatment is given to the inferior rectus of the hypotropic (lower) eye. Examples:

- Following inadvertent anaesthetic injection to a vertical rectus muscle during retrobulbar/peribulbar anaesthesia for ocular surgery, usually cataract.

Local anaesthetics are myotoxic and cause an initial paresis of the injected muscle, most often the inferior rectus. This produces a hypertropia of the affected eye. Healing is associated with fibrosis and a secondary small-angle hypotropia. A trial of treatment with botulinum toxin to the inferior rectus of the hypotropic eye is indicated before considering definitive surgery. This condition is now rare due to the widespread adoption of sub tenons and topical anaesthesia for cataract surgery.

- *Thyroid ophthalmopathy.* It is important to recognize that in most cases of thyroid eye disease all the extraocular muscles are involved, but some are characteristically more involved than others. The medial and inferior rectus muscles are generally the most enlarged on orbital imaging, with limitation of outward and upward movement of the eye. The condition may be symmetric or asymmetric.

In the active inflammatory phase of the disorder extraocular muscle surgery is contraindicated, and systemic immunosuppression may not be considered appropriate for the individual. High doses of systemic steroids are justifiable for the short term control of sight threatening complications, but not for the long term management of the condition when other modalities, such as orbital decompression should be considered.

Active thyroid eye disease may cause double vision with both horizontal and vertical elements. Mechanical tethering of the globes results in an increase in neuronal drive to the elevators, which in turn leads to overaction of the levator muscles and upper lid retraction and also to raised intraocular pressure[9].

Botulinum toxin treatment of extraocular muscles can be beneficial in these circumstances by:

- Reducing or abolishing a horizontal deviation (usually esotropia) allowing restoration of binocularity with or without smaller prism assistance.
- When injected to the inferior rectus muscles, reducing or helping in the prism control of a vertical deviation as well as allowing the eyes to move upwards, reducing upper lid retraction. Intraocular pressure control may also be improved.

There are other potential uses for botulinum toxin in thyroid eye disease — see eyelid position below.

- Muscle adherence syndrome following inferior oblique recession. A rare complication of inferior oblique recession is reduced elevation of the operated eye presumed to be due to either post-surgical fibrosis, or possibly damage to the nerve to the inferior oblique. Surgical treatment is not always successful.

Injecting the inferior rectus/inferior oblique complex with botulinum toxin may improve elevation of the affected eye[10].

• Restrictive strabismus following orbital myositis (horizontal or vertical deviation). In most cases successful treatment of orbital myositis with steroidal or non-steroidal anti-inflammatory drugs leads to a complete resolution of the ocular deviation. In some cases a residual tethering of the eye by the previously inflamed muscle is evident and binocularity can be restored by injecting this muscle.

5. *Paralytic strabismus*[11]:

• *VIth nerve palsy.* Botulinum toxin treatment to the ipsilateral medial rectus may be indicated:

(a) Acutely to retain binocularity in the primary position for patient comfort and rehabilitation whilst anticipating spontaneous resolution of the palsy. In many cases, for example after microvascular occlusion causing lateral rectus palsy, recovery of function in this muscle will match the post botulinum recovery in the medial rectus with the gradual restoration of a normal area of binocular single vision.

(b) In recovered VIth nerve palsy with persistent esotropia due to medial rectus contracture when an injection alone may restore normal eye movements. Why contracture develops in the medial rectus in some cases following acute VIth nerve palsy but not others is not understood. Myofibrilar shortening occurs as a response in the unopposed medial rectus muscle. A traction test can be carried out under the topical anaesthesia used to perform the botulinum injection to confirm the presence of contracture. Also an EMG on the lateral rectus will establish if there has been restoration of innervation to that muscle.

(c) Unrecovered lateral rectus palsy presents a difficult management problem, involving surgical attempts to redistribute the forces generated by the medial, superior and inferior rectus muscles to straighten the eye in the orbit without interfering with the anterior segment circulation. Paralysis of the medial rectus with botulinum toxin, before surgically transposing the superior and inferior rectus muscles temporally alongside the lateral rectus, produces a sufficient abducting vector to produce an exotropia. As the medial rectus recovers, the exotropia resolves and binocularity should be re-established without recurrence of the esotropia. In the event of the esotropia recurring the medial rectus can either be re-injected or surgically recessed once the anterior segment circulation has recovered from the initial intervention.

- This procedure will not restore normal movement to the affected eye, but will maximize the field of binocular single vision.
- *IVth nerve palsy.* Theoretically the principles outlined above in the management of VIth nerve palsy may be applied to IVth nerve palsy. The difference is that the overacting ipsilateral antagonist of the paralysed muscle is the inferior oblique, and it is difficult to selectively weaken this muscle without spread to the inferior rectus. An alternative strategy in unrecovered IVth nerve palsy is to inject the contralateral agonist of the paralysed muscle (the inferior rectus). Again benefit may be compromised by spread to the inferior oblique. Note that this is unlike the situation in thyroid ophthalmopathy where the inferior rectus is markedly enlarged, making it easier to confine the effect of an injection to this muscle alone without spread.
- *IIIrd nerve palsy.* In a persistent partial IIIrd nerve palsy with a good vertical alignment, no ptosis and a reasonable range of medial rectus activity but persistent divergent strabismus, botulinum toxin treatment to the ipsilateral lateral rectus may restore binocularity. The injection may have to be repeated to maintain binocularity but provided there is no other ocular co-morbidity, once binocular function is achieved, the area of binocular single vision often progressively enlarges.
- Vertical squint due to a disruption of brainstem prenuclear inputs (skew deviation) can be due to a variety of causes such as brainstem, inflammatory and vascular disease. If it persists, and the angle between the visual axes is not more than 10–15 prism dioptres, then treatment of the inferior rectus of the hypotropic (lower) eye may be helpful. The caveat in relation to spread to the inferior oblique (see above) applies.

In a persisting internuclear ophthalmoplegia, double vision and oscillopsia due to secondary overaction of the lateral rectus muscle or muscles may be reduced by an injection of botulinum toxin into that muscle.

6. *Nystagmus.* There are a number of reports of the use of either retrobulbar or intramuscular botulinum toxin in the management of nystagmus and other disorders of fixation. In nystagmus the slow phase is the abnormal movement (the fast phase being corrective) so theoretically reducing activity in the muscle responsible for the slow phase may be beneficial. Alternatively in pendular nystagmus the muscles responsible for the abnormal movements in each direction can be treated.

There are a number of practical difficulties which limit the benefits of this treatment. For example downbeat nystagmus cannot be treated as it is not possible to treat the superior rectus without also inducing a ptosis. Attempts to treat horizontal nystagmus by symmetric injections to agonist muscles in both eyes very often have an unequal effect on the two eyes resulting in double vision. Because of these problems attempts have been made to damp extraocular muscle activity generally with retrobulbar injections, which can produce generalized ophthalmoparesis. Again double vision, due to an asymmetric effect, and asymmetric ptosis can be problems.

The ophthalmoparesis produced by retrobulbar botulinum toxin, as well as damping nystagmus or other abnormal ocular movements, will also prevent normal eye movements including the vestibulo ocular response. The absence of this normal reflex eye movement in response to acceleration and deceleration of the head or body can itself produce a disconcerting illusory movement of the environment.

A further problem, particularly in patients with multiple sclerosis and pendular nystagmus, is of a co-existent optic neuropathy such that even when the eyes are relatively still, visual function remains disappointingly poor.

It is usually the case that if patients find a particular treatment helpful they will return for repeat treatments. Very few individuals who have been treated with botulinum toxin for oscillopsia request a second treatment, but there are a small number who find this intervention helpful on a long term basis[12].

13.5   Facial movement disorders

As noted above Scott commented with admirable foresight in 1973 regarding the 'possible extension of the technique of local muscle paralysis to the management of such conditions as blepharospasm'. The treatment of patients with blepharospasm by botulinum toxin injection began in the United States in the early 1980s and in the United Kingdom in 1983. The first reports of its often spectacular efficacy appeared in 1985, and since then there has been a steady increase in its usage in the management of both facial and other focal movement disorders (Table 13.2).

Table 13.2. Treatment of facial movement disorders

Dystonic blepharospasm
Hemifacial spasm
Post facial palsy problems
Facial myokymia

13.5.1   Idiopathic blepharospasm

The introduction of botulinum toxin injections has dramatically improved measures of practical visual function, and health-related quality of life in a high proportion of patients with this previously untreatable disorder. It has also stimulated medical ascertainment of the condition and research into the characteristics and pathogenesis. As a result of studying large numbers of patients with blepharospasm we have improved information on the incidence, natural history and factors exacerbating and improving the condition which may help in management. For example, patients are often concerned that the abnormal movements may spread to other parts of the body, but studying large numbers of patients has indicated that although cranial dystonia may develop, usually within 2–3 years of the onset of the blepharospasm, other muscle groups will not be affected unless there is an underlying specific cause. We also have insights into possible genetic factors in the pathogenesis.

It is now recognized that there are two principle variants of idiopathic blepharospasm. Typical blepharospasm involves forceful eye closure via all components of the orbicularis oculi muscle, i.e. the pretarsal, the preseptal and orbital parts. The brows are lowered. By contrast in atypical or pretarsal blepharospasm (5–10 per cent of cases), the brows are elevated and the spasm is confined to or predominant in the pretarsal section of the muscle. Attempts to activate the levator muscles appear to exacerbate the contraction in the pretarsal orbicularis oculi, and there is EMG evidence of co-contraction in these two muscles. Atypical blepharospasm should be differentiated from 'apraxia of eye opening' (see below).

Up to 90 per cent of patients with blepharospasm report some symptomatic improvement with botulinum toxin injections, and in approximately 75 per cent long term maintenance of a degree of symptomatic relief is possible by repeat injections at 2–3 monthly intervals. Informed consent to the procedure requires an explanation of the risks and benefits and an attempt to give an insight into how the treatment works. It is important for patients to realize that it is not a specific cure for the condition, and that weakening the orbicularis oculi has no effect on the fundamental underlying neurological disorder[13].

In the doses used for the treatment of blepharospasm, antibodies to botulinum toxin do not develop. Therefore if a response can be obtained it is usually repeatable indefinitely. Secondary treatment failure, i.e. the development of an apparent resistance to the beneficial effects of botulinum toxin is unusual and probably indicates a worsening of the underlying disorder[14].

Injections into the pretarsal orbicularis oculi alone (in both typical and atypical cases) allow lower total dose usage than orbital injections with better relief and fewer side effects[15]. Injections are given subcutaneously using a 1 ml syringe and a 30-gauge needle. In some cases pretarsal injections will need to be augmented by additional orbital treatment. The force, amplitude and frequency of blinking is reduced. Up to 50 per cent of patients with idiopathic blepharospasm have mid- and lower-facial dystonia (Meige syndrome) and many have some symptomatic relief from these muscle spasms when the blinking is controlled or reduced. Some individuals consciously or unconsciously use facial grimacing or yawning as a means of keeping the eyes open better when blepharospasm is bad. Improvement of the blepharospasm reduces the need for this category of abnormal facial movement.

The side effects of treatment are predictable — partial ptosis, double vision, paralytic entropion and corneal exposure — but usually short-lived and well tolerated. Mid-facial and upper-lid mobility problems may follow medial injections on the lower lids, which for this reason are sometimes omitted. This location of injection may also interfere with the lower-lid tear drainage mechanism and cause epiphora (see also below). EMLA cream may be used pre-treatment to relieve injection pain[16].

Not all the patients benefit from long term treatment, and it is important to recognize that even in those who do symptoms are usually reduced but not abolished. Health related quality of life measures (HR-QoL) indicate continuing problems and depression is also common[17]. Long term remission is very rare. Adjunctive treatment may be helpful — in particular ptosis props or a spectacle attachment to apply pressure around the eyes. Systemic drug treatment is rarely helpful. Many different categories of drug have been used in individual cases of blepharospasm, but there is no consistent pharmacological profile, which would help determine a rational choice of treatment.

13.5.2 Apraxia of eye opening

The term 'apraxia of eye opening' is used to designate the condition in which the eyes appear to be passively closed and there is an inability or difficulty in initiating eye opening. Once the eyes are open, however, they remain normally open with normal reflex blinking. This may be a feature of progressive supranuclear palsy when the periodic blink rate is often low. The condition needs to be differentiated from pretarsal blepharospasm (see above) in which there is active contraction in that portion of orbicularis oculi. The difficulty in eye opening that may be seen in Parkinson's disease is usually due to pretarsal blepharospasm rather than apraxia of eye opening.

Apraxia of eye opening rarely responds to pretarsal injections of botulinum toxin. It may improve with brow (frontalis) suspension surgery[18]. The combination of botulinum toxin treatment to orbicularis oculi and brow suspension surgery may also be useful in some cases of resistant pretarsal blepharospasm. Other eyelid surgeries may also be helpful in some individuals with typical blepharospasm, including the removal of excess skin (blepharochalasis surgery) and advancement of the levator muscle when there is a secondary levator dehiscence type ptosis.

13.5.3 Hemifacial spasm

In contrast to blepharospasm, which is associated with centrally determined facial nuclear hypersensitivity, hemifacial spasm is due to chronic low grade damage to the extra axial facial nerve. Hemifacial spasm characteristically begins insidiously with myokymia type contractions in orbicularis oculi, but these persist and extend to involve increasing numbers of the ipsilateral facial nerve innervated muscles. Spasms are of variable frequency and intensity from short-lived twitches to sustained clonic contractions. They occur spontaneously at a variable rate and are also triggered by the normal use of facial muscles in talking, eating, etc. and may be exacerbated by anxiety. Hemifacial spasm continues in sleep and may interrupt it[19].

Most cases are secondary to microvascular compression of the facial nerve in the root exit zone, but occasionally other pathology, e.g. vascular anomalies or lipoma – are responsible. Again unlike blepharospasm, an alternative reportedly effective, definitive treatment exists for many cases – surgical decompression of the facial nerve in the posterior fossa. However, most patients with hemifacial spasm are middle aged to elderly and vascular co-morbidity, e.g. systemic hypertension is common. Microvascular decompression of the facial nerve requires intracranial surgery, and the potential risks of this treatment mean that botulinum injections are the primary treatment option. Systemic drug treatment is generally ineffective.

Provided the examination of an individual with hemifacial spasm does not reveal any evidence of other cranial neuropathy (e.g. trigeminal sensory dysfunction), there is no indication for neuro-imaging unless surgery is to be contemplated. Hemifacial spasm very rarely occurs in children and, except in those cases which are familial (and probably due to an inherited vascular anomaly), these cases are generally due to a structural, usually vascular, cause which should be established by neuro-imaging. Characteristically the spasms of the face involve eye closure (orbicularis oculi) but brow elevation (frontalis) laterally-pulling mid-facial contractions as well as contractions in the superficial neck muscle (platysma). Some patients complain of synchronous clicking in the ipsilateral ear due to stapedius contraction.

Most patients with hemifacial spasm appreciate the partial symptomatic relief that repeated botulinum toxin injections in the brows, lids and upper face laterally (also the platysma) can give[20]. The mid and lower face is generally avoided because of side effects of mouth droop and gum biting. Some patients benefit from injections to the contralateral brow and lower lid to achieve a more symmetric result (very rarely hemifacial spasm is bilateral). The injection schedule in hemifacial spasm needs to be tailored to suit the individual patient.

The period of relief is usually longer than that seen in blepharospasm averaging around 3 months, sometimes up to 6 months. Partial ptosis is the commonest side effect occurring in 10 per cent of patients over 12 treatments at one centre. As with the treatment of blepharospasm, the side effects include eyelid malposition or malfunction giving entropion or watering.

13.5.4 Post facial palsy problems

A number of problems that can develop following facial palsy of any aetiology may be amenable to botulinum toxin treatment.

- In unrecovered facial palsy the lid elevating action of the levator muscle is unopposed by the normal tonic orbicularis oculi contraction. This in some cases leads to upper lid retraction and corneal exposure. As a temporary measure the upper lid can be lowered by an injection of botulinum toxin either via the skin or conjunctiva into the levator.
- Post facial palsy misdirection regeneration can lead to unwanted synkinetic movements in the face, for example partial eye closure on smiling or talking. Low dose (because of persistent facial weakness) botulinum injections into the orbicularis oculi may be helpful. Synkinetic contractions in platysma can also be dealt with this way.
- Crocodile tears (gustatory hyperlacrimation) may develop and can be treated as below.

13.5.5 Other facial movement disorders

Facial muscle myokymia is usually a focal short-lived annoyance that requires no active intervention. Occasionally it persists for days or weeks and can be stopped by appropriate focal botulinum injections. Rarely widespread facial myokymia occurs secondary to an intrinsic pontine lesion affecting the facial nucleus or intra-axial nerve, most commonly demyelination. This condition may respond to systemic steroid treatment but if reasonably localized in the face can be treated with botulinum injections[21].

Orbicularis oculi neuromyotonia is a rare disorder that may be isolated or associated with neuromyotonia in muscles elsewhere (Isaac's syndrome). The symptom is difficulty opening the eyes after forceful lid closure, for example after sneezing. This may be embarrassing or even dangerous — for example when driving or operating machinery. Systemic drug treatment is usually ineffective, but botulinum injections provide symptomatic relief.

13.5.6   Other ophthalmic indications

Eyelid position

- *Ptosis induction.* Botulinum toxin can be injected into the levator palpebrae to induce a ptosis. EMG guidance is not required — an injection into the superior orbit behind the globe is effective. The extent and duration of the ptosis is dose dependent. This is a useful adjunct in the management of refractory corneal pathology with non-healing epithelial defects, where otherwise a temporary surgical tarsorrhaphy would be considered. It is also effective in the combination of anaesthetic cornea and facial palsy (e.g. after acoustic neuroma surgery) when corneal exposure is a threat[22].

  The advantages of a botulinum or medical tarsorrhaphy as against a surgical one are that there is no damage to the eyelid margins and that the passively closed lid is easier to open to inspect the corneal surface. Because the palpebral aperture is not shortened horizontally it is usually easier to instil drops needed for the corneal pathology and there is evidence from impression cytology studies that corneal healing is faster and more permanent. A medical tarsorrhaphy is repeatable, if necessary, and may obviate the need for a permanent surgical tarsorrhaphy, otherwise required in about 20 per cent of cases. The cosmetic outcome once the cornea has healed is likely to be better after a botulinum than a temporary surgical tarsorrhaphy.

- After an injection into the levator, there is inevitably spread of paralytic effect to the superior rectus, producing a vertical deviation (hypotropia) of the eye. This potential side effect needs to be explained in detail before this treatment is carried out. This will usually resolve spontaneously as the ptosis recovers, but may persist for some weeks or even indefinitely. Occasionally ocular muscle surgery is required.

- *Entropion.* Spastic lower lid entropion may be relieved by an injection into the pretarsal orbicularis oculi, which is responsible for everting the lid in this situation. This is usually a temporizing measure only, but sometimes relieving the corneal irritation of the in-turning lashes allows the situation to resolve[23].

- *Lid retraction.* Upper lid retraction, associated with thyroid eye disease (if not due to globe tethering, see above) may be relieved by injecting the levator complex at the upper border of the tarsal plate. Both percutaneous and subconjunctival approaches are described and produce lid lowering for between one to four months[24]. Injections into the secondarily overactive accessory muscles of eyelid closure — the glabellar muscles, corrugator supercilli and procerus — relieves furrowing frown lines, which contribute to the unsightly thyroid facial appearance.

Asymmetry of eyebrow position — which follows, for example, partly recovered facial palsy with a brow ptosis — may respond to reducing frontalis muscle function on the contralateral brow.

Tear function

- *Gustatory hyperlacrimation ('crocodile tears')*. This may follow aberrant VIIth nerve regeneration after facial palsy, due to unwanted secretor motor drive to the lacrimal gland from the superior salivatory nucleus. Direct transconjunctival injection of botulinum into the lacrimal gland, under topical anaesthesia, results in partial or complete resolution for up to 4—5 months. Partial ptosis is the obvious potential side effect, but is generally reported inconsistently as 'mild'[25].
- *Functional epiphora*. Some individuals, with a patent lacrimal drainage system and normal eyelid position and function, have persistent watery eye(s), a situation designated 'functional epiphora'. Reducing tear output by trans-conjunctival botulinum injection of the lacrimal gland may be helpful symptomatically[26].
- *Dry eyes*. Injecting botulinum into the medial pretarsal orbicularis oculi on both upper and lower eyelids reduces the force of the blink medially, and impairs the normal tear drainage mechanism. Patients with dry eye report improved eye comfort after this treatment[27].

Facial scars

Scars following facial trauma may be exacerbated by underlying muscle contraction tending to disrupt the aposition of tissue edges. Immediate injection of botulinum toxin into the muscles underlying a wound after suturing can improve the cosmetic outcome of the facial cutaneous scar (Table 13.3)[28].

Table 13.3. Other ophthalmic indications

Ptosis induction
Entropion
Lid retraction
Brow asymmetry
Crocodile tears
Functional epiphora
Dry eyes
Facial scarring

REFERENCES

1. Scott, A. B., Rosenbaum, A. and Collins, C. C. (1973). Pharmacological weakening of extra-ocular muscles. *Invest. Ophthalmol. Vis. Sci.*, **12**, 924–7.

2. Lennerstrand, G., Nordbo, O. A., Tian, S., Eriksson-Derouet, B. and Ali, T. (1998). Treatment of strabismus and nystagmus with botulinum toxin type A. An evaluation of effects and complications. *Acta Ophthalmol. Scand.*, **76**(1), 27.

3. McNeer, K. W., Tucker, M. G., Guerry, C. H. and Spencer, R. F. (2003). Incidence of stereopsis after treatment of infantile esotropia with botulinum toxin A. *J. Pediatr. Ophthalmol. Strabismus*, **40**(5), 288–92.

4. Campos, E. C., Schiavi, C. and Bellusci, C. (2000). Critical age of botulinum toxin treatment in essential infantile esotropia. *J. Pediatr. Ophthalmol. Strabismus*, **37**(6), 328–32.

5. Tejedor, J. and Rodriguez, J. M. (1999). Early retreatment of infantile esotropia: comparison of reoperation and botulinum toxin. *Br. J. Ophthalmol.*, **83**(7), 783–7.

6. Rayner, S. A., Hollick, E. J. and Lee, J. P. (1999). Botulinum toxin in childhood strabismus. *Strabismus*, **7**(2), 103–11.

7. Dawson, E. L., Marshman, W. E. and Adams, G. G. (1999). The role of botulinum toxin A in acute-onset esotropia. *Ophthalmology*, **106**(9), 1727–30.

8. Maurino, V., Kwan, A., Khoo, B. K., Gair, E. and Lee, J. P. (1998). Ocular motility disturbances after surgery for retinal detachment. *J. AAPOS*, **2**(5), 285–92.

9. Kikkawa, D. O., Cruz, R. C. Jr., Christian, W. K., Rikkers, S., Weinreb, R. N., Levi, L. and Granet, D. B. (2003). Botulinum A toxin injection for restrictive myopathy of thyroid-related orbitopathy: effects on intraocular pressure. *Am. J. Ophthalmol.*, **135**(4), 427–31.

10. Ozkan, S. B., Kir, E., Dayanir, V. and Dundar, S. O. (2003). Botulinum toxin A in the treatment of adherence syndrome. *Ophthalmic Surg. Lasers Imaging*, **34**(5), 391–5.

11. Repka, M. X., Lam, G. C. and Morrison, N. A. (1994). The efficacy of botulinum neurotoxin A for the treatment of complete and partially recovered chronic sixth nerve palsy. *J. Pediatr. Ophthalmol. Strabismus*, **31**(2), 79–83.

12. Repka, M. X., Savino, P. J. and Reinecke, R. D. (1994). Treatment of acquired nystagmus with botulinum neurotoxin A. *Arch. Ophthalmol.*, **112**(10), 1320–4.

13. Hallett, M. (2002). Blepharospasm: recent advances. *Neurology*, **59**(9), 1306–12.

14. Calace, P., Cortese, G., Piscopo, R., Della Volpe, G., Gagli, V., Magli, A. and De Berardinis, T. (2003). Treatment of blepharospasm with botulinum neurotoxin type A: long-term results. *Eur. J. Ophthalmol.*, **13**(4), 331–6.

15. Price, J., Farish, S., Taylor, H. and O'Day, J. (1997). Blepharospasm and hemifacial spasm. Randomized trial to determine the most appropriate location for botulinum toxin injections. *Ophthalmology*, **104**(5), 865–8.

16. Soylev, M. F., Kocak, N., Kuvaki, B., Ozkan, S. B. and Kir, E. (2002). Anesthesia with EMLA cream for botulinum A toxin injection into eyelids. *Ophthalmologica*, **216**(5), 355–8.

17. Muller, J., Kemmler, G., Wissel, J., Schneider, A., Voller, B., Grossman, J., Diez, J., Homann, N., Wenning, G. K., Schni, P. and Poewe, W. (2002). The impact of

blepharospasm and cervical dystonia on health-related quality of life and depression. *J. Neurol.*, **249**(7), 842–6.

18. De Groot, V., De Wilde, F., Smet, L. and Tassignon, M. J. (2000). Frontalis suspension combined with blepharoplasty as an effective treatment for blepharospasm associated with apraxia of eye opening. *Ophthal. Plast. Reconstr. Surg.*, **16**(1), 34–8.

19. Wang, A. and Jankovic, J. (1998). Hemifacial spasm: clinical findings and treatment. *Muscle Nerve*, **21**(12), 1740–7.

20. Jitpimolmard, S., Tiamkao, S. and Laopaiboon, M. (1998). Long term results of botulinum toxin type A (Dysport) in the treatment of hemifacial spasm report of 175 cases. *J. Neurol. Neurosurg. Psychiatry*, **64**(6), 751–7.

21. Sedano, M. J., Trejo, J. M., Macarron, J. L., Polo, J. M., Bercian, J. and Calleja, J. (2000). Continuous facial myokymia in multiple sclerosis treatment with botulinum toxin. *Eur. Neurol.*, **43**(3), 137–40.

22. Ellis, M. F. and Daniell, M. (2001). An evaluation of the safety and efficacy of botulinum toxin type A (BOTOX) when used to produce a protective ptosis. *Clin. Experiment. Ophthalmol.*, **29**(6), 394–9.

23. Steel, D. H., Hoh, H. B., Harrad, R. A. and Collins, C. R. (1997). Botulinum toxin for the temporary treatment of involutional lower lid entropion: a clinical and morphological study. *Eye*, **11**, 472–5.

24. Uddin, J. M. and Davies, P. D. (2002). Treatment of upper eyelid retraction associated with thyroid eye disease with subconjunctival botulinum toxin injection. *Ophthalmology*, **109**(6), 1183–7.

25. Montoya, F. J., Riddell, C. E., Caesar, R. and Hague, S. (2002). Treatment of gustatory hyperlacrimation (crocodile tears) with injection of botulinum toxin into the lacrimal gland. *Eye*, **16**(6), 705–9.

26. Whittaker, K. W., Matthews, B. N., Fitt, A. W. and Sandramouli, S. (2003). The use of botulinum toxin A in the treatment of functional epiphora. *Orbit*, **22**(3), 193–8.

27. Sahlin, S., Chen, E., Kaugesaar, T., Almqvist, H., Kjellberg, K. and Lennerstrand, G. (2000). Effect of eyelid botulinum toxin injection on lacrimal drainage. *Am. J. Ophthalmol.*, **129**(4), 481–6.

28. Sherris, D. A. and Gassner, H. G. (2002). Botulinum toxin to minimize facial scarring. *Facial Plast. Surg.*, **18**(1), 35–9.

Bladder and bowel indications

Giuseppe Brisinda, Federica Cadeddu and Giorgio Maria

Department of Surgery, Catholic School of Medicine, University Hospital Agostino Gemelli, Rome, Italy

14.1 Introduction

Botulinum neurotoxin (BoNT) inhibits neuromuscular transmission and it has become a drug with many indications[1-3]. The range of clinical applications has grown to encompass several neurological and non-neurological conditions. Over the years, the number of primary clinical publications has grown exponentially, and continues to increase every year. Although BoNT blocks cholinergic nerve endings in the autonomic nervous system, it has also been shown that it does not block non-adrenergic non-cholinergic responses mediated by nitric oxide (NO)[4]. This has promoted further interest in using BoNT as a treatment for overactive smooth muscles and sphincters (Table 14.1).

Recent clinical experience of BoNT in urological impaired patients will be described in this chapter. Moreover, understanding the anatomical and functional organization of gastrointestinal tract (GIT) innervation is necessary to understand many features of BoNT action on the GIT and the effect of injecting specific sphincters. This chapter presents current data on the use of BoNT to treat GIT diseases and summarizes recent knowledge on the pathogenesis of GIT disorders due to a dysfunction of the enteric nervous system (ENS).

14.2 Urinary bladder indications

14.2.1 Anatomy and physiology of micturition

The two functions of lower urinary tract (LUT) are storage and active expulsion of urine. The LUT consists of the bladder (detrusor muscle bundles) and the urethra. The urethra contains a dual sphincter mechanism. The internal sphincter is a smooth muscle part of the vesical neck and posterior urethra with both adrenergic and cholinergic innervation. It is closed during bladder filling by constant

Clinical Uses of Botulinum Toxins, eds. Anthony B. Ward and Michael P. Barnes. Published by Cambridge University Press. © Cambridge University Press 2007.

Table 14.1. Target site for the injection of BoNT in different LUT and GIT clinical conditions

Site of injection	Condition
Lower esophageal sphincter	Achalasia
	Diffuse esophageal spasm
	Isolated hypertensive LES
	Esophageal diverticula
Cricopharyngeal muscle	Cricopharyngeal dysphagia
Pylorus	Delayed gastric emptying
	Infantile hypertrophic pyloric stenosis
Sphincter of Oddi	Sphincter of Oddi dysfunction
Internal anal sphincter	Chronic anal fissure
External anal sphincter	Chronic anal fissure
	Outlet-type constipation
	Anterior rectocele
Puborectalis muscle	Outlet-type constipation
	Anterior rectocele
External urethral sphincters	Detrusor-sphincter dyssynergia
	Urinary retention
	Chronic prostatic pain
	Chronic prostatitis
Detrusor muscle	Neurogenic detrusor overactivity
	Idiopathic detrusor overactivity
Prostate	Benign prostatic hyperplasia

BoNT: botulinum toxin; GIT: gastrointestinal tract; LES: lower esophageal sphincter; LUT: lower urinary tract.

background adrenergic tone. The external sphincter has two components: muscle intrinsic to the urethra, mainly under autonomic control, and muscle around the membranous urethra made of striated muscle under voluntary control via the pudendal nerve[5].

Within the detrusor muscle, a single nerve innervates several muscle fibres, which produces coordinated bladder contraction. Cholinergic fibres predominate in the body of the bladder, whereas adrenergic fibres are present in both the body and bladder neck (Table 14.2).

The LUT is innervated by three groups of peripheral nerves: sacral parasympathetic, lumbar sympathetic, and sacral somatic nerves (Figure 14.1). Urine is stored when the external urethral sphincter muscle (somatic) and the internal urethral sphincter muscle (sympathetic) are contracted and the detrusor muscle and sacral parasympathetic activity are inhibited through sympathetic mediation. Sympathetic integrity is not essential for the performance of micturition.

Table 14.2. Receptors for putative transmitters in LUT

Tissue	Cholinergic		Adrenergic		Other	
	Excitatory	Inhibitory	Excitatory	Inhibitory	Excitatory	Inhibitory
Bladder body	M2, M3	–	α1	β2	Purinergic [P2x], PG, Substance P	VIP
Bladder base	M2, M3	–	α1	–	Purinergic [P2x]	VIP
Ganglia	N, M1	–	α1, β	α2	Purinergic [P1, P2x], Substance P	Enkephalinergic [δ]
Urethra	M	–	α1, α2	β2	Purinergic [P2x]	NO, VIP
Parasympathetic terminals	M1	M4	α1	α2	5-HT	NPY
Afferent neurons	–	–	–	–	CAPS, PG, Purinergic [P2x]	–
Sphincter striated muscle	N	–	–	–	–	–

5-HT: 5-hydroxytryptamine; CAPS: capsaicin; LUT: lower urinary tract; M: muscarinic; N: nicotinic; NO: nitric oxide; NPY: neuropeptide Y; PG: prostaglandins; VIP: vasoactive intestinal polypeptide.

However, experimental evidence suggests that sympathetic input causes tonic inhibitory input to the bladder and excitatory input to the urethra. During micturition, descending pathways originating from the pontine micturition centre inhibit external urethral sphincter activity, inhibit sympathetic outflow (inhibition of the vesicosympathetic reflex), activate parasympathetic outflow to the bladder, and activate parasympathetic outflow to the urethra[5].

The neural pathways controlling LUT function are organized as simple on–off switching circuits (Figure 14.2) that maintain a reciprocal relationship between the urinary bladder and urethral outlet. The principal reflex components of these switching circuits are listed in Table 14.3.

14.2.2 Detrusor-sphincter dyssynergia

Detrusor-sphincter dyssynergia (DSD) is defined as inappropriate contractions of the urethral sphincter coincident with detrusor contractions[6]. DSD is a major cause of morbidity in spinal cord injury patients. The resulting high intravesical

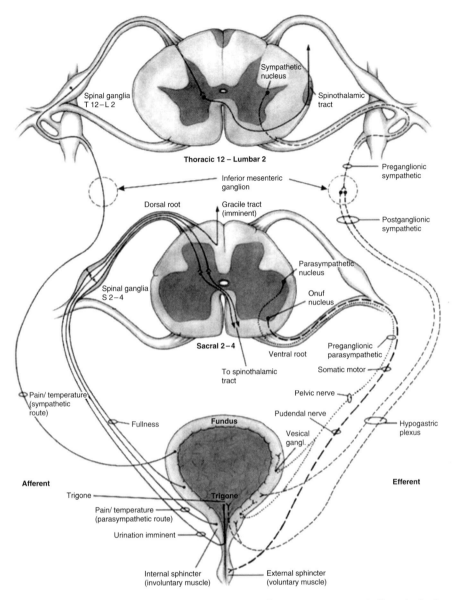

Figure 14.1 Micturition is controlled by a region of the ponto-mesencephalic reticular formation at the level of the trigeminal motor nucleus referred to as the pontine micturition centre. This is the only centre that is able to coordinate detrusor contraction and sphincter relaxation. This occurs through reticulospinal pathways. Anteromedial portion of the frontal lobes, anterior vermis and basal ganglia. There are direct connections between frontal centres and pontine centre. Autonomic centres in the spinal cord include sympathetic (T9 – L1) and parasympathetic (S2 – S3). Control of external sphincter striated muscle by neurons in Onuf's nucleus in the sacral cord. Receive voluntary input from frontal lobes via pyramidal tracts. A control system was based on functional arcs. An alternate functional classification also exists that defines four distinct control loops which provide for coordinated detrusor-sphincter function during urine storage and evacuation.

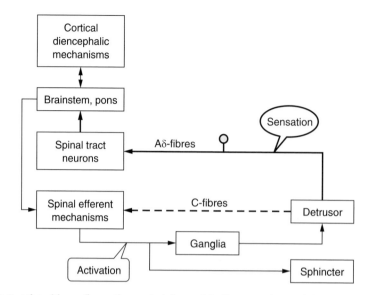

Figure 14.2 Micturition reflex pathway. A alpha and C afferent pathways initiate micturition. A alpha fibres exhibit graded response to passive distension, while C fibres have a much higher threshold, being activated by inflammation and noxious stimuli. Fullness of the bladder is detected by receptors in the bladder wall, which send impulses through the sacral parasympathetic nerves. Impulses reach the cortex through the spinothalamic tracts. The act of micturition is both reflex and voluntary. When a normal person is asked to void, there is first a voluntary relaxation of the perineum, the increased tension of the abdominal wall with a slow contraction of the detrusor and an associated opening of the internal sphincter. The external sphincter must also relax. When the bladder is filling, impulses from sensory receptors in the peripheral nerves ascend to the brainstem nuclei. The brainstem sends descending tracts to prevent micturition by inhibiting the detrusor nucelus and stimulating the pudendal nucleus (holding reflex). The sympathetic fibres cause relaxation of the bladder body (beta adrenergic) and tightening of the bladder neck (alpha adrenergic). When the bladder reaches a certain volume, the impulses start reaching the cerebral cortex and the desire to micturate is perceived. At the same time, the sympathetic tone is decreased, and parasympathetic tone increased causing detrusor contraction and inhibition of smooth muscle tone of the urethral sphincter. Striated muscle relaxation is done voluntarily via the pudendal nerve. Voiding is characterized by increased parasympathetic discharges to stimulate detrusor contraction, and decreased sympathetic discharges to relax outlet sphincters. Increased sympathetic tone leads to detrusor relaxation and bladder outlet contraction.

pressures and poor bladder emptying may lead to autonomic dysreflexia, severe urinary tract infections, renal damage and premature death. DSD is typically managed with medication, condom or indwelling catheters, intermittent catheterization and electrical stimulation, or surgery to destroy sphincter function.

Table 14.3. Reflex to the LUT

Afferent pathway	Efferent pathway	Central pathway
Urine storage	1. External sphincter contraction (somatic nerves)	Spinal reflex
Low-level vesical afferent activity (pelvic nerve)	2. Internal sphincter contraction (sympathetic nerves)	
	3. Detrusor inhibition (sympathetic nerves)	
	4. Ganglionic inhibition (sympathetic nerves)	
	5. Sacral parasympathetic outflow inactive	
Micturition	1. Inhibition of external sphincter activity	Spinobulbospinal reflex
High level vesical afferent activity (pelvic nerve)	2. Inhibition of sympathetic outflow	
	3. Activation of parasympathetic outflow to the bladder	Spinal reflex
	4. Activation of parasympathetic outflow to the urethra	

LUT: lower urinary tract.

All of these treatments have associated complications. The possibility to induce a reversible sphincterotomy with BoNT injections in spinal cord injured patients have first been described by Dykstra et al[7]. Thereafter, other authors reported on the technique and its results (Table 14.4). BoNT has been either injected transurethrally via cystoscope or transperineally under electromyographic control. However, the dose, dilution volume and intervals between two injections vary from author to author[8-14].

Main parameters to assess BoNT effect were the urethral pressure profile and the post-void residual volume. Using an initial dose of 140 units of toxin injected transurethrally via cystoscope, and subsequent weekly doses of 240 units, an average of three injections was needed to produce maximum decrease in post-void residual volume. Eight out of 11 patients improved. Urethral pressure profile decreased on an average by 27 cmH$_2$O, residual urine volume decreased by an average of 146 ml. Duration of effect was about 50 days, and side effects were not observed[15].

In a prospective study on 24 spinal cord injury patients, the effect of one single injection (100 BOTOX® units) versus three repeated injections at monthly intervals has been compared[6,16]. In 87.5 per cent of patients, the maximum

Table 14.4. BoNT and DSD. Published results

	Dykstra et al., 1988	Dykstra et al., 1990	Schurch et al., 1996	Beleggia et al., 1997	Petit et al., 1998	Gallien et al., 1998	de Seze et al., 2002
Number of patients	11	5	24	5	17	5	13
Name of drug/dose	BOTOX®/140–240	BOTOX®/140–240	BOTOX®/100	Nr	Dysport/150	Nr	BOTOX®/100
Method of injections	Transurethral/transperineal	Transurethral/transperineal	Transurethral/transperineal	Transurethral	Transurethral	Transperineal	Transperineal
Urethral pressure	Decrease	Decrease	Decrease	Decrease	Decrease	Not significant	Decrease
Post void residual volume	Decrease	Decrease	Decrease	Decrease	Decrease	Not significant	Decrease
Bladder pressure during voiding or uninhibited bladder contraction	—	Decrease	Decrease	Decrease	Decrease	Decrease	Decrease
Mean maximum urethral pressure during DSD	—	—	Decrease	—	—	—	Decrease
Duration of DSD	—	—	Decrease	—	—	—	—
Functional detrusor capacity	—	—	—	—	—	Increase	—
Autonomic dysreflexia	—	Decrease	Not improved	—	—	Decrease	—
Duration of effects (days)	50	65	60–90	60	60–90	90	Not reported

BoNT: botulinum toxin; —: no measurement; DSD: detrusor-sphincter dyssynergia. Dysport is the trade name of the type A botulinum toxin preparation manufactured by Ipsen (Maidenhead, UK); BOTOX® is the trade name of the type A preparation manufactured by Allergan (Irvine, CA, USA).

urethral pressure during DSD, duration of DSD and basic urethral pressure significantly decreased by 48, 47, and 20 per cent, respectively. The main point observed was a longer lasting effect of the repetitive injections on the voiding dysfunction (9–13 months), versus one single injection (2–3 months).

In patients with lesion above T6, transurethral BoNT injections into the urethral sphincter may require general anaesthesia because of the high risk of autonomic dysreflexia. Schurch *et al.* reported on the same results of both techniques (transurethral versus transperineal), when using the same BoNT amount of toxin[6]. Similarly, Gallien *et al.*[10] reported on good results using the transperineal approaches.

Recently, in a double-blind study on 13 spinal cord injury patients with DSD, de Seze *et al.*[9] compared the efficacy and tolerance of BoNT (100 units of BOTOX®) versus lidocaine (4 ml at 0.5%) applied into the external urethral sphincter with a single transperineal injection. They found a significant improvement in all parameters in BoNT group but not in the lidocaine group.

According to these reports, BoNT injections into the external urethral sphincter appear to be efficient to treat DSD in spinal cord injured patients. However, randomized studies comparing the effects of this treatment against placebo are still lacking. Clinical effects begin within 7 days and last up to 6 months; thereafter, patients have to be re-injected to maintain efficacy of the treatment. The reversibility of the treatment might raise controversies, especially in high complete tetraplegic patients, where a surgical sphincterotomy might appear more secure and appropriate. By contrast, BoNT into the external urethral sphincter appears to be a worthwhile option in acute incomplete spinal cord injured patients with DSD and high residual volume. This indication can be extended to multiple sclerosis patients[6].

14.2.3   Neurogenic detrusor overactivity

This condition causes high intravesical pressure, reduced capacity, low compliance of the bladder and can lead to upper urinary tract damage. Current treatment options rely mainly on clean intermittent catheterization and anticholinergic medication. However, side effects of oral anticholinergic medication are troublesome and reduce patient compliance. Other treatment options (functional stimulation of the pudendal nerve afferents, implantation of a sacral root nerve stimulator, sacral root rhizotomy, enterocystoplasty and ileal conduit, intravesical application of vanilloid-antagonists) are controversially discussed or have still to be evaluated.

Effect of 200–400 BOTOX® units injected into detrusor muscle in spinal cord injured patients, suffered from severe detrusor overactivity and incontinence resistant to anticholinergic drugs, was first reported by Schurch *et al*[13,17]. A total of 19 patients were regularly observed over a period of 9 months by clinical and urodynamic checks. Six weeks follow-up after injections showed a significant increase in the reflex volume and in the maximum cystometric bladder capacity, associated a decrease in the maximum detrusor voiding pressure (Figure 14.3). At 36 weeks follow-up, ongoing improvement occurred. The amount of anticholinergics could be reduced or even completely abolished. The actual experience of the European group increased to approximately 200 patients with the same results[18].

Furthermore, Schulte-Baukloh *et al.*[19-21] tested the efficacy of 85–300 BOTOX® units in 17 children with neurogenic detrusor overactivity due to myelomeningocele. Urodynamic checks were done 2–4 weeks after injection (Figure 14.4). All results were significant and continence could be restored for at least the 4 weeks follow-up. Recently, long-term efficacy of BoNT injection was demonstrated with significantly improved urodynamic situation[22].

According to data, BoNT injections into the detrusor muscle seem to be indicated in spinal cord injured patients with incontinence due to neurogenic detrusor overactivity. This treatment option seems to establish its indication in

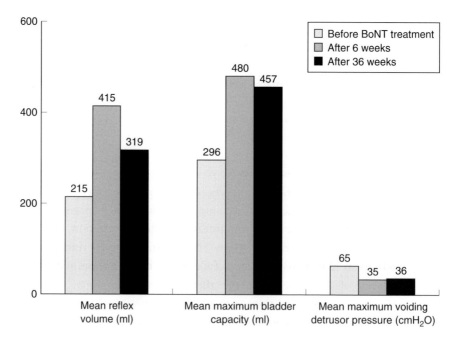

Figure 14.3   Effect of BoNT injections into the overactive detrusor muscle in spinal cord injured patients. The bladder filling was stopped as soon as the rise in detrusor pressure was constant and at maximum level. This value was then compared to the maximum detrusor voiding pressure prior to the treatment. (Modified from Schurch *et al., J. Urol.*, 2000, 164 (3 Pt. 1), 692–7.)

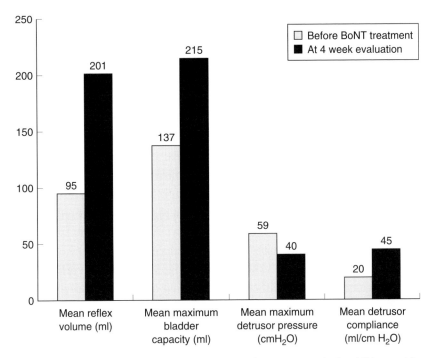

Figure 14.4 Effect of BoNT injections into the overactive detrusor muscle in children with myelo-meningocele. (Modified from Schulte-Baukloh *et al.*, *Urology*, 2002, 59, 325–7.)

cases where anticholinergic medication fails or is intolerable and appears to be a valuable alternative to surgery.

14.2.4 Idiopathic detrusor overactivity or sensor urge

Recently, effect of injections of 200 BOTOX® units into the detrusor muscle in 30 patients with severe detrusor overactivity has been reported. Of the patients reported, 67 per cent improved continence, lasting 8 months[6]. However, high residual volume and one acute retention, that might be explained by the high amount of toxin used for this indication, have been also noted. As opposed, Radzieszweski and Borkowski observed marked improvement of bladder over-activity in 12 patients at 1 month follow-up without change in the residual volume by using 300 Dysport units[23]. In another prospective study, BoNT was tested on 16 patients suffering from incontinence with motor (9 patients) or sensory urge (7 patients) with or without a neurological impairment. After treatment with 200 BOTOX® units into the detrusor muscle, 13 patients were dry and 3 patients with sensory incontinence remained incontinent. Nine of the treated patients were free of urge symptoms. Seven patients (one with motor and six with sensory urge) noted no clinical improvement.

14.2.5 Urinary retention

Recent reports clearly demonstrated that BoNT might be effective in reducing urethral resistance and facilitate voiding efficiency in patients who had either cauda equina lesion or peripheral neuropathy, as well as in those with detrusor failure and poor relaxing urethral sphincter. The role of BoNT injections into the external urethral sphincter for a variety of bladder outlet obstructions and to decrease outlet resistance in patients with a contractile detrusor wishing to void by Valsalva manoeuvre has been studied by Phelan et al[24]. After injection of 100 BOTOX® units, 20 patients were able to void without catheterization.

Kuo et al.[25] repeated the experience in 20 patients with dysuria or urinary retention due to detrusor underactivity and non-relaxing urethral sphincter, who were refractory to conservative treatment. After treatment, spontaneous voiding resumed in 11 patients and significantly improved in five. As opposed to Kuo and Phelan reports, Fowler et al.[6] found no significant improvement of micturition in six women who had difficulties in voiding or complete urinary retention due to abnormal myotonic-like activity in the striated urethral sphincter and who were treated with transperineal BoNT injection.

However, the actual controversial results strongly suggest that further studies are necessary to clarify the exact therapeutic role of BoNT injections in these cases.

14.3 Male genitourinary dysfunction

14.3.1 Chronic prostatic pain

Chronic prostatic pain is a common situation confronting the practising urologist. Up to now, the different therapies of this syndrome and their longstanding results are mostly frustrating. Recently, four consecutive men with chronic non-bacterial prostatitis and poor bladder emptying because of spastic external urethral sphincter (mean duration of symptoms 18 ± 3 months), who failed to respond to tamsulosin 0.4 mg once daily for more than 4 months were treated with 30 BOTOX® units. All the patients had uroflowmetric studies to assess times of urinary flow (TQ) and maximum urinary flow (TQ_{max}), maximum flow (Q_{max}), average flow (Q_{ave}), and total urinary volume (V_{comp}). An increased value of TQ and TQ_{max} with a normal value of Q_{max} was taken to be indicative of incomplete relaxation of bladder neck. Within 1 week of injection all patients had a striking improvement in their voiding; none complained of urinary incontinence. At 4 weeks, three patients showed a continuing improvement. At 8 weeks, the same three patients were satisfied with the therapy and none of them complained of urinary incontinence. The patients were followed up for a mean of 12 months. No relapse occurred in the three patients who improved. Uroflowmetric study showed a decrease in TQ and TQ_{max} values at 1, 4, and 8 weeks compared with baseline values[26]. Similar results have been reported in a placebo-controlled, randomized paper (Brisinda, G. and Maria, G., unpublished report — Table 14.5).

Table 14.5. AUA symptoms score and uroflowmetric data before and after BoNT treatment in men with voiding dysfunction due to non-bacterial prostatitis

	BoNT group	Saline group
AUA symptoms score		
Baseline	13 ± 6.1	12.7 ± 5.4
At 4 weeks	$3 \pm 0.7^{a,b}$	13 ± 4.8
At 8 weeks	$2.7 \pm 1.1^{a,b}$	12.4 ± 3.1
TQ (sec)		
Baseline	48.7 ± 13.2	47.6 ± 14
At 4 weeks	$16.7 \pm 10.9^{a,b}$	41.9 ± 20
At 8 weeks	$20.1 \pm 11.9^{a,b}$	42.1 ± 19.7
TQ_{max} (sec)		
Baseline	18.6 ± 6.4	19 ± 5.6
At 4 weeks	$8.8 \pm 1.2^{a,b}$	17.1 ± 3
At 8 weeks	$10.3 \pm 3.1^{a,b}$	18.2 ± 3.1
Q_{max} $(ml\,s^{-1})$		
Baseline	17.3 ± 5.5	16.9 ± 6
At 4 weeks	14.1 ± 2.8	15 ± 4.1
At 8 weeks	15.2 ± 8.7	16.1 ± 3.7
Q_{ave} $(ml\,s^{-1})$		
Baseline	10.2 ± 4.2	11 ± 3.8
At 4 weeks	9.7 ± 1.2	11 ± 2.7
At 8 weeks	10.2 ± 3.8	10.3 ± 3.1
V_{comp} (ml)		
Baseline	364.7 ± 157.5	348.2 ± 180
At 4 weeks	290.5 ± 89	344.6 ± 156.8
At 8 weeks	342.3 ± 58.2	348.4 ± 141.6

[a]$P < 0.05$ versus baseline values; [b]$P < 0.05$ versus saline group.

AUA: American Urological Association; BoNT: botulinum toxin; Q_{max}: Maximal flow; Q_{ave}: Average flow; TQ: Time of urinary flow; TQ_{max}: Time of maximal urinary flow; V_{comp}: Total urinary volume.

In 11 patients with chronic prostatic pain, urodynamic investigation, pelvic floor function and cystoscopy were conducted before and after a transurethral perisphincteric injection of 200 BOTOX® units. Nine of 11 patients reported subjective pain relief; average pain level on a visual analogue scale decreasing from 7.2 to 1.6 after the injection. The pre-post-injection comparison of the urodynamic findings showed a decrease of the functional urethral length and the urethral closure pressure, decrease of postvoidal residual volume and an increase of peak and average uroflow[27].

In these patients, BoNT into the external urethral sphincter seem to reduce the sphincter activity and improve the LUT symptoms. However, large controlled trials are needed.

14.3.2   Benign prostatic hyperplasia (BPH)

Benign prostatic hyperplasia is a non-malignant enlargement of the prostate that involves both the stromal and the epithelial elements of the gland[28−34]. Symptoms stem from urethral obstruction and gradual loss of bladder function, which results in incomplete bladder emptying, and can lead to complications, including acute urinary retention[30,35,36]. It rarely causes symptoms before age 40, but more than half of men in their sixties and as many as 90 per cent in their seventies and eighties have some symptoms of disease[37].

The goal of therapy is to reduce or alleviate LUT symptoms, to prevent complications, and to minimize adverse effects of treatment[29]. Few treatments are without any adverse consequences, and this is particularly so with treatments with BPH, where there is a delicate balancing act between benefits and demerits of the available treatments[37]. There are several treatment options, that include medical therapies and various surgical procedures[30−32,38]. Although transurethral prostatic resection is an effective treatment for symptomatic BPH, it is by no means perfect. Approximately 25 per cent of patients who undergo surgical treatment do not have satisfactory long-term outcomes[39]. Analysis of data found that mortality in the 30 days after transurethral resection for BPH ranged from 0.4 per cent for men aged 65−69 to 1.9 per cent for men aged 80−84, and has fallen in recent years. Furthermore, the procedure was associated with immediate surgical complications in 12 per cent of patients, bleeding requiring intervention in 2 per cent, erectile dysfunction in 14 per cent, retrograde ejaculation in 74 per cent, and incontinence in about 5 per cent[35]. Because of these problems, as well as desire of patients to avoid surgery whenever possible, there has been much interest in alternative treatments[37]. Recent studies have reported that both finasteride, a 5α-reductase inhibitor, and long-acting α1-adrenergic antagonist drugs, such as terazosin, doxazosin, and tamsulosin, are safe and effective treatments for BPH[30,36,40−42]. It has also documented that the combination of terazosin and finasteride was no more effective than terazosin alone[41]. Although these drugs represent an attractive options for men with BPH, they have adverse effects. However, a systematic review found that withdrawals attributed to adverse events were similar for alfusozin, tamsulosin, and placebo[40,42,43]. A higher withdrawal rate was found with doxazosin and terazosin.

Recently, it has been documented that BoNT injection into the rat prostate induces selective denervation and subsequent atrophy of the gland[44]. A placebo-controlled study has been recently performed. Men 50−80 years of age who had symptomatic BPH were enrolled in the study. All the patients underwent a digital rectal examination. The symptoms were assessed with the American Urological Association (AUA) symptom index[45,46]. In addition, uroflowmetry was performed, and residual urinary volume was determined ultrasonographically[35,47]. Serum concentrations of prostate-specific antigen (PSA) were measured, and transrectal ultrasonography was performed to determine prostatic volume[35]. The primary end point was evaluation of symptomatic improvement after treatment, as measured by means of AUA symptoms score and peak urinary flow rates. The secondary end point was evaluation of prostatic volume, serum PSA concentration, and residual urinary volume. Each of the participants received 4 ml of solution injected in the prostate gland, divided into two injections of equal volume (2 ml) on each lobe of the gland. Patients in the control group received just saline solution; patients in the treated group received 200 BOTOX® units.

Thirty patients were randomized; 15 received BoNT, and 15 received placebo. No statistical difference were found regarding to age, AUA symptoms score, serum PSA concentration, prostatic volume, peak urinary flow rate, and residual urine volume at base-line between the two groups (Table 14.6). No local complications during the procedure or post-injection systemic side effects were observed in any patient.

At 2 months evaluations, no local or systemic side effects were reported. Thirteen BoNT patients and 3 in the control group had symptomatic relief ($P = 0.0007$). In patients who received BoNT, AUA symptoms score was reduced by 65 per cent ($P = 0.00001$) as compared with base-line values, and significantly vary from 1-month values ($P = 0.0001$). In the same patients, serum PSA concentration was reduced by 51 per cent ($P = 0.00001$) from baseline, and did not vary from a 1-month value. In patients who received saline, AUA symptoms score and serum PSA concentration were not significantly changed, as compared with base-line and 1-month values in the same patients, and significantly differ from values in treated patients.

In treated patients, as compared with base-line values, prostatic volume and residual urine volume were reduced by 68 per cent ($P = 0.00001$) and 83 per cent

Table 14.6. Base-line characteristics and results at 1 and 2 months evaluations in the 30 patients with BPH. Values are mean $\pm$ SD. All patients were included in all evaluations

Characteristics	BoNT group	Saline group
Number of patients	15	15
Age (yr)	69.4 $\pm$ 4.9	68.2 $\pm$ 3.9
Base-line		
AUA symptoms score (points)	23.2 $\pm$ 4.1	23.3 $\pm$ 3.9
Serum PSA (ng per ml)	3.7 $\pm$ 0.9	3.5 $\pm$ 1.0
Prostatic volume (ml)	52.6 $\pm$ 10.6	52.3 $\pm$ 10.0
Peak urinary flow (ml per second)	8.1 $\pm$ 2.2	8.8 $\pm$ 2.5
Residual urinary volume (ml)	126.3 $\pm$ 38.3	118.0 $\pm$ 39.7
One month evaluation		
AUA symptoms score (points)	10.6 $\pm$ 1.7	23.4 $\pm$ 3.5
Serum PSA (ng per ml)	2.1 $\pm$ 0.7	3.4 $\pm$ 0.8
Prostatic volume (ml)	23.8 $\pm$ 6.2	50.5 $\pm$ 8.1
Peak urinary flow (ml per second)	14.9 $\pm$ 2.1	8.8 $\pm$ 2.3
Residual urinary volume (ml)	49.6 $\pm$ 13.4	116.7 $\pm$ 33.1
Two months evaluation		
AUA symptoms score (points)	8.0 $\pm$ 1.6	23.3 $\pm$ 3.3
Serum PSA (ng per ml)	1.8 $\pm$ 0.7	3.4 $\pm$ 0.8
Prostatic volume (ml)	16.8 $\pm$ 7.8	50.3 $\pm$ 7.9
Peak urinary flow (ml per second)	15.4 $\pm$ 1.7	8.7 $\pm$ 2.3
Residual urinary volume (ml)	21.0 $\pm$ 16.2	116.7 $\pm$ 31.0

AUA: American Urological Association; BoNT: botulinum toxin; BPH: benign prostatic hyperplasia; PSA: prostatic specific antigen.

($P=0.00001$), respectively; mean peak urinary flow rate was significantly increased from baseline value ($P=0.00001$). In patients who received saline, these values were not significantly changed as compared with base-line and with 1-month values, and significantly differ from values in treated patients.

A rescue treatment was proposed to the 14 patients: 10 of them refused and underwent medical or surgical therapy. The other four patients, all of whom had been receiving saline, received 200 BOTOX® units each. All the 17 patients who received botulinum toxin injections were periodically evaluated. Follow-up averaged 19.6 $\pm$ 3.8 months. Six and twelve months after botulinum toxin injections, the patients underwent the same evaluations performed as the baseline (Table 14.7).

This study demonstrates that botulinum toxin can be used to treat BPH. A symptomatic improvement has been observed in 86 per cent of BoNT patients[48].

Table 14.7. Long-term results in 17 patients with BPH who received BoNT. Values are mean $\pm$ SD. All patients were included in all evaluations

Characteristics	Six-months evaluation	Twelve-months evaluation
AUA symptoms score (points)	9.1 ± 3	8.9 ± 3.2
Serum PSA (ng per ml)	2.1 ± 1.1	2.3 ± 1.4
Prostatic volume (ml)	2.1 ± 7.1	20.5 ± 8
Peak urinary flow (ml per second)	14.6 ± 4.1	15 ± 2.9
Residual urinary volume (ml)	24.2 ± 17	24 ± 18

AUA: American Urological Association; BoNT: botulinum toxin; BPH: benign prostatic hyperplasia; PSA: prostatic specific antigen.

The BoNT benefit was evident within 1 month after the treatment, and it continued throughout the follow-up period. A decrease of AUA symptoms score and improvement of peak urinary-flow rate have been observed after BoNT injections: at 2-month evaluation, AUA symptoms score was reduced as compared with base-line values, and, in the same patients, mean peak urinary flow rate was significantly increased from pre-treatment evaluation. It has also documented that BoNT induces a decrease in the mean residual urinary volume (at 2-month evaluation, ultrasonography not showed residual urinary volume in six treated patients) and a reduction in prostate volume, as documented by both ultrasonography and serum PSA concentration.

The prostatic growth has been considered to be controlled by endocrine means[49–51]. However, abundance of adrenergic and muscarinic receptors and nerve fibres suggests that the autonomic nervous system may play a role in the growth and secretory function of the gland[50–53]. It has been also found that a subtype of muscarinic receptors is present in BPH and was the predominant subtype there. In the human prostate, it has been proposed that these muscarinic receptors stimulate growth of the gland[53]. It seems conceivable that BoNT, blocking these receptors at which acetylcholine is the transmitter, induces denervation and atrophy in human prostate. In fact, prostatic volume and serum PSA concentration were reduced in treated patients, without signs of either systemic or local toxicity. Furthermore, use of α-adrenergic blockade to treat symptomatic BPH is based on the hypothesis that the disease arises from bladder-outlet obstruction and that 40 per cent of the cellular volume of the hyperplastic gland is made up of smooth muscle[50], whose tension is mediated by $\alpha 1$-adrenoceptors. BoNT may induce directly smooth muscle relaxation or by means of neuronal NO.

14.4 Female sexual dysfunction

Female sexual dysfunction includes desire, arousal, orgasmic, and sex pain disorders (dyspareunia and vaginismus). It can be associated with a number of conditions, which may be unrelated to the sexual act and chronic general medical conditions can contribute. These include physical conditions, such as gynaecological problems and ill-health, as well as psychological conditions, such as physical and sexual abuse.

14.4.1 Vaginismus

Botulinum toxin has been proposed as a treatment for vaginismus, whose aetiology is unclear. It is described as a vaginal pain disorder, but more recently, has been conceptualized as an aversion/phobia of vaginal penetration[54]. There is no doubt, however, that anecdotal reports suggest the benefit of muscle relaxation in allowing easier penetration, which thus contributes to easing the fear. BoNT has thus been used, as skeletal muscle is involved and its mechanism of action is the same as for muscle relaxation elsewhere.

There are no controlled trials of BoNT in the treatment of vaginismus, but a number of reviews of the management of bladder, bowel and pelvic floor disorders have included this condition[55]. BoNT is injected into the pelvic floor muscle around the distal vagina. The effect, like elsewhere, is dose-dependent, but 50–80 U BOTOX® is recommended in the first instance. The effect is to diminish the tension in the pelvic floor by allowing the main effect of the muscle to be raised cranially. This mechanism is thought to decrease pain and allow easier access. No reports have indicated whether there is any adverse effect on vaginal secretions, as BoNT could possibly reduce them.

14.5 Bowel and anal problems

14.5.1 Anatomy and physiology of anal sphincters

The complex anatomy and physiology of the anal canal and rectum account for their important role in continence and for their susceptibility to diseases. The main component of the pelvic floor is the *levator ani* muscle (Figure 14.5). The anorectal angle indicates bending of the rectum by the sling-shaped fibres of the puborectalis at the level of the anorectal junction; it is important to maintain gross faecal continence (Figure 14.6)[3,56,57].

At the anal level, the sphincter complex consists of two overlapping sphincters (Figure 14.7). The external anal sphincter (EAS), that forms the outer layer, is composed of a voluntary, skeletal muscle. The internal anal sphincter (IAS) is

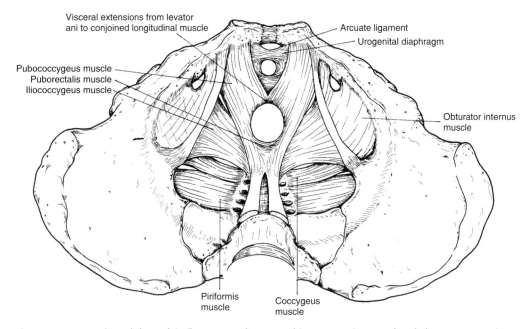

Figure 14.5 Drawing of the pelvic floor musculature and its connections to the skeleton as seen from inside the abdomen. The *levator ani* muscle is composed by the iliococcygeous, the pubococcygeous and the puborectalis. The puborectalis is a U-shaped strong loop of striated muscle that pulls the anorectum junction to the back of the pubis. It represent the most medial portion of the *levator ani* muscle and is situated immediately cephalad to the deep component of the external anal sphincter.

the involuntary, smooth muscle component of the sphincter complex. Being in a state of continuous maximal contraction, the IAS is a natural barrier to the involuntary loss of stool and gas. This is due to a combination of intrinsic myogenic and extrinsic autonomic neurogenic properties[58]. The IAS is responsible for 50–85 per cent of resting anal tone. Being of visceral origin, it is supplied both by sympathetic and parasympathetic nerves; in addition, the ENS modulates its tonic activity. Noradrenergic sympathetic nerves are considered excitatory and the parasympathetic inhibitory to the IAS. Sympathetic neurons that supply the IAS are noradrenergic. Vagal neurons do not act directly, but rather form synaptic connections with neurons whose cell bodies are in the intrinsic GIT ganglia. This transmission is principally mediated by ACh acting on nicotinic receptors[57]. Recently, it has been shown that the longitudinal layer and the circular smooth muscle in the human rectum receive an intrinsic NO-mediated inhibitory innervation[59–61]. The exact site of involvement remains to be determined, but recent data suggest that carbon monoxide and heme oxygenase pathway may have a role in neurally mediated relaxation of the IAS[62,63].

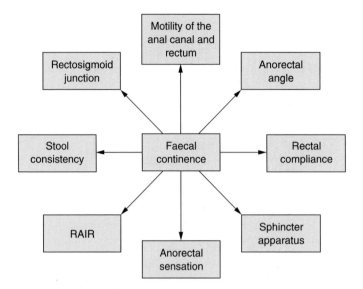

Figure 14.6 Factors contributing to the maintenance of faecal continence. Continence is maintained by normal rectal sensation and tonic contraction of the internal anal sphincter and the puborectalis muscle, which wraps around the anorectum, maintaining an anorectal angle between 80 and 110 degrees. During defecation, the pelvic-floor muscles (including the puborectalis) relax, allowing the anorectal angle to straighten by at least 15 degrees, and the perineum descends by 1.0–3.5 cm. The external anal sphincter also relaxes and reduces pressure on the anal canal. A faecal bolus in the rectum results in reflex relaxation of the IAS, the so-called rectoanal inhibitory reflex (RAIR). There is agreement on the local intramural nature of the reflex, and morphologic data provide compelling anatomic evidence that NO mediates RAIR.

14.5.2 Neuromyogenic properties of the GIT smooth muscles

Motility of a gut segment depends on its extrinsic and intrinsic innervation[58,64]. Preganglionic parasympathetic nerves and postganglionic sympathetic nerves, which constitute the autonomic nervous system, provide extrinsic innervation; the ENS is a highly complex system, responsible for the coordination of motility, secretion, and microcirculation in the GIT and for the regulation of the local response to immune inflammatory processes. The ENS can function independently of the central nervous system (CNS), which nevertheless maintains a coordinating role for diverse functions of GIT neurons via sympathetic and parasympathetic motor and sensory pathways[58,65].

Functional organization of the ENS

ENS is composed of nerve cell bodies and their processes embedded in the gut wall, which form two main ganglionated plexuses: Auerbach's myenteric plexus and Meissner's sub-mucous plexus. Other, non-ganglionated, plexuses supply GIT layers[57].

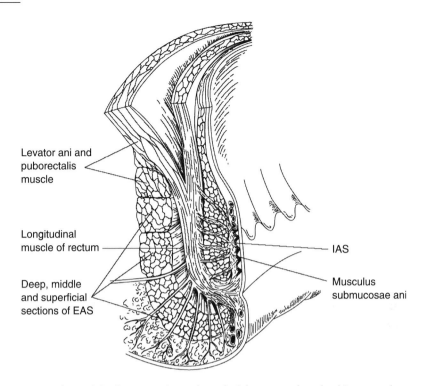

Figure 14.7 Connections of the *levator ani* muscle and of the external anal sphincter to the rectum and the perineum.

In the ENS, intraparietal neurons encompass motor neurons (excitatory and inhibitory), interneurons and intrinsic sensory neurons (Figure 14.8). Sympathetic and parasympathetic neurons also innervate the GIT. Excitatory motor neurons innervate longitudinal and circular muscles and the muscularis mucosae. Their primary transmitter is acetylcholine (ACh), but they also release tachykinins, substance P, neurokinin A, neuropeptide K, and neuropeptide Y. Inhibitory motor neurons relax smooth muscles and are involved in reflexes that facilitate the passage of food along the GIT. Inhibitory neurons release a combination of at least three transmitters: NO, adenosine triphosphate (ATP), and vasoactive intestinal polypeptide (VIP). In most neurons, NO is the primary transmitter, while the roles played by VIP and ATP may vary. A neuronal NO synthase is expressed in ENS neurons where it is usually co-localized with VIP[65].

Sympathetic pathways to the GIT are noradrenergic; they inhibit motility, constrict the sphincters and in general inhibit contractile activity, by means of a presynaptic action on the myenteric plexus. The vagus nerve includes the axons of neurons located in the brainstem. A variety of central effects (relaxation of

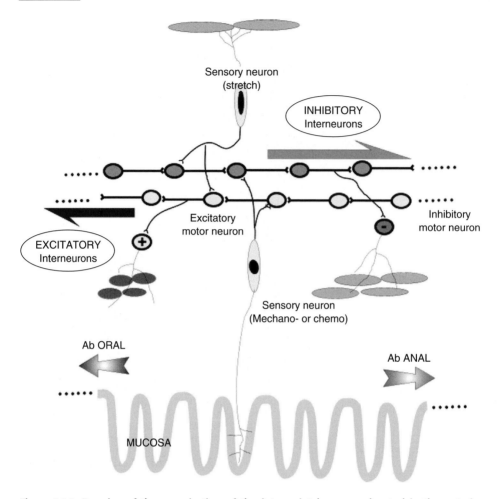

Figure 14.8 Drawing of the organization of the intraparietal neurons located in the enteric nervous system.

the proximal stomach, enhancement of gastric peristalsis, secretion of acid) are mediated by the vagus nerve[58,66]. Vagal neurons are involved in complex circuits integrating various enteric reflexes with signals that derive from the CNS and from other GIT regions; ACh principally mediates this transmission (Figure 14.9)[58].

Smooth muscle contraction

This function is regulated by changes in cytosol calcium levels. Calcium regulation is affected by a variety of regulatory proteins (myosin light chains, calmodulin, and calponin). The precise mechanisms responsible for the maintenance of smooth muscle tone are still not entirely known. These functions depend on the intrinsic electrical and mechanical properties of GIT smooth muscles and are regulated by

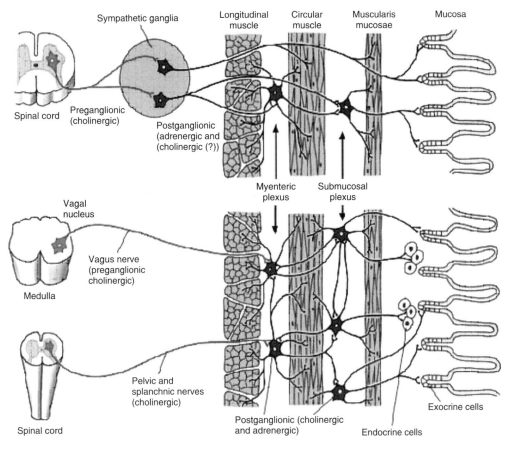

Figure 14.9 Schematic view of sympathetic, vagal, and pelvic and splanchnic pathways that regulate functions of the gastrointestinal tract.

the ENS and by sympathetic and parasympathetic influences. An increase in cellular calcium can be produced by the influx of calcium through membrane channels or by stimulation of α1 adrenoceptors, resulting in a release of calcium from the sarcoplasmic reticulum mediated by inositol triphosphate. Stimulation of β2 adrenoceptors brings about cAMP-mediated return of calcium to the sarcoplasmic reticulum. Stimulation of NO induces cGMP-mediated decrease in cellular calcium.

14.6 Bowel and anal treatment indications

14.6.1 Chronic anal fissure

A chronic fissure is a cut or crack in the anal canal or anal verge (Figure 14.10). The fissure can be seen as the buttocks are parted (Figure 14.11). It is often

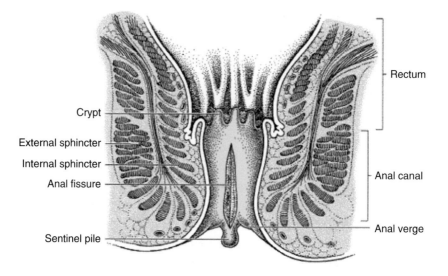

Figure 14.10 Drawing of anal fissure. It is a cut or crack in the anal canal or anal verge that may extend from the muco-cutaneous junction to the dentate line. Classic symptoms are pain on or after defecation that is often severe and may last from minutes to several hours. Often there is bright blood on the toilet paper. The majority of fissures occur in the posterior midline of the anal canal.

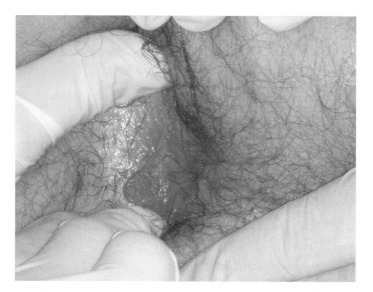

Figure 14.11 Direct observation of a chronic anal fissure, with sharp borders and exposure of fibres of the internal anal sphincter.

suspected because there is marked spasm of the anus making examination difficult. IAS spasm has been noted in association with chronic fissure and for many years treatment has focused on alleviating IAS hypertonia (Figure 14.12).

Pathophysiology of chronic fissure

The cause of chronic fissures and the reasons for their failure to heal remain unclear. Also unexplained are the main characteristics of this painful condition, including the predilection for posterior midline and the lack of granulation tissue at the fissure site. Several theories have been advanced to unravel the underlying cause of anal fissure. Most of them are conflicting and none gives a satisfactory explanation for the characteristic features of chronic fissure.

The passage of a hard stool bolus has traditionally been thought to cause anal fissure. Fibres of the superficial EAS decussate to form a Y shape posteriorly; the overlying skin has been said to be poorly supported and to be prone to tear on passage of a large stool. However, a history of constipation preceding the onset of anal fissure is obtained only in one of four cases and diarrhoea is seen to be a predisposing factor in about 6 per cent of patients[67].

IAS spasm has been noted for many years in association with anal fissure. It has been found that the IAS of patients with anal fissure is fibrotic, compared with that of controls[68]. It was then postulated that a myositis might occur early in the course of a fissure and that this is the underlying cause of both spasm and fibrosis. Although the cause of the spasm remains obscure, it has been consistently found that resting anal pressure is higher in the patients with anal fissure than in normal controls, suggesting that the high resting pressure be related to IAS hypertonicity.

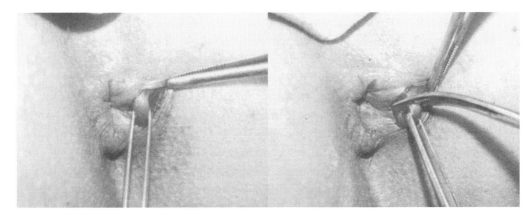

Figure 14.12 Intraoperative photographs of a lateral internal sphincterotomy.

It has been postulated that the increased incidence of fissure in the anterior and posterior midline positions is related to the distribution of vessels supplying blood to the anal canal[69,70]. Relief of symptoms and healing induced by treatment could be attributed to a decrease in anal pressure, that would increase the mucosal blood flow and relieve ischaemia. The predilection of anal fissures for the posterior midline and the lack of granulation tissue seen in the base of a chronic fissure may be explained by ischaemia.

Decreased anodermal blood flow may be promoted by endothelial cells dysfunction associated with reduced NO synthesis, which is known to be involved in the regulation of local blood flow. Activation of the endothelium may express antigens as the endothelial cells can act as antigen-presenting cells. Anti-endothelial cell antibodies have been found in many patients with anal fissure, but not in healthy controls[71]. In antibody-positive patients, higher resting anal tone has been observed. This supports a role of the endothelium in the pathogenesis of anal ischaemia. Circulating antibodies may activate the endothelium to produce vasoactive autacoids, which could contribute to the increased basal tone and aggravate the ischaemia at the level of the posterior commissure[72].

A primary IAS disturbance may be a contributing etiologic factor. IAS supersensitivity to β2-agonists has been observed in chronic fissure[73]. This may be induced by a prolonged absence of the neurotransmitter, by abnormalities at neurotransmitter or metabolic level, or by a modification of cholinergic and adrenergic receptors.

Results of BoNT treatment

BoNT can be used to treat anal fissure, particularly when a patient is at high risk of incontinence (Table 14.8)[1–3,74–107]. With the patient lying on a side (usually the left side when the operator is right-handed), the IAS can be easily palpated and injected. The lower rounded edge of the IAS can be felt on physical examination about 1–1.5 cm to the dentate line. The groove between the internal and the external sphincters can be visualized or easily palpated.

BoNT appears as a safe treatment for patients with chronic anal fissure. It is easier to perform than surgical treatment and does not require anaesthesia. It is also more efficacious than nitrate therapy. In the patients with a posterior chronic fissure better results are achieved when toxin is injected anteriorly into the IAS. No adverse effects or permanent IAS damage have resulted from BoNT injection.

The therapeutic efficacy of different BoNT-A doses in chronic fissure have been reported recently[1–3,97,98,102,103]. It has been found that the healing rate does not differ significantly when the total dose and the number of injection sites are varied. In a recent experience, patients with a posterior chronic fissure have better results,

Table 14.8. Comparison of published results on the treatment of patients with anal fissure

Author/Year	No. cases	Units/injection's site	Healing rate (%) 1 m	Healing rate (%) 2 m	Reinjection (%)/dose	Complete healing rate (%)	Temporary incontinence (%)	Recurrence (%)	Reduction in RAP (%) 1 m	Reduction in RAP (%) 2 m	Reduction in MVC (%) 1 m	Reduction in MVC (%) 2 m
Gui et al., 1994	10	15 B/IAS	60	70	40/20 B	90	10	10	23.9	7.8	0	+13.1
Jost et al., 1994	12	5 B/EAS	Nr	83.3	—	83.3	0	8.3	Within normal limits in 3 months		Within normal limits	
Jost et al., 1995	54	5 B/EAS	Nr	78	—	78	6	6	Nr	Nr	Nr	Nr
Mason et al., 1996	5	Nr D/IAS	Nr	60	—	60	0	Nr	Nr	Nr	Nr	Nr
Jost, 1997	100	2.5–5 B/EAS	Nr	82	—	82	7	8	Normal limits	Normal limits		
Espi et al., 1997	36	10 B/IAS	65	—	—	65	0	0	Nr	Nr	Nr	Nr
		15 B/IAS	81			81		0				
Maria et al., 1998	15	20 B/IAS	53.3	73.3	26.6/25 B	100	4	6.7	27	25.7	15.5	9.9
	15	Saline	13.3	13.3					3.9	4.9	0	0
Maria et al., 1998	23	15 B/IAS	21.7	43.5	8.7/20 B	100	0	0	27.7	15.9	18.2	12.1
	34	20 B/IAS	50	67.6	20.6/25 B	100	0	0	27.9	28.8	14.3	11.9
Minguez et al., 1999	23	10 B/IAS	48	Nr	52	83	0	37–52	4.9	Nr	16.9	
	27	15 B/IAS	74		30	78			13.1		18.4	
	19	21 B/IAS	100		37	90			16.1		34.2	
Jost and Schrank, 1999	25	20 D/EAS	Nr	76	—	76	4	4	Nr	Nr	Nr	Nr
	25	40 D/EAS		80		80	12	8				
Brisinda et al., 1999	25	20 B/IAS	88	96	—	96	0	0	26.3	28.9	5.7	4.6
	25	0.2% GTN	40	60		60	0	0	16.7	13.8	+2.3	+8.5
Fernandez et al., 1999	76	40 B/IAS	56	67	45.2/40 B	67	3	0	Nr	Nr	Nr	Nr

Table 14.8. (*Cont.*) Comparison of published results on the treatment of patients with anal fissure

Author/Year	No. cases	Units/injection's site	Healing rate (%) 1 m	Healing rate (%) 2 m	Reinjection (%)/dose	Complete healing rate (%)	Temporary incontinence (%)	Recurrence (%)	Recurrence	Reduction in RAP (%) 1 m	Reduction in RAP (%) 2 m	Reduction in MVC (%) 1 m	Reduction in MVC (%) 2 m
Madalinski et al., 1999	13	20 B/EAS	84.6	Nr	–	–	Nr	15.4	Nr	Nr	Nr	Nr	Nr
Khademi and Feldman*, 2000	11	25 B/IAS	Nr	82	–	82	0	0	0	Nr	Nr	Nr	Nr
Maria et al., 2000	25	20 B/IAS PI	48	60	24/25 B	80	0	0	0	22.6	22.4	4.6	4.8
	25	20 B/IAS AI	88	88	12/25 B	100				30.9	31.9	1.8	1.8
Lysy et al., 2001	15	20 B+ID/IAS	66	73	–	73	0	0	0	24.2	Nr	4.8	Nr
	15	20 B/IAS	20	60		60				20.6		4.4	
Madalinski et al.*, 2001	14	25–50 B/EAS	Nr	54	–	54	0	8	0	Nr	Nr	Nr	Nr
Tilney et al., 2001	10	Nr D/IAS	Nr	Nr	10.7/30 B		Nr	Nr	20	Nr	Nr	Nr	Nr
Jost, 2001	10	200 NB/EAS	Nr	70 improved	Nr	0	Nr	Nr	Nr	Nr	Nr	Nr	Nr
Brisinda et al., 2002	75	20 B/IAS	73	89	10.7/30 B	100	0	0	0	30	30	3.5	0
	75	30 B/IAS	87	96	4/50 B	100	3	4		32.6	34.3	15	7.8
Brisinda et al., 2003	6	150 D/IAS	100	Nr	–	100	0	0	0	34.9	Nr	1	Nr
Mentes et al., 2003[†]	61	20–30 B/IAS	62.3	73.8	–	86.9	0	11.4	0	Nr	Nr	Nr	Nr
	50	LIS	82	98		98	16	0					

| Siproudhis et al., 2003‡ | 22 | 100 D/IAS | 50 | 32 | Nr | Nr | Nr | Nr | 22.7 | Nr | Nr | Nr |
| | 22 | Saline | 45 | 32 | | | | | 22.7 | | | |

*Plus topical nitrates. AI: injection in anterior midline; B: BOTOX® (trade name of the type A preparation manufactured by Allergan, Irvine, CA, USA); D: Dysport (trade name of the type A botulinum toxin preparation manufactured by Ipsen, Maidenhead, UK); EAS: external anal sphincter; GTN: glyceryl trinitrate; IAS: internal anal sphincter; ID: isosorbide dinitrate; LIS: lateral internal sphincterotomy; MVC: maximum voluntary contraction; NB: Neurobloc (trade name of the type B preparation manufactured by Elan Pharma International Ltd, Ireland); Nr: Not reported; PI: injection in posterior midline; RAP: resting anal pressure.

†The authors conducted a randomized, prospective trial to compare BoNT with LIS as definitive management for chronic anal fissure. It has been shown in botulinum group A complete healing, after a single injection, in 45 of the 61 patients (73.8%) at the second month. Of the 16 failures, six patients refused further treatment, and 10 were treated with a second injection, which resulted in an overall healing rate of 86.9 per cent (53/61) at 6 months. In the sphincterotomy group, the success rate was 82 per cent (41/50) at 1 month and 98 per cent (49/50) at 2 months. At 6 months, two patients who had undergone LIS developed recurrences, and the healing rate was similar to that of BoNT group. At 12 months, the success rate of the BOTOX® group fell to 75.4 per cent (46/61) with seven recurrences, whereas it remained stable in the sphincterotomy group (94%). Furthermore, the authors have also documented that sphincterotomy was associated with a significantly higher complication rate (eight cases of anal incontinence), and they suggested that BoNT injection is inferior to LIS in the treatment of anal fissure, regarding healing rates within the time limits of their study. However, we have noted that at 12-months evaluation in LIS group healing rate (78% − 39 patients) was similar to that of BoNT group (75%); we believe that anal incontinence after LIS should be considered as a failure of surgical treatment. Furthermore, no manometric study of both the IAS and EAS were performed to demonstrate hypertonia; virtually every article in the literature impugning BoNT as a treatment of chronic anal fissure has manometric data demonstrating the efficacy of toxin in inducing reduction of resting tone and fissure healing.

‡This study addresses the lack of efficacy of botulinum toxin in the treatment of patients with chronic anal fissure. The work is commended for prospective, randomized, double-blind study design. The authors find no benefit from botulinum toxin as assessed by a 100 mm visual analogue scale. Together these facts make this an interesting article with results worth reporting. However, every procedure needs a learning curve: 44 patients in six ambulatory care clinics (7.3 patients for each ambulatory care clinic) is a small number.

represented by a lowering of resting anal tone and early development of a healing scar, when BoNT is injected anteriorly into the IAS. The practice of anteriorly placed injections induces a higher fall in resting pressure and improves the clinical outcome. Fibrosis of the IAS, that is more prominent in the site of the fissure than elsewhere in the smooth muscle, may reduce IAS compliance and limit BoNT diffusion. It is known that the myenteric plexus with myenteric ganglia is located between the circular and longitudinal smooth muscle layers along the entire extent of the IAS. A chronic reduction of perfusion in the posterior part of the anus may affect the myenteric nervous fibres at this location and make them less sensitive to the action of BoNT.

It has been observed that BoNT injections into the EAS are also effective for treating fissure. The mechanism is probably mediated by diffusion to the IAS, as shown by the observation that maximum squeeze pressure and resting pressure are both reduced with this procedure. Since the fundamental pathogenic event in chronic fissure is the IAS spasm, the injection into the EAS is not the first choice for treatment. In addition, the IAS is readily visible and easier to inject than the EAS.

Complications of the treatment have been reported by several authors. Reported side effects, other than mild and transitory incontinence for flatus or faeces, encompass perianal thrombosis and haematoma[100]. However, the development of the potential complications[106,107] does not seem to influence the overall efficacy of the treatment[76–79,81,84,85,87,88,101,110–112]. To evaluate safety of this treatment, six patients, without detectable cardiovascular or autonomic diseases, who underwent treatment with 150 Dysport units for chronic anal fissure have been studied. Ewing protocol (measurement of heart rate changes during deep breathing, Valsalva manoeuvre, and during standing up; blood-pressure measurement during handgrip and during standing up) in basal condition (before treatment) and repeated the tests within 96 hours and within 30 days after treatment has been conducted. To classify the severity of the effect on the ANS, a score (0 = normal response; 1 = borderline; 2 = abnormal) is given to each test; an ending score can change from 0/10–1/10 (normal pattern), to 2/10–4/10 (borderline pattern), to 5/10–10/10 (abnormal pattern). No patient had worsening of test scores after BoNT injections. In particular, before treatment a borderline pattern (2/10 score) was found in four patients. At 96-hour evaluation, a borderline pattern (2/10 score) was found in one patient; at 30 days evaluation, all patients who had previously an abnormal score no longer had such a score, and a normal pattern (0/10) was found in all treated patients[102].

Minguez and co-workers[98] analysed the long-term outcome (42 months) of 57 patients in whom an anal fissure had healed after BoNT injections.

The authors state that the late recurrence rate of chronic fissure is high when the BoNT effect disappears. A fissure recurrence has been noted in 22 patients (41.5%). Furthermore, they showed that the highest risk of recurrence is associated with anterior location of the fissure, prolonged illness, a need for reinjection and for high doses to achieve healing.

14.6.2 Other applications in the lower GIT

Pelvic floor dysfunction

Pelvic floor dysfunction is characterized by a failure of the puborectalis muscle to relax during efforts to defecate, or by its paradoxical contraction. With an effort to evacuate the rectum, the puborectalis and the EAS normally relax to straighten the anorectal angle and open the anal canal. The diagnosis is suggested by the demonstration of a persistent impression of the puborectalis on the posterior surface of the anal canal during attempted evacuation of barium paste and, more reliably, by EMG evidence of increased electrical activity in the puborectalis muscle during straining.

The etiology of pelvic floor dysfunction is unclear. As in other forms of constipation, the patients are commonly females, who developed constipation as adolescents or young adults. Prolonged efforts to empty the rectum may aggravate the condition. It has been suggested that paradoxical puborectalis contraction during straining represents a focal dystonia.

BoNT-A has been used to selectively weaken the EAS and puborectalis muscle in constipated patients[113,114]. It has been observed that BoNT-A relaxes the puborectalis muscle[115,116]; as a consequence, the anorectal angle increases during straining and evacuation becomes possible (Table 14.9). However, despite good results, the effect of BoNT-A injections is fairly short term.

Outlet-type constipation may also occur in Parkinson's disease (PD)[117]. We performed a prospective study to identify the prevalence of this condition among PD out-patients. Patients with a diagnosis of PD filled an inventory of gastro-intestinal function and received a proctological evaluation. A total of 138 patients met the inclusion criteria for chronic constipation; 18 of them (13%) had isolated or prominent outlet-type constipation. Ten patients (one woman and nine men, mean age $\pm$ SD 69.1 $\pm$ 9.2 years, mean duration of PD 70 $\pm$ 53 months, mean duration of constipation 35.3 $\pm$ 11 months) were studied. BoNT was injected in the puborectalis muscle (two sites on either side of the muscle) under transrectal ultrasonography guidance; the total dose per session was 100 units in each patient. This observation indicates that outlet obstruction is the main cause for constipation in a minority of PD patients and provides evidence that BoNT-A may be a remedy for them (Figure 14.13). The duration of efficacy of the injections

Table 14.9. Published results of treatment of outlet type constipation with BoNT

Author/Year	Number of patients	Name of drug/dose (units)	Results	Complications
Hallan et al., 1988	7	Dysport – Dose: Nr	Maximum voluntary contraction from 70 to 28 cmH$_2$O. Anorectal angle from 96 to 124°. Symptomatic improvement in four patients.	Incontinence in two patients
Joo et al., 1996	4	BOTOX® – 6–15 U	Symptomatic improvement in all treated patients. Two patients relapsed.	0
Shafik et al., 1998	15	BOTOX® – 25 U	Symptomatic improvement in 13 patients, on average 4.8 months after the first treatment.	0
Bentivoglio et al., 2000	10 PD	BOTOX® – 30 to 100 U	Anal tone during straining from 95 mmHg to 38 mmHg at 8 weeks. Increment of anorectal angle.	Nr
Maria et al., 2000	4	BOTOX® – 30 U	75 per cent were improved at 8 weeks. Anal tone during straining from 96.2 mmHg to 42.5 mmHg at 4 weeks, and to 63.2 mmHg at 8 weeks. Anorectal angle from 94° to 114°.	0
Maria et al., 2000	14 AR	BOTOX® – 30 U	At 2-month evaluation, a symptomatic improvement was found in nine patients. At defecography, the rectocele depth was reduced from 4.3 ± 0.6 cm to 1.8 ± 0.5 cm ($P<0.001$) and the rectocele area was reduced from 9.2 ± 1.3 cm^2 to 2.8 ± 1.6 cm^2 ($P<0.001$). The anorectal angle measured during straining increased from a mean of 98 ± 15° before treatment to a mean of 121 ± 19° ($P=0.001$)[116]. At one-year evaluation, there was no report of digitally assisted rectal voiding and rectocele was not found at physical examination.	0

Ron et al., 2001	25	BOTOX® – 20 U	Symptomatic improvement in 75 per cent of the patients.	Perineal pain in three patients
Madalinski et al., 2002	39	BOTOX® – 25 U Dysport – 150 U	Nr	Perineal pain in four patients
Albanese et al., 2003	10 PD	BOTOX® – 100 U	Following treatment, anal tone during straining was reduced from 97.4 ± 19.6 mmHg at baseline to 40.7 ± 11.5 mmHg one month after treatment ($P = 0.00001$); no further change was observed at the two-month evaluation (38.2 ± 10.4 mmHg; $P = 0.00001$ vs. baseline values). The anorectal angle during straining (as measured with defecography) increased from a mean of $99° \pm 7.9$ before treatment to $122.2° \pm 15$ ($P = 0.0004$); nine patients evacuated the barium paste without the need for laxatives or enemas.	0

Nr: not reported. Dysport is the trade name of the type A botulinum toxin preparation manufactured by Ipsen (Maidenhead, UK); BOTOX® is the trade name of the type A preparation manufactured by Allergan (Irvine, CA, USA). AR: anterior rectocele; BoNT: botulinum toxin; PD: Parkinson's disease.

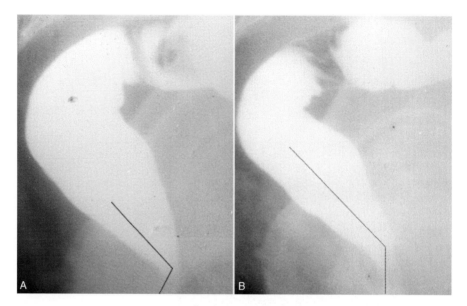

Figure 14.13 Treatment of outlet-type constipation in patient with Parkinson's disease by injection of 100 BOTOX® units in the puborectalis muscle, before (A) and after (B) toxin treatment. Defecographies A and B have been taken during straining. Following treatment, during straining the pelvic floor descends about 3 cm and the anorectal angle becomes obtuse.

remains to be measured, and repeated treatments are probably necessary[118]. Optimal dose also remains to be determined; a placebo controlled study with long-term follow-up is warranted.

Rectocele is a hernia of the anterior rectal wall into the lumen of the vagina (Figure 14.14)[119,120]. It has been suggested that in some instances the rectocele is caused by failure of relaxation or paradoxical contraction of the puborectalis muscle occurring during attempted evacuation, but the reason for its establishment is not clear. A wide variety of surgical approaches have been proposed with the aim of assuring rectal emptying by reducing the dimension of the rectocele. However, the results of surgery are often disappointing with regard to emptying difficulties. Surgical repair, either vaginal, transperineal, or transanal, does not always alleviate symptoms, and in some patients causes impaired faecal continence. Furthermore, transanal repair may compromise anal sphincter pressures and an alternative approach should be considered when the anal sphincter is lax. Recently, 14 women (mean age of 55 ± 11 years) were treated with a total of 30 BOTOX® units evenly divided into three sites, two on either side of the puborectalis muscle and the third anteriorly in the EAS[119].

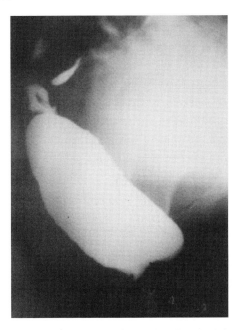

Figure 14.14 Anterior rectocele at defecography taken during straining. Anterior rectocele is a frequent finding in women and its clinical relevance is questionable: from 20 to 81 per cent of non-symptomatic women and of constipated people may present a rectocele. If less than 2 cm in diameter, rectocele is considered a normal finding in constipated or healthy subjects. When the diameter increases beyond 2 cm, the rectocele can cause outlet obstruction and rectal emptying difficulties.

Chronic idiopathic anal pain

Chronic idiopathic anal pain is part of a rather ill-defined group of disorders termed chronic idiopathic perineal pain, which also includes proctalgia fugax and coccygodynia. The main feature of these syndromes is that no objective abnormalities are found on clinical examination, and the distinction between the different groups of perineal pain is based solely on the patient's description of the pain and location of tenderness by palpation.

A feeling of obstructed defecation has also been described. The cause and pathogenesis of the syndrome are unknown. There is no satisfactory treatment for anal pain; nonetheless, anal stretch and LIS are still used in several patients on the assumption that the pain might be caused by a hypertonic IAS, because no objective changes can be demonstrated. Recently, injections of BoNT (20 units placed intersphincterically in four quadrants and/or at the lower rim of the puborectalis muscle under ultrasonographic guidance) resulted in improvement in four patients with chronic anal pain that persisted during a follow-up of 12–24 months[121].

Other anorectal conditions

BoNT into the IAS has been applied both diagnostically and therapeutically after pull-though surgery for Hirschsprung's disease in which it is postulated that IAS spasm can result in persistent obstructive symptoms. Minkes and Langer[122,123] prospectively evaluated 18 such children who underwent BoNT injection (total dose 15–60 units) into four quadrants of the sphincter. Twelve patients (67%) improved for at least 1 month; improvement was sustained beyond 6 months in five patients. These investigators advocated BoNT, not only as an alternative to myectomy in such cases, but also as a diagnostic trial, with persistent symptoms after injection, despite a decrease in sphincter pressure, suggesting another etiology for the constipation.

Pain after haemorrhoidectomy appears to be multifactorial and dependent on individual pain tolerance, mode of anaesthesia, postoperative analgesia, and surgical technique. IAS spasm is believed to play an important role. The BoNT role in reducing pain after haemorrhoidectomy has been assessed in a double-blind study on 50 consecutive patients undergoing Morgan haemorrhoidectomy and assigned to an IAS injection of 0.4 ml of solution containing either 20 BOTOX® units or normal saline. Those patients who had botulinum toxin had significantly less pain towards the end of the first week after surgery[124]. Reduction in IAS spasm is the presumed mechanism of action.

14.7 Pancreato-biliary system

14.7.1 Sphincter of Oddi

Sphincter of Oddi (SO) dysfunction has been a subject of controversy ever since its original description. Its very existence as a distinct anatomic or physiological entity has been disputed[125]. Treatment for its dysfunction is therefore perhaps not unsurprisingly a little contentious. There is no doubt, however, that the terminal biliary duct is involved in the control of bile flow and pancreatic juices into the second part of the duodenum. This coincides with the passage of stomach contents through the pylorus and the SO prevents reflux of duodenal contents in the biliary tree[126].

Dysfunction of the biliary tree and pancreas covers the motor disorders of the gall bladder and SO. Two forms are recognized where there are structural changes and alterations in function[127]. SO and gall bladder dysfunction produce similar symptoms of biliary pain and is characterized by episodes of severe continuous pain in the epigastrium and right hypochondrium, which may last for 30 minutes or more. Not all biliary–pancreatic pain is due to this, as functional abdominal pain may also have to be considered. However, physicians and surgeons not wishing to contemplate surgery now have other medical interventions to consider. The investigations should determine whether the patient has biliary obstruction due to cholelithiasis or neoplasia or due to pancreatic disease, where elevated pancreatic enzymes would be found. SO dysfunction can occur following cholecystectomy and three types are described[127]. Manometry of both the biliary and pancreatic sphincters should be carried out in the absence of a structural abnormality. This is supported by a Cochrane review of the effect of sphincter-otomy for biliary SO dysfunction, where surgery for patients with an elevated SO basal pressure of >40 mmHg appeared effective, but was no better than placebo in patients with a normal basal pressure[128]. Further studies are therefore required, but the principle is established that relaxing the terminal pressure is beneficial for the relief of symptoms.

A hypothesis has been proposed that chronic alcoholic patients damage their muscarinic receptors in the pancreas, duodenum and SO, which produce a heightened response to acetylcholine and ultimately duodeno-pancreatic reflux and acute pancreatitis in humans and experimental animals[129]. This may take 10 years or so, but its symptoms of chronic pancreatitis are characteristic.

Available treatments

If functional obstruction of the biliary tract and smooth muscle of the SO is the mechanism of pain production, then smooth muscle relaxants should be worthwhile therapy. However, the benefits of calcium channel blockers and other drugs have not been shown in studies and not only are they associated with side effects in a significant number of patients, but they are only short-acting[130]. Anticholinergic drugs are similarly limited, but BoNT has been shown to be effective in dealing with SO dysfunction in a small number of open label trials. Wehrmann *et al.* studied 15 consecutive patients with recurrent attacks of acute pancreatitis, in whom BoNT was used to predict the success of endoscopic sphincterotomy[131]. They injected the papilla of Vater in the pancreatic aspect of the SO. These patients had been shown to have elevated SO pressures on manometry, indicating dysfunction and 100 units BOTOX® was injected. Twelve of the 15 patients (80%) became asymptomatic after the treatment. Three symptomatic patients continued to have raised pancreatic sphincter pressure at manometry and proceeded to pancreatic sphincterotomy, but only one gained benefit. However, 11 of the 12 successfully treated patients developed a relapse after 4–8 months of BoNT treatment and achieved long-term remission (at least 15 months) after pancreatic or combined sphincterotomy. The conclusion is that BoNT provides short-term relief in patients and is a safe procedure. There were no adverse events. The study does not, however, discuss whether the patients would have benefited similarly from a primary sphincterotomy procedure and whether the BoNT was justified. Both the drug and the surgery were carried out endoscopically and the latter had a longer-term outcome. The fact that only one out of the three non-responders gained benefit from surgery probably does not tell us much, as the numbers are too small. The procedure was nonetheless safe and may be of value in patients unable to tolerate immediate sphincterotomy. However, the procedure is no less invasive.

The use of BoNT does gain further support, as Gorelick et al.[132] propose that endoscopic biliary sphincterotomy is risky in patients with SO dysfunction and should not be undertaken unless the pancreas is protected by a relaxation of the SO. They point out that the procedure is associated with a high risk of post-ERCP pancreatitis. They also suggest that it is the endoscopic retrograde pancreatography (ERCP) that causes the problem, but that this is significantly diminished after BoNT injection into the residual pancreatic sphincter at the time of the surgery. In their randomized placebo-controlled study of 98 patients referred for ERCP, 26 had elevated baseline SO pressures. Twelve were injected with 50 U BOTOX® and 14 received injections of 0.5 ml saline. Three of the treated group (25%) developed procedure-induced pancreatitis compared to six of the placebo group (43%) ($P = 0.34$). A larger study is required to confirm these findings and the procedure requires validation, but a significant mortality and morbidity exists with this complication.

The safety of BoNT was once again demonstrated and supports the notion that the treatment of choice is pharmacological with patients receiving the drug and only being submitted to endoscopic sphincterotomy, if they fail to respond adequately[133]. BoNT has also been tried in other conditions, such as achalasia and oesophageal spasm.

REFERENCES

1. Brisinda, G. and Maria, G. (2003). Botulinum toxin for spastic GI disorders. *Gastrointest. Endosc.*, **58**, 472–3.
2. Brisinda, G. and Maria, G. (2003). Botulinum toxin in the treatment of chronic anal fissure. *Dis. Colon. Rectum*, **46**, 1144–7.
3. Brisinda, G., Civello, I. M., Albanese, A. and Maria, G. (2003). Gastrointestinal smooth muscles and sphincters spasms: treatment with botulinum neurotoxin. *Curr. Med. Chem.*, **10**, 603–23.
4. MacKenzie, I., Burnstock, G. and Dolly, J. O. (1982). The effects of purified botulinum neurotoxin type A on cholinergic, adrenergic and non-adrenergic, atropine-resistant autonomic neuromuscular transmission. *Neuroscience*, **7**, 997–1006.

5. Mathias, C. J. and Bannister, R. (1999). Investigation of autonomic disorders. In C. J. Mathias and R. Bannister, eds., *Autonomic Failure. A Textbook of Clinical Disorders of the Autonomic Nervous System.* New York: Oxford University Press, pp. 169–95.

6. Leippold, T., Reitz, A. and Schurch, B. (2003). Botulinum toxin as a new therapy option for voiding disorders: current state of the art. *Eur. Urol.,* **44**, 165–74.

7. Dykstra, D. D., Sidi, A. A., Scott, A. B., Pagel, J. M. and Goldish, G. D. (1988). Effects of botulinum A toxin on detrusor-sphincter dyssynergia in spinal cord injury patients. *J. Urol.,* **139**, 919–22.

8. Beleggia, F., Beccia, E., Imbriani, E., Basciani, M., Intiso, D., Cioffi, R., Simone, P. and Ricci, B. V. (1997). The use of type A botulin toxin in the treatment of detrusor-sphincter dyssynergia. *Arch. Ital. Urol. Androl.,* **69**(Suppl. 1), 61–3.

9. de Seze, M., Petit, H., Gallien, P., de Seze, M. P., Joseph, P. A., Mazaux, J. M. and Barat, M. (2002). Botulinum A toxin and detrusor sphincter dyssynergia: a double-blind lidocaine-controlled study in 13 patients with spinal cord disease. *Eur. Urol.,* **42**, 56–62.

10. Gallien, P., Robineau, S., Verin, M., Le Bot, M. P., Nicolas, B. and Brissot, R. (1998). Treatment of detrusor sphincter dyssynergia by transperineal injection of botulinum toxin. *Arch. Phys. Med. Rehabil.,* **79**, 715–17.

11. Parratte, B., Bonniaud, V., Tatu, L., Metton, G., Michel, F., Cosson, A. and Monnier, G. (2003). Detrusor-sphincter dyssynergia and botulinum toxin. *Ann. Readapt. Med. Phys.,* **46**, 319–25.

12. Petit, H., Wiart, L., Gaujard, E., Le Breton, F., Ferriere, J. M., Lagueny, A., Joseph, P. A. and Barat, M. (1998). Botulinum A toxin treatment for detrusor-sphincter dyssynergia in spinal cord disease. *Spinal Cord,* **36**, 91–4.

13. Schurch, B., Stohrer, M., Kramer, G., Schmid, D. M., Gaul, G. and Hauri, D. (2000). Botulinum-A toxin for treating detrusor hyperreflexia in spinal cord injured patients: a new alternative to anticholinergic drugs? Preliminary results. *J. Urol.,* **164**, 692–7.

14. Schurch, B., Hodler, J. and Rodic, B. (1997). Botulinum A toxin as a treatment of detrusor-sphincter dyssynergia in patients with spinal cord injury: MRI controlled transperineal injections. *J. Neurol. Neurosurg. Psychiatry,* **63**, 474–6.

15. Dykstra, D. D. and Sidi, A. A. (1990). Treatment of detrusor-sphincter dyssynergia with botulinum A toxin: a double-blind study. *Arch. Phys. Med. Rehabil.,* **71**, 24–6.

16. Schurch, B. (1998). Botulinum A toxin in spinal cord injury. *Arch. Phys. Med. Rehabil.,* **79**, 1481.

17. Schurch, B., Schmid, D. M. and Stohrer, M. (2000). Treatment of neurogenic incontinence with botulinum toxin A. *N. Engl. J. Med.,* **342**, 665.

18. Reitz, A., Stohrer, M., Kramer, G., Del Popolo, G., Chartier-Kastler, E., Panneck, J., Burgdorfer, H., Gocking, K., Madersbacher, H., Schumacher, S., Richter, R., Von Tobel, J. and Schurch, B. (2003). European experience of 200 cases treated with botulinum-A toxin injections into the detrusor muscle for neurogenic incontinence. *Eur. Urol. Supplements,* **2**(1), 140.

19. Schulte-Baukloh, H., Michael, T., Sturzebecher, B. and Knispel, H. H. (2003). Botulinum-A toxin detrusor injection as a novel approach in the treatment of bladder spasticity in children with neurogenic bladder. *Eur. Urol.,* **44**, 139–43.

20. Schulte-Baukloh, H., Knispel, H. H. and Michael, T. (2002). Botulinum-A toxin in the treatment of neurogenic bladder in children. *Pediatrics*, **110**, 420−1.

21. Schulte-Baukloh, H., Michael, T., Schobert, J., Stolze, T. and Knispel, H. H. (2002). Efficacy of botulinum-A toxin in children with detrusor hyperreflexia due to myelomeningocele: preliminary results. *Urology*, **59**, 325−7.

22. Staehler, M., Sauter, T. and Miller, K. (2003). Long term results prove botulinum toxin A injection in the m. detrusor vesicae to be an alternative to surgery in children with myelomeningocele. *Eur. Urol. Supplements*, **2**(1), 140.

23. Radziszewski, P. and Borkowski, A. (2003). Botulinum toxin type A intravesical injections for intractable bladder overactivity. *Eur. Urol. Supplements*, **2**(1), 134.

24. Phelan, M. W., Franks, M., Somogyi, G. T., Yokoyama, T., Fraser, M. O., Lavelle, J. P., Yoshimura, N. and Chancellor, M. B. (2001). Botulinum toxin urethral sphincter injection to restore bladder emptying in men and women with voiding dysfunction. *J. Urol.*, **165**, 1107−10.

25. Kuo, H. C. (2003). Botulinum A toxin urethral injection for the treatment of lower urinary tract dysfunction. *J. Urol.*, **170**, 1908−12.

26. Maria, G., Destito, A., Lacquaniti, S., Bentivoglio, A. R., Brisinda, G. and Albanese, A. (1998). Relief by botulinum toxin of voiding dysfunction due to prostatitis. *Lancet*, **352**, 625.

27. Zermann, D., Ishigooka, M., Schubert, J. and Schmidt, R. A. (2000). Perisphincteric injection of botulinum toxin type A. A treatment option for patients with chronic prostatic pain? *Eur. Urol.*, **38**, 393−9.

28. Hollander, J. B. and Diokno, A. C. (1996). Prostatism: benign prostatic hyperplasia. *Urol. Clin. North Am.*, **23**, 75−86.

29. Barry, M. J. and Roehrborn, C. G. (2001). Benign prostatic hyperplasia. *BMJ*, **323**, 1042−6.

30. Clifford, G. M. and Farmer, R. D. (2000). Medical therapy for benign prostatic hyperplasia: a review of the literature. *Eur. Urol.*, **38**, 2−19.

31. Oesterling, J. E. (1995). Benign prostatic hyperplasia. Medical and minimally invasive treatment options. *N. Engl. J. Med.*, **332**, 99−109.

32. Djavan, B., Madersbacher, S., Klingler, H. C., Ghawidel, K., Basharkhah, A., Hruby, S., Seitz, C. and Marberger, M. (1999). Outcome analysis of minimally invasive treatments for benign prostatic hyperplasia. *Tech. Urol.*, **5**, 12−20.

33. Roehrborn, C. G., Bartsch, G., Kirby, R., Andriole, G., Boyle, P., de la Rosette, J., Perrin, P., Ramsey, E., Nordling, J., De Campos, F. G. and Arap, S. (2001). Guidelines for the diagnosis and treatment of benign prostatic hyperplasia: a comparative, international overview. *Urology*, **58**, 642−50.

34. Kaplan, S. A., Holtgrewe, H. L., Bruskewitz, R., Saltzman, B., Mobley, D., Narayan, P., Lund, R. H., Weiner, S., Wells, G., Cook, T. J., Meehan, A. and Waldstreicher, J. (2001). Comparison of the efficacy and safety of finasteride in older versus younger men with benign prostatic hyperplasia. *Urology*, **57**, 1073−7.

35. McConnell, J. D., Barry, M. J. and Bruskewitz, R. C. (1994). Benign prostatic hyperplasia: diagnosis and treatment. Agency for Health Care Policy and Research. *Clin. Pract. Guidel. Quick Ref. Guide Clin.*, 1−17.

36. McConnell, J. D., Bruskewitz, R., Walsh, P., Andriole, G., Lieber, M., Holtgrewe, H. L., Albertsen, P., Roehrborn, C. G., Nickel, J. C., Wang, D. Z., Taylor, A. M. and Waldstreicher, J. (1998). The effect of finasteride on the risk of acute urinary retention and the need for surgical treatment among men with benign prostatic hyperplasia. Finasteride Long-Term Efficacy and Safety Study Group. *N. Engl. J. Med.*, **338**, 557–63.

37. Walsh, P. C. (1996). Treatment of benign prostatic hyperplasia. *N. Engl. J. Med.*, **335**, 586–7.

38. de la Rosette, J. J., Alivizatos, G., Madersbacher, S., Perachino, M., Thomas, D., Desgrandchamps, F. and de Wildt, M. (2001). EAU Guidelines on benign prostatic hyperplasia (BPH). *Eur. Urol.*, **40**, 256–63.

39. Lu-Yao, G. L., Barry, M. J., Chang, C. H., Wasson, J. H. and Wennberg, J. E. (1994). Transurethral resection of the prostate among Medicare beneficiaries in the United States: time trends and outcomes. Prostate Patient Outcomes Research Team (PORT). *Urology*, **44**, 692–8.

40. Boyle, P., Robertson, C., Manski, R., Padley, R. J. and Roehrborn, C. G. (2001). Meta-analysis of randomized trials of terazosin in the treatment of benign prostatic hyperplasia. *Urology*, **58**, 717–22.

41. Lepor, H., Williford, W. O., Barry, M. J., Brawer, M. K., Dixon, C. M., Gormley, G., Haakenson, C., Machi, M., Narayan, P. and Padley, R. J. (1996). The efficacy of terazosin, finasteride, or both in benign prostatic hyperplasia. Veterans Affairs Cooperative Studies Benign Prostatic Hyperplasia Study Group. *N. Engl. J. Med.*, **335**, 533–9.

42. Narayan, P. and Lepor, H. (2001). Long-term, open-label, phase III multicenter study of tamsulosin in benign prostatic hyperplasia. *Urology*, **57**, 466–70.

43. Lepor, H. (1990). Role of long-acting selective alpha-1 blockers in the treatment of benign prostatic hyperplasia. *Urol. Clin. North Am.*, **17**, 651–9.

44. Doggweiler, R., Zermann, D. H., Ishigooka, M. and Schmidt, R. A. (1998). Botox-induced prostatic involution. *Prostate*, **37**, 44–50.

45. Barry, M. J., Fowler, F. J., Jr., O'Leary, M. P., Bruskewitz, R. C., Holtgrewe, H. L. and Mebust, W. K. (1992). Correlation of the American Urological Association symptom index with self-administered versions of the Madsen-Iversen, Boyarsky and Maine Medical Assessment Program symptom indexes. Measurement Committee of the American Urological Association. *J. Urol.*, **148**, 1558–63.

46. Barry, M. J., Fowler, F. J., Jr., O'Leary, M. P., Bruskewitz, R. C., Holtgrewe, H. L., Mebust, W. K. and Cockett, A. T. (1992). The American Urological Association symptom index for benign prostatic hyperplasia. The Measurement Committee of the American Urological Association. *J. Urol.*, **148**, 1549–57.

47. Barry, M. J., Girman, C. J., O'Leary, M. P., Walker-Corkery, E. S., Binkowitz, B. S., Cockett, A. T. and Guess, H. A. (1995). Using repeated measures of symptom score, uroflowmetry and prostate specific antigen in the clinical management of prostate disease. Benign Prostatic Hyperplasia Treatment Outcomes Study Group. *J. Urol.*, **153**, 99–103.

48. Maria, G., Brisinda, G., Civello, I. M., Bentivoglio, A. R., Sganga, G. and Albanese, A. (2003). Relief by botulinum toxin of voiding dysfunction due to benign prostatic hyperplasia: results of a randomized, placebo-controlled study. *Urology*, **62**, 259–64.

49. Doehring, C. B., Sanda, M. G., Partin, A. W., Sauvageot, J., Juo, H., Beaty, T. H., Epstein, J. I., Hill, G. and Walsh, P. C. (1996). Histopathologic characterization of hereditary benign prostatic hyperplasia. *Urology*, **48**, 650–3.

50. Farnsworth, W. E. (1999). Prostate stroma: physiology. *Prostate*, **38**, 60–72.

51. McVary, K. T., McKenna, K. E. and Lee, C. (1998). Prostate innervation. *Prostate Suppl.*, **8**, 2–13.

52. Gup, D. I., Shapiro, E., Baumann, M. and Lepor, H. (1990). Autonomic receptors in human prostate adenomas. *J. Urol.*, **143**, 179–85.

53. Ruggieri, M. R., Colton, M. D., Wang, P., Wang, J., Smyth, R. J., Pontari, M. A. and Luthin, G. R. (1995). Human prostate muscarinic receptor subtypes. *J. Pharmacol. Exp. Ther.*, **274**, 976–82.

54. Reissing, E. D., Brink, Y. M. and Khalife, S. (1999). Does vaginismus exist? A critical review of the literature. *Journal of Nervous and Mental Disease*, **187**(5), 261–74.

55. Maria, G., Cadeddu, F., Brisinda, D., Brandara, F. and Brisinda, G. (2005). Management of bladder, prostatic and pelvic floor disorders with botulinum neurotoxin. *Current Medicinal Chemistry*, **12**(3), 247–65.

56. Brisinda, G., Maria, G., Bentivoglio, A. R. and Albanese, A. (2002). The role of botulinum toxin in gastrointestinal disorders. In M. F. Brin, M. Hallett and J. Jankovic, eds., *Scientific and Therapeutic Aspects of Botulinum Toxin*. Philadelphia: Lippincott Williams & Wilkins, pp. 269–85.

57. Brisinda, G., Maria, G. and Albanese, A. (2002). Anisme, fissure anale. In D. Ranoux and C. Gury, eds., *Manuel d'utilisation pratique de la toxine botulique*. Marseille: Solal, editeur, pp. 201–17.

58. Albanese, A., Brisinda, G. and Mathias, C. J. (2001). The autonomic nervous system and gastrointestinal disorders. In O. Appenzeller, ed., *The Autonomic Nervous System*. Part II. Dysfunctions. Amsterdam: Elsevier, pp. 613–63.

59. Stebbing, J. F. (1998). Nitric oxide synthase neurones and neuromuscular behaviour of the anorectum. *Ann. R. Coll. Surg. Engl.*, **80**, 137–45.

60. Stebbing, J. F., Brading, A. F. and Mortensen, N. J. (1997). Role of nitric oxide in relaxation of the longitudinal layer of rectal smooth muscle. *Dis. Colon Rectum*, **40**, 706–10.

61. Stebbing, J. F., Brading, A. F. and Mortensen, N. J. (1996). Nitric oxide and the rectoanal inhibitory reflex: retrograde neuronal tracing reveals a descending nitrergic rectoanal pathway in a guinea-pig model. *Br. J. Surg.*, **83**, 493–8.

62. Battish, R., Cao, G. Y., Lynn, R. B., Chakder, S. and Rattan, S. (2000). Heme oxygenase-2 distribution in anorectum: colocalization with neuronal nitric oxide synthase. *Am. J. Physiol. Gastrointest. Liver Physiol.*, **278**, G148–G155.

63. Chakder, S., Cao, G. Y., Lynn, R. B. and Rattan, S. (2000). Heme oxygenase activity in the internal anal sphincter: effects of nonadrenergic, noncholinergic nerve stimulation. *Gastroenterology*, **118**, 477–86.

64. Albanese, A., Bentivoglio, A. R., Cassetta, E., Viggiano, A., Maria, G. and Gui, D. (1995). Review article: the use of botulinum toxin in the alimentary tract. *Aliment. Pharmacol. Ther.*, **9**, 599–604.

65. Goyal, R. K. and Hirano, I. (1996). The enteric nervous system. *N. Engl. J. Med.*, **334**, 1106–15.

66. Mathias, C. J. and Bannister, R. (1999). *Autonomic Failure. A Textbook of Clinical Disorders of the Autonomic Nervous System*. New York: Oxford University Press.

67. Lund, J. N. and Scholefield, J. H. (1996). Aetiology and treatment of anal fissure. *Br. J. Surg.*, **83**, 1335–44.

68. Brown, A. C., Sumfest, J. M. and Rozwadowski, J. V. (1989). Histopathology of the internal anal sphincter in chronic anal fissure. *Dis. Colon Rectum*, **32**, 680–3.

69. Lund, J. N., Binch, C., McGrath, J., Sparrow, R. A. and Scholefield, J. H. (1999). Topographical distribution of blood supply to the anal canal. *Br. J. Surg.*, **86**, 496–8.

70. Schouten, W. R., Briel, J. W., Auwerda, J. J. and De Graaf, E. J. (1996). Ischaemic nature of anal fissure. *Br. J. Surg.*, **83**, 63–5.

71. Maria, G., Brisinda, D., Ruggieri, M. P., Civello, I. M. and Brisinda, G. (1999). Identification of anti-endothelial cell antibodies in patients with chronic anal fissure. *Surgery*, **126**, 535–40.

72. Maria, G. and Brisinda, G. (2003). Chronic anal fissure: advances and insights in pathophysiology and treatment. *Gastroenterology*, **125**, 995–6.

73. Regadas, F. S., Batista, L. K., Albuquerque, J. L. and Capaz, F. R. (1993). Pharmacological study of the internal and sphincter in patients with chronic anal fissure. *Br. J. Surg.*, **80**, 799–801.

74. Atienza, P. (1998). Effect of botulinum toxin in the treatment of chronic anal fissure. *Gastroenterol. Clin. Biol.*, **22**, 654–5.

75. Baron, K. (2000). Anal fissure: unclear causes but promising new treatments. *JAAPA*, **13**, 45–55.

76. Espi, A., Melo, F., Minguez, M., Garcia-Granero, E., Mora, F., Esclapez, P., Benages, A. and Lledo, S. (1997). Therapeutic use of botulinum toxin in anal fissure. *Int. J. Colorectal. Dis.*, **12**, 163.

77. Fernandez, L. F., Conde, F. R., Rios, R. A., Garcia, I. J., Cainzos, F. M. and Potel, L. J. (1999). Botulinum toxin for the treatment of anal fissure. *Dig. Surg.*, **16**, 515–18.

78. Gui, D., Cassetta, E., Anastasio, G., Bentivoglio, A. R., Maria, G. and Albanese, A. (1994). Botulinum toxin for chronic anal fissure. *Lancet*, **344**, 1127–8.

79. Jost, W. H. and Schrank, B. (1999). Repeat botulin toxin injections in anal fissure: in patients with relapse and after insufficient effect of first treatment. *Dig. Dis. Sci.*, **44**, 1588–9.

80. Jost, W. H. (1999). Incidence of anal fissure in nonselected neurological patients. *Dis. Colon Rectum*, **42**, 828.

81. Jost, W. H. (1997). One hundred cases of anal fissure treated with botulin toxin: early and long-term results. *Dis. Colon Rectum*, **40**, 1029–32.

82. Jost, W. H., Schanne, S., Schimrigk, K. and Mlitz, H. (1995). Therapy of anal fissure using botulinum toxin: perianal thrombosis as a complication. *Dtsch. Med. Wochenschr.*, **120**, 665.

83. Jost, W. H., Schimrigk, K. and Mlitz, H. (1995). Riddle of the sphincters in anal fissure. *Dis. Colon Rectum*, **38**, 555.

84. Jost, W. H. and Schimrigk, K. (1995). Botulinum toxin in therapy of anal fissure. *Lancet*, **345**, 188–9.

85. Jost, W. H. and Schimrigk, K. (1994). Therapy of anal fissure using botulin toxin. *Dis. Colon Rectum*, **37**, 1340.

86. Jost, W. H. and Schimrigk, K. (1993). Use of botulinum toxin in anal fissure. *Dis. Colon Rectum*, **36**, 974.

87. Khademi, A. and Feldman, D. M. (2000). A comparison of combination of botox (botulinum toxin) and nitroglycerin in the treatment of chronic anal fissure. *Am. J. Gastroenterol.*, **95**, 2538.

88. Lindsey, I., Jones, O. M., Cunningham, C., George, B. D. and Mortensen, N. J. (2003). Botulinum toxin as second-line therapy for chronic anal fissure failing 0.2 per cent glyceryl trinitrate. *Dis. Colon Rectum*, **46**, 361–6.

89. Lock, G. and Holstege, A. (1999). Botulinum toxin in treatment of chronic anal fissure. *Z. Gastroenterol.*, **37**, 253–5.

90. Lysy, J., Israelit-Yatzkan, Y., Sestiery-Ittah, M., Weksler-Zangen, S., Keret, D. and Goldin, E. (2001). Topical nitrates potentiate the effect of botulinum toxin in the treatment of patients with refractory anal fissure. *Gut*, **48**, 221–4.

91. Madalinski, M., Jagiello, K., Labon, M., Adrich, Z. and Kryszewski, A. (1999). Botulinum toxin injection into only one point in the external anal sphincter: a modification of the treatment for chronic anal fissure. *Endoscopy*, **31**, S63.

92. Madalinski, M. H. (1999). Nonsurgical treatment modalities for chronic anal fissure using botulinum toxin. *Gastroenterology*, **117**, 516–17.

93. Madalinski, M. H. and Slawek, J. (2003). The higher doses of botulinum toxin and the potentiate effect of its action after nitric oxide donors application for the treatment of chronic anal fissure. *Surgery*, **133**, 455–6.

94. Madalinski, M. H. (2003). Higher or lower doses of botulinum toxin for the treatment of chronic anal fissure? *Gastroenterology*, **124**, 1165.

95. Madoff, R. D. and Fleshman, J. W. (2003). AGA technical review on the diagnosis and care of patients with anal fissure. *Gastroenterology*, **124**, 235–45.

96. McCallion, K. and Gardiner, K. R. (2001). Progress in the understanding and treatment of chronic anal fissure. *Postgrad. Med. J.*, **77**, 753–8.

97. Minguez, M., Melo, F., Espi, A., Garcia-Granero, E., Mora, F., Lledo, S. and Benages, A. (1999). Therapeutic effects of different doses of botulinum toxin in chronic anal fissure. *Dis. Colon Rectum*, **42**, 1016–21.

98. Minguez, M., Herreros, B., Espi, A., Garcia-Granero, E., Sanchiz, V., Mora, F., Lledo, S. and Benages, A. (2002). Long-term follow-up (42 months) of chronic anal fissure after healing with botulinum toxin. *Gastroenterology*, **123**, 112–17.

99. Minguez, M., Herreros, B. and Benages, A. (2003). Chronic anal fissure. *Curr. Treat. Options Gastroenterol.*, **6**, 257–62.

100. Nelson, R. L. (2003). Treatment of anal fissure. *BMJ*, **327**, 354–5.

101. Tilney, H. S., Heriot, A. G. and Cripps, N. P. (2001). Complication of botulinum toxin injections for anal fissure. *Dis. Colon Rectum*, **44**, 1721–4.

102. Brisinda, D., Maria, G., Fenici, R., Civello, I. M. and Brisinda, G. (2003). Safety of botulinum neurotoxin treatment in patients with chronic anal fissure. *Dis. Colon Rectum*, **46**, 419–20.

103. Brisinda, G., Maria, G., Sganga, G., Bentivoglio, A. R., Albanese, A. and Castagneto, M. (2002). Effectiveness of higher doses of botulinum toxin to induce healing in patients with chronic anal fissures. *Surgery*, **131**, 179–84.

104. Brisinda, G., Maria, G., Bentivoglio, A. R., Cassetta, E., Gui, D. and Albanese, A. (1999). A comparison of injections of botulinum toxin and topical nitroglycerin ointment for the treatment of chronic anal fissure. *N. Engl. J. Med.*, **341**, 65–9.

105. Maria, G., Brisinda, G., Bentivoglio, A. R., Cassetta, E., Gui, D. and Albanese, A. (2000). Influence of botulinum toxin site of injections on healing rate in patients with chronic anal fissure. *Am. J. Surg.*, **179**, 46–50.

106. Maria, G., Brisinda, G., Bentivoglio, A. R., Cassetta, E., Gui, D. and Albanese, A. (1998). Botulinum toxin injections in the internal anal sphincter for the treatment of chronic anal fissure: long-term results after two different dosage regimens. *Ann. Surg.*, **228**, 664–9.

107. Maria, G., Cassetta, E., Gui, D., Brisinda, G., Bentivoglio, A. R. and Albanese, A. (1998). A comparison of botulinum toxin and saline for the treatment of chronic anal fissure. *N. Engl. J. Med.*, **338**, 217–20.

108. Mentes, B. B., Irkorucu, O., Akin, M., Leventoglu, S. and Tatlicioglu, E. (2003). Comparison of botulinum toxin injection and lateral internal sphincterotomy for the treatment of chronic anal fissure. *Dis. Colon Rectum*, **46**, 232–7.

109. Siproudhis, L., Sebille, V., Pigot, F., Hemery, P., Juguet, F. and Bellissant, E. (2003). Lack of effficacy of botulinum toxin in chronic anal fissure. *Aliment. Pharmacol. Ther.*, **18**, 515–24.

110. Jost, W. H. and Schrank, B. (1999). Chronic anal fissure treated with botulinum toxin injections: a dose-finding study with Dysport. *Colorectal Dis.*, **3**, 26–8.

111. Mason, P. F., Watkins, M. J., Hall, H. S. and Hall, A. W. (1996). The management of chronic fissure in ano with botulinum toxin. *J. R. Coll. Surg. Edinb.*, **41**, 235–8.

112. Madalinski, M. H., Slawek, J., Zbytek, B., Duzynski, W., Adrich, Z., Jagiello, K. and Kryszewski, A. (2001). Topical nitrates and the higher doses of botulinum toxin for chronic anal fissure. *Hepatogastroenterology*, **48**, 977–9.

113. Joo, J. S., Agachan, F., Wolff, B., Nogueras, J. J. and Wexner, S. D. (1996). Initial North American experience with botulinum toxin type A for treatment of anismus. *Dis. Colon Rectum*, **39**, 1107–11.

114. Ron, Y., Avni, Y., Lukovetski, A., Wardi, J., Geva, D., Birkenfeld, S. and Halpern, Z. (2001). Botulinum toxin type-A in therapy of patients with anismus. *Dis. Colon Rectum*, **44**, 1821–6.

115. Shafik, A. and El Sibai, O. (1998). Botulin toxin in the treatment of nonrelaxing puborectalis syndrome. *Dig. Surg.*, **15**, 347–51.

116. Hallan, R. I., Williams, N. S., Melling, J., Waldron, D. J., Womack, N. R. and Morrison, J. F. (1988). Treatment of anismus in intractable constipation with botulinum A toxin. *Lancet*, **2**, 714–17.

117. Albanese, A., Brisinda, G., Bentivoglio, A. R. and Maria, G. (2003). Treatment of outlet obstruction constipation in Parkinson's disease with botulinum neurotoxin A. *Am. J. Gastroenterol.*, **98**, 1439–40.

118. Albanese, A., Maria, G., Bentivoglio, A. R., Brisinda, G., Cassetta, E. and Tonali, P. (1997). Severe constipation in Parkinson's disease relieved by botulinum toxin. *Mov. Disord.*, **12**, 764–6.

119. Maria, G., Brisinda, G., Bentivoglio, A. R., Albanese, A., Sganga, G. and Castagneto, M. (2001). Anterior rectocele due to obstructed defecation relieved by botulinum toxin. *Surgery*, **129**, 524–9.

120. Sailer, M., Bussen, D., Debus, E. S., Fuchs, K. H. and Thiede, A. (1998). Quality of life in patients with benign anorectal disorders. *Br. J. Surg.*, **85**, 1716–19.

121. Christiansen, J., Bruune, E., Skjoldbye, B. and Hagen, K. (2001). Chronic idiopathic anal pain. *Dis. Colon Rectum*, **44**, 661–5.

122. Langer, J. C. and Birnbaum, E. (1997). Preliminary experience with intrasphincteric botulinum toxin for persistent constipation after pull-through for Hirschsprung's disease. *J. Pediatr. Surg.*, **32**, 1059–61.

123. Minkes, R. K. and Langer, J. C. (2000). A prospective study of botulinum toxin for internal anal sphincter hypertonicity in children with Hirschsprung's disease. *J. Pediatr. Surg.*, **35**, 1733–6.

124. Davies, J., Duffy, D., Boyt, N., Aghahoseini, A., Alexander, D. and Leveson, S. (2003). Botulinum toxin (botox) reduces pain after hemorrhoidectomy: results of a double-blind, randomized study. *Dis. Colon Rectum*, **46**, 1097–102.

125. Kalloo, A. N. and Pasricha, P. J. (1996). Therapy of sphincter of Oddi dysfunction. *Gastrointestinal Endoscopy Clinics of North America*, **6**(1), 117–25.

126. Toouli, J. and Craig, A. (1999). Clinical aspects of sphincter of Oddi function and dysfunction. *Current Gastroenterology Reports*, **1**(2), 116–22.

127. Corazziari, E., Shaffer, E. A., Hogan, W. A., Sherman, S. and Toouli, J. (1999). Functional disorders of the biliary tree and pancreas. *Gut*, **45**(Suppl. 2), II48–54.

128. Craig, A. and Toouli, J. (2001). Sphincterotomy for biliary sphincter of Oddi dysfunction. *Cochrane Database of Systematic Reviews*, **3**, CD001509.

129. McCutcheon, A. D. (2000). Neurological damage and duodeno-pancreatic reflux in the pathogenesis of alcoholic pancreatitis. *Archives of Surgery*, **135**(3), 278–85.

130. Craig, A. and Toouli, J. (2002). Sphincter of Oddi dysfunction: is there a role for medical therapy? *Current Gastroenterology Reports*, **4**(2), 172–6.

131. Wehrmann, T., Schmitt, T. H., Arndt, A., Lembcke, B., Caspary, W. F. and Seifert, H. (2000). Endoscopic injection of botulinum toxin in patients with recurrent acute pancreatitis due to pancreatic sphincter of Oddi dysfunction. *Alimentary Pharmacology and Therapeutics*, **14**(11), 1469–77.

132. Gorelick, A., Barnett, J., Chey, W., Anderson, M. and Elta, G. (2004). Botulinum toxin after biliary sphincterotomy. *Endoscopy*, **36**(2), 170–3.

133. Piccinni, G., Angrisano, A., Testini, M. and Bonomo, G. M. (2004). Diagnosing and treating sphincter of Oddi dysfunction: a critical literature review and re-evaluation. *Journal of Clinical Gastroenterology*, **38**(4), 350–9.

Cosmetic uses of botulinum toxin A

Kenneth Beer[1], Joel L. Cohen[2] and Alastair Carruthers[3]

[1]Palm Beach Esthetic Center, West Palm Beach, Florida, USA
[2]AboutSkin Dermatology and Dermsurgery, Englewood, Colorado, USA
[3]Department of Dermatology, University of British Columbia, Vancouver BC, Canada

15.1 Introduction

The cosmetic uses of botulinum toxin (BoNT) are the most commonly used of its applications. Interest started after the effect of BoNT was shown in the treatment of blepharospasm and the first description of botulinum toxin for treatment of glabellar frown lines was in 1992[1]. At that time, the use of this potent neurotoxin for cosmetic indications was an interesting footnote to treatments for strabismus, torticollis and other dystonias. Subsequently, physicians began to study and use the botulinum toxins for a variety of cosmetic indications. Today, BoNT is the most commonly performed cosmetic procedure in the world. Understanding how these toxins are used in this arena is essential to any discussion of the botulinum toxins.

15.1.1 Dilution of the toxin for cosmetic purposes

For the purposes of this chapter, the dilution of BoNT will be described in units of the BOTOX® brand of type A toxin. Oculoplastic specialists usually inject using a 1 ml dilution per 100 units of BOTOX®, whereas dermatologists and plastic surgeons vary in their practice towards a general range from 1 ml to 4 ml per 100 units. Variations in concentration affect the concentration gradient between the toxin and its environment. In the forehead, for instance, a dilute concentration may be preferable in order to increase migration, but, in general, clinicians use lower volumes to minimize the risk of this getting into unplanned areas. Since there is no standardized recipe for dilution and no exact way to identify precise injection sites, it is necessary to understand the principles of BoNT injections before treating patients[1,2].

Although the package insert for BOTOX® recommends dilution with sterile *non-preserved* saline, studies have demonstrated that *preserved* saline provides

Clinical Uses of Botulinum Toxins, eds. Anthony B. Ward and Michael P. Barnes. Published by Cambridge University Press. © Cambridge University Press 2007.

increased patient comfort without decreasing efficacy[3]. The medical literature has also reported the adding of lidocaine to the toxin[4], but, although there was no significant decrease in efficacy, this practice was abandoned following a probable unrelated death. There is, in addition, a case report of adding hyaluronidase to BOTOX® in an effort enhance efficacy in the treatment of axillary hyperhidrosis[5].

15.2   Cosmetic use of botulinum toxins

15.2.1   General tips

Physicians should know the regional facial anatomy and understand the various interactions between the muscle groups of the face. A precise injection technique is critical when using BoNT-A, particularly when injecting the lower face, where minor variations may result in significant facial asymmetry and speech impediments. Treatment of the mid-face, lower-face and neck is best reserved for experienced injectors and for patients who have been successfully treated in the upper face.

The use of pre-treatment photography is highly recommended, as any pre-existing asymmetry that is not documented is likely to be ascribed to treatment. Written informed consent is therefore mandatory for this procedure and, included in this, patients should be notified that the use of BOTOX® in any area other than the glabella constitutes an 'off label' indication (in the USA). A proper informed consent should be specific to the areas of treatment and should mention complications, such as headache, flu-like symptoms, bruising, infection, eyelid drooping, smile asymmetry, speech enunciation changes and, although rare, dysphagia.

During the patient consultation, it is wise to explain the dose–response curve for botulinum toxin A and the estimation of the correct dose. Since each person has different anatomy, it is possible that a given individual may require more or less. In the event that more is required, a waiting period of approximately 14 days is recommended. It is important to study the patient's anatomy prior to treatment and it may be helpful to demonstrate the muscles involved through a mirror. Most experienced physicians do not routinely see patients back for post-treatment follow-up except when treating the lips, neck, blepharochalasis or hyperhidrosis, when patients are reviewed at 2–2½ weeks.

Applying ice to the injection sites before and after treatment vasoconstricts and may decrease the pain of injection and the risk of swelling, oozing and bruising. This is especially useful when treating the crow's feet and infraorbital areas. One additional method of reducing swelling is to advise patients, if medically feasible, to discontinue aspirin, vitamin E and non-steroidal anti-inflammatory drugs at least one week prior to treatment. Some patients may benefit from topical medication such as lidocaine. When applying topical anaesthetics, it is important to identify patients with sulfa allergies. With the exception of cocaine, most topical anesthetics are vasodilators and this may reduce the efficacy of BOTOX®, thereby potentially increasing its migration to unintended areas.

Prior to any facial injection, it is important to cleanse the area of any makeup and lipstick and prepare the sites with alcohol. Makeup is a foreign substance that may contain dyes and thorough removal of this is needed to avoid any introduction into the injection sites. Be sure however, to allow the alcohol to dry completely prior to injection, as there is a theoretical concern over the alcohol inactivating the botulinum toxin.

Botulinum toxin A is commonly injected with a B-D 0.3 cm^3 insulin syringe with a short hub 31 g needle. The short needle minimizes the dead space of the syringe and decreases waste. Other syringes designed to minimize dead space may also be utilized. When using a syringe that has an integrated needle, fill it with enough material to inject at six sites. When using a syringe that has interchangeable needles, simply change the needle after about six injections to avoid using a blunt needle to penetrate the skin. A novice injector may wish to mark anticipated injection sites with a water-soluble pen, as this can be helpful for the planning and accuracy of injections.

Patients are instructed to 'exercise' the muscles treated after treatment for 1.5 hours and to avoid bending, lying down, going to sleep, or physically exercising for 1.5 hours to avoid the theoretical risk of diffusion.

15.3   BOTOX® in the glabella

15.3.1   General tips for treatment of the glabella

The glabella is currently the only FDA-approved site for cosmetic injection of BOTOX® in the USA. As such, it is the most common site for patients and physicians to begin treatment with BoNT-A. Injections of the small muscles in this area are technically simple to perform and they result in a high degree of patient satisfaction. Close attention should be paid to the eyelid and eyebrow for possible ptosis and redundant eyelid skin that, if not identified and discussed, can be a source for patient dissatisfaction following treatment. When static rhytids are present, it is important to discuss the need for adjunctive fillers, such as Restylane®, if the patient wants to eliminate all lines in this area. Stretching the skin in this area will demonstrate that, even after treatment with BoNT-A, skin creases may still be present at rest. Prior to treatment, the physician must explain that repeated treatments, performed at 3–4 month intervals, may further reduce wrinkles in the areas treated. Patients need to be evaluated for medial recruitment from the mid-brow area. When this occurs, the contribution this makes to frown lines may be significant. Failure to discuss this and/or treat this component will result in patients thinking that BOTOX® was ineffective. In reality, some of these medial brow adductors should not be treated, as to do so might risk depression of the medial and lateral brow. Medial recruitment is caused by hyper-functional orbicularis oculi fibers just below the mid-eyebrow. Evaluation of the length and direction of the corrugators and the prominence of the procerus and nasalis muscles should also be performed prior to injection. A clear plan should be devised and discussed that addresses the individual's anatomy and concerns.

One recent study has shown that glabellar treatment may help convey positive and relaxed emotions more accurately[6] and that BoNT-A injections of the glabella can be beneficial for patients, who believe their faces are not communicating their emotions properly, want to delay the outward appearance of aging, or simply want to look their best.

15.3.2 Glabellar anatomy

The anatomy of the glabellar area must be understood not as a group of independent muscles but rather as a complex of inter-related muscles that must be addressed in concert. Muscles between the brows depress the medial brow. Reduction of these depressors results in a medial brow lift that is cosmetically desirable. This effect is separate and distinct from reduction of the 'scowl' lines associated with activity of these muscles. Due to the proximity of the forehead musculature, treatment of the glabella may result in diffusion to the inferior fibers of the frontalis – resulting in some degree of relaxation of lower and medial aspects of this muscle. If significant diffusion to the frontalis occurs, the medial brow lift may disappear as the brow elevators are weakened. Typically, weakening of the inferomedial frontalis results in a compensatory overactivity of the superior frontalis. This provides increased tone and a nice brow lift. This compensatory activity may be the most important mechanism in producing the brow lift recognized after glabella injection of BoNT.

Relevant brow anatomy is considered in two distinct aspects: the medial brow and lateral brow. Medial brow anatomy includes depressor supercilii, procerus, corrugator supercilii, frontalis (Figure 15.1). Lateral brow anatomy includes the lateral portion of the orbicularis oculi and the frontalis muscles (Figure 15.2) and it will be considered with the periorbital area.

The depressor supercilii originates on the nasal bridge and inserts into the skin of the mid-brow area. It draws the middle and medial portions of the brow inferiorly and medially. Corrugator supercilii also draws the mid and medial

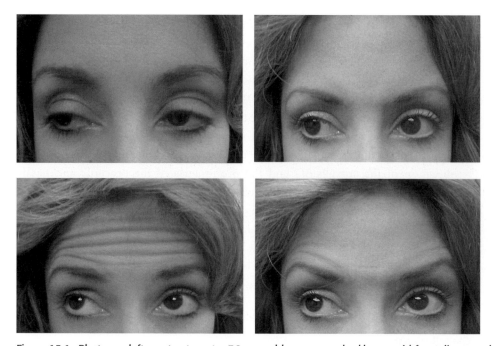

Figure 15.1 Photos on left: pre-treatment, a 36-year-old woman, arched brow, mid-frontalis musculature most prominent, and muscular lines do not extend all the way up to the hairline. Photos on right: 12 days after 18 U BOTOX® using five injection sites, −4 units midline, 4 units about 2 cm lateral to midline (all three being about 4 cm above brow) and −3 units injected laterally on each side (about 1.5 cm higher than medial injection points, and about 1.5 cm medial to temporal fusion line). Note the preservation of the arched brow at repose and the inferior frontalis musculature, which remains after treatment − allowing maintenance of brow shape and position as well as expression. Photos: Joel L. Cohen, MD.

brow in these directions. It originates on the nasal bone and inserts into the skin of the brow above the pupil. Variations in anatomy mean that the insertion point into the brow may be more lateral in some people than in others. This variation is occasionally responsible for movement of the brow even after the glabella has been correctly injected. In addition to these two muscles, the third muscle that forms the medial brow complex is the procerus. Unlike the other two muscles, which tend to form vertical lines by drawing the skin medially, the procerus tends to form horizontal lines by drawing the skin inferiorly. As these muscles contract they form etched-in lines perpendicular to the direction of their action. The procerus muscle originates on the nasal bridge and inserts into the skin of the mid-glabella directly above it. Treatment of this area with botulinum toxins typically addresses the muscles in concert. Opposing these depressors is the frontalis muscle, which is a brow elevator and may be a solitary wispy sheet that invests the entire forehead or it may be two muscles separated by a thin fascial component in the mid-forehead.

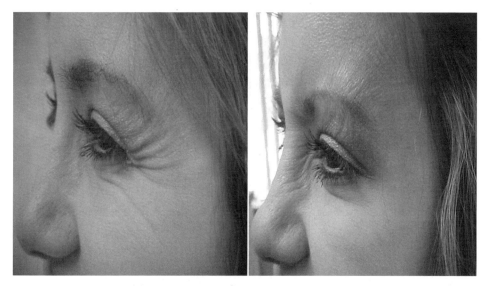

Figure 15.2 Crow's feet photos: 9 U BOTOX® into the crow's feet — four at superior aspect, two mid, two lower and one lateral lower lid. Photos: Joel L. Cohen, MD.

15.3.3   Injection technique for the glabella

Variations in technique exist between expert injectors in the approach to the medial brow complex. Many injectors will inject using 20–30 U in five injection sites[7]. Other injectors will inject this site with three injections, allowing diffusion to treat the adjacent areas. Differences in muscle mass affect the amount of toxin needed for relaxation of the muscles. Patients with hypertrophic muscles in this area require higher doses of toxin and men will require more material than women[8].

The most frequent sites of injection are the following: upper procerus (one injection), medial corrugator (one on each side) and lateral corrugator muscles (one injection on each side). The lateral corrugator injection is placed at least 1 cm above the orbital rim, in order to avoid diffusion to the adjacent orbital septum. Diffusion to the levator palpebrae superioris muscle may cause ptosis.

Adjustments may be made for prominent medial recruitment require 2–3 U about 1.5 cm above the bony supraorbital rim and for prominent procerus activity (5–7 U). The supraorbital rim is a reliable landmark and it, rather than the eyebrow, should be used to identify locations for injections. Avoid forceful injections in this area as this may increase the risk of diffusion as well as increase the risk of bruising and headaches. During the injection, patients are asked to frown, so that the length and direction of the corrugator can be followed.

15.3.4 Complications from glabella injections

Complications from injections of toxins to the brow area are rare. The most common complications include headache, respiratory infection, a flu-like syndrome, temporary eyelid droop and nausea[9,10]. Others include bruising or temporary periorbital oedema (the incidence of which increases with increased volumes of injection). When evaluating the actual incidence of complications, it is worth noting that for BOTOX®, many of the complications listed in the package insert were comparable to reactions seen with placebo. The management of complications is critical to patient safety and satisfaction. Most complications resolve spontaneously and require only patient reassurance.

Ptosis is the most unsettling complication seen with treatment of the glabellar complex and its management is subject to debate. Oculoplastic surgeons recommend treatment of ptosis with over-the-counter Naphcon A or apraclonidine hydrochloride (IOPIDINE® 0.5% Ophthalmic Solution), an alpha adrenergic agonist. Beware however, that Iopidine may unmask an underlying glaucoma, so this should be reserved for refractory cases. Untreated, the ptosis will resolve over the span of a few weeks.

15.4 Prominent forehead lines

15.4.1 General tips

Prior to treatment, it is crucial to note the brow position, shape, degree of blepharochalasis/dermatochalasis or scars using photographs, as post treatment asymmetry or eyelid redundancy is much more easily explained with pre-existing photos.

Women tend to have an arched brow whereas men tend to have a more horizontal brow orientation. A female arched-brow may be preserved by avoiding treatment of the lateral brow elevators and a weakening of the lateral brow depressors. Since the lower 3 cm of frontalis elevates and shapes the brow, the lateral 1/3 of this zone should be avoided in women to avoid brow heaviness.

15.4.2 Anatomy of the forehead musculature

The frontalis muscle normally varies significantly. The vertical orientation of the frontalis muscle fibers allows it to function as a brow elevator. Knowledge of its interaction with musculature of the medial brow and lateral brow allows the skilled physician to tailor his or her technique to fit the goals and anatomy of each patient. To activate the frontalis muscle, have the patient elevate their brows.

The frontalis muscle is continuous with the galea aponeurotica in its superior aspect. Inferiorly, it invests the skin of the brow. Contraction of this muscle not only raises the brow but also creates transverse rhytids across the forehead. The lateral border of the frontalis muscle is the temporal fusion plane. This plane is the boundary between the frontal and temporal bones and is easily palpated in most people. Inferior and slightly lateral to the temporal fusion line, the downward pull from the orbicularis muscle counteracts the upward pull of the frontalis. Understanding the interaction between these two muscles is critical when creating a brow lift using botulinum toxins (Figure 15.3).

15.4.3   Injection technique: forehead

Injecting the frontalis muscle takes account of the anatomy and goals of the individual being treated. Some patients desire to be wrinkle free. However this should be avoided, as eliminating every wrinkle of the forehead can increase the length of the forehead and neutralize the elevation needed by the brow to avoid sagging. In order to preserve the lateral brow lift in a woman, a different injection technique is required to that for a horizontal brow for a man. In a woman, injecting near the temporal fusion plane should be avoided, allowing the lateral brow to lift. In a man, one may inject a small amount of BOTOX® in the lateral aspect of the forehead to produce a horizontal brow. In addition, injection of the depressor component of the orbicularis should not be performed in a man, as it will accentuate the brow lift by reducing the depressor action on the lateral brow. When injecting the brow, it is best to avoid the most inferior rhytid in older

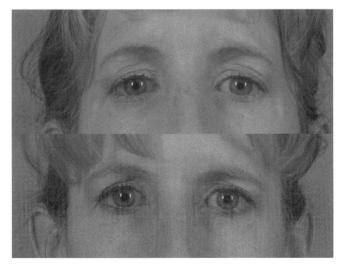

Figure 15.3   Lateral brow lift. Bottom: Pre-injection, note the upper eyelid redundancy ('hooding') present just below the lateral brow. Top: Post-injection of 5 U BOTOX® at a single point (described above) at the lateral and inferior aspect of the lateral brow on each side. Photos: Joel L. Cohen, MD.

women, as this musculature elevates the brow. Removing this results in a 'heavy' brow that will need to be manually suspended for makeup to be applied. Finally, for all forehead treatments, inject superficially, causing a bleb, rather than injecting at the depth of the periosteum. Gently massage each of the blebs for a few seconds after the treatment to facilitate some mild diffusion to these large muscles.

When injecting a woman with minimal skin laxity, several injections are made into the frontalis in a row that uses between five and nine injections. Consideration must be given to particularly wide or tall foreheads as well as to preferred hairstyles. Patients with tall foreheads will benefit from a second row of injections superior to the first one. Wider foreheads require more injections to cover the expanse. Failure to extend the injections laterally will result in a 'Mr. Spock' brow, caused by untreated lateral frontalis musculature.

As one injects the horizontal lines, one should inject higher moving laterally. In most patients, one should remain about 1.5 cm medial to temporal fusion line. Medial injection points should be at least 3–3.5 cm above the brow. A 1 or 2 cm dilution is appropriate and this dilution will reduce the chance of spread to unintended muscles. Doses vary depending on size of forehead and muscle mass. Treatment of the glabella can be accomplished at the same visit as the frontalis treatment. Alternatively, injectors can first treat the glabella and have patients follow-up 2 weeks later – which may potentially allow lower dosages to then be used in the forehead as there will be some degree of spread to the frontalis after the glabellar treatment. Pre-treatment marking during animation will avoid injecting too inferiorly. Average doses for frontalis treatment in women typically range from 10 to 30 units, whereas a man may require 20–40 units. One study has shown that higher dosages in the forehead are clearly associated with a longer duration of efficacy in this area[10].

Inactivation of the medial frontalis causes a compensatory elevation resulting in a rise of the lateral brow. This may be augmented when combined with an injection of the depressor aspect of the orbicularis. When treating men, injections of the brow should be more horizontal in men and should extend to the lateral aspect of the brow (in contrast to injections of female brow where injections tend to become more superior as the lateral brow is treated). Males recruit more laterally than most women and are more likely to require an injection of BoNT vertically above the lateral canthus at the orbital rim.

15.4.4 Complications: forehead

Complications that arise from injecting the frontalis include haematoma, brow drooping and headache. One problem that is encountered is the 'Mr. Spock' brow that results when the lateral aspects of the frontalis elevate the lateral brow producing a quizzical look. This situation is easily rectified with about 2 units in the lateral temporalis. Another situation unique to frontalis injections is an electrical shock sensation that occurs when the supraorbital nerve is hit by the needle. Patients report a sharp pain that radiates along the distribution of this nerve on frontal scalp. This situation is easily solved by avoiding injections in the mid-pupillary line or avoiding injecting too deeply.

15.5   Crow's feet and infraorbital rhytids

15.5.1   Anatomy of the periorbital area and of the eyelids

Variations of the lateral crow's feet exist among patients[11]. The major muscle affecting the orbital area is the orbicularis oculi, which is a thin band surrounding the eye. Its action is to constrict the skin surrounding the eye. Since it is a circular muscle, its action is different in different areas. For example, inferior to the lateral brow it works as a brow depressor. Its portion superior and lateral to the pupil may potentiate frowning and, at times, be responsible for patients that are able to frown after adequate injection of the glabella complex. The pretarsal component of this muscle has important actions for maintaining the shape of the periorbital areas. Without the actions of the orbicularis, there is a risk of festooning[12].

15.5.2   Injection technique for the periorbital areas

The single most popular injection of the orbicularis muscle is to prevent and treat the lateral canthal rhytids commonly known as crow's feet. Treatment for these wrinkles has high patient satisfaction and is technically simple. Using between 10–12 units of BOTOX® on each side, three or four injections are made[13]. The injections should be made at least 1 cm lateral to the orbital rim to avoid any unintended treatment of the ophthalmic muscles (which would produce diplopia). Since the muscles are very superficial, injections may be made by raising a wheal. At the inferior aspect of the treatment zone, care must be taken not to treat every last wrinkle as this will treat the zygomaticus minor and major, impairing the ability to raise the corners of the mouth and lips.

One of the most interesting and technically challenging aspects of injecting the periorbital area is the brow lift for women seeking this treatment. Performing this injection involves injecting approximately 3–6 units of BOTOX® into the portion of the orbicularis that tugs the lateral brow down[14]. When done in conjunction with injection of the medial frontalis, significant lateral brow elevation may be achieved. In severe cases of eyelid redundancy, surgical blepharoplasty is the treatment of choice.

The lower eyelid may be treated using 2 units of BOTOX® placed subdermally in the mid-pupillary line approximately 3—4 mm below the lid margin[15]. When this injection was administered in conjunction with treatment of crow's feet, the results were an improvement of infraorbital rhytids and a widening of the palpebral aperture, especially on smiling. This treatment should be reserved for those patients with minimal lower eyelid laxity.

15.5.3 Complications from injection of the orbital area

The most common complication from injections in this area is small hematomas and bruises due to the rich vasculature of this area. More serious complications include ptosis which occurs from injections that affect the levator palpebrae superioris. Injections placed too inferiorly on the zygomatic arch may lead to inability to raise the corners of the mouth or raise the lips and this can be most unsettling for both physician and patient alike. Diplopia may occur from either direct injection or diffusion that brings toxin in contact with the extraocular musculature. Photophobia has also been reported.

15.5.4 BOTOX® for lateral brow lift

Elevation of the lateral brow tends to give the patient a more alert, open-eyed look — one of the hallmarks of a youthful brow. Precise injections of BoNT-A into the superior and lateral aspect of orbicularis oculi can impart an arch to many brows. Specific injection sites are essential to locate and require some patient participation to elicit the correct musculature on each side. The first step in this procedure is to ask the patient to elevate their brow and find the temporal fusion plane (where the lateral frontalis ends). Then ask the patient to close their eyes forcefully and mark the site that the orbicularis oculi maximally pulls the lateral brow inward and downward. Inject 4—6 units just inferior to the point of maximal pull — making sure this point is at least 1.5 cm away (lateral-inferior) from temporal fusion area elicited in step one[14]. This technique can achieve a 2—3 mm elevation of lateral brow. Fillers such as Restylane® may be injected into the lateral aspect of the brow to alleviate upper lid redundancy. Combination therapy with BoNT-A and filler may increase the duration of response, as has been documented in other areas of combination therapy such as the glabella.

15.5.5 'Bunny lines'

The upper nasalis muscle is responsible for the formation of 'bunny lines' at the bridge of the nose that extend horizontally toward the medial canthus. These lines may form a sharp contrast to a perfectly smooth glabellar area, and may be seen as a sign of someone who has had glabellar and crow's feet

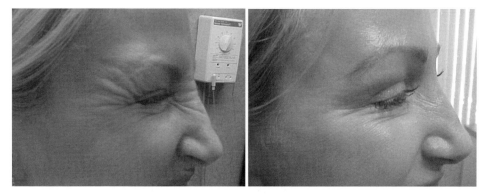

Figure 15.4   A 40-year-old woman with prominent bunny lines treated with 4 U BOTOX® to each lateral nasal side wall (in addition, patient was treated in the crow's feet with 12 units to each lateral aspect of the orbicularis oculi). Photos: Joel L. Cohen, MD.

treated with botulinum toxin A. It is recommended that the nasalis be injected in concert with the glabella. This muscle can be isolated for injection by having the patient frown, smile or squint. The nasalis muscle is injected with approximately 3–5 units of botulinum toxin A superficially at each medial proximal sidewall of the bridge of the nose (Figure 15.4). Insertion of the needle must be gentle and should be in the subcutaneous but not periosteal plane. Caution must be exercised when injecting this area as an injection that is placed lateral to the nasal sulcus may affect the levator labii superioris aleque nasi, resulting in a drooping of the lateral lip. To complete this cosmetic unit, it is best to also treat the procerus with 5–7 units as well to complement the glabella and nasalis regions[16].

15.6   Lower face

Treatment of the lower face requires more advanced knowledge of injection techniques as well as of the relevant anatomy. When considering the anatomy of the lower- and mid-face, it is helpful to think about how injections will affect the position of the mouth and how they will affect the contour of the lips. It is also important to consider treatment of these areas in conjunction with soft tissue augmentation.

15.6.1   General anatomy of the lower face

The corners of the mouth are moved by two sets of opposing muscles: elevators and depressors (Figure 15.5). The major elevator of the lateral mouth and cheek is the zygomaticus major. Medial elevation is accomplished by the zygomaticus minor as well as the levator labii superioris and minor.

The orbicularis oris is a sphincter-like muscle surrounding the mouth. It is responsible for pursing the lips resulting in perioral rhytids. Women frequently

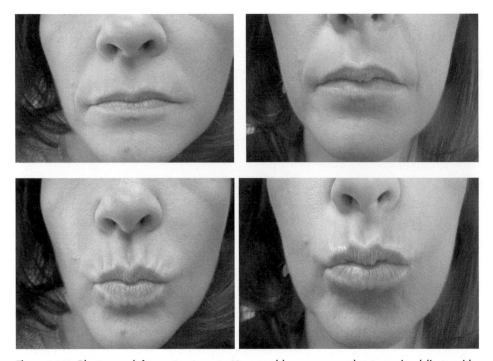

Figure 15.5 Photos on left: pre-treatment, 42-year-old woman, moderate perioral lines with pursing lips, no significant baseline imprinted superficial lines at repose. Photos on right: 14 days post-treatment with 8 U BOTOX® (10 injection sites, as diagrammed below). Note: post-treatment lips appear fuller, especially with movement − likely a pseudo-augmentation appearance due to upward pull of the remaining superior aspect of the orbicularis oris from the levator labii superioris aleque nasi and zygomaticus insertions. In addition, there is preservation of Cupid's bow symmetry as midline philtrum is maintained. Photos: Joel L. Cohen, MD.

complain that lipstick 'bleeds' into these lines and any improvement is greatly welcomed by patients.

The position of the lips is also controlled by depressors that counteract the elevator muscles. The depressor anguli oris will, over time, cause the lateral aspects of the mouth and lips to turn inferiorly. This imparts a negative impression and is a frequent impetus for patients seeking cosmetic improvement. The explosion of filler substances available to use in conjunction with the toxins has greatly enhanced our ability to treat these marionette lines.

The mentalis muscle lies at the most inferior portion of the face. It originates in the incisive fossa and inserts into the skin of the chin and is responsible for the appearance of lines in the chin area that are variously described as 'pebble chin' or the more dreaded 'scrotal chin.' Treatment of this muscle relaxes the mentalis and leads to significant improvement of the appearance of the chin.

15.6.2   Lips

General tips for lips

The lips are a popular site for BoNT-A treatment in women. Patients seeking correction of lip rhytids typically have many questions from the common misconception that botulinum toxin A should not be used in the lower face. Treatment with botulinum toxin A not only softens vertical lip lines, but also provides the appearance of fuller lips. This results from diminishing the hollowing appearance within the vertical muscular bands, offering a 'pseudo-augmentation.' Smokers tend to have more dramatic results than non-smokers. Patients with deep perioral rhytids should combine botulinum toxin A with fillers, such as collagen or hyaluronic acid. CO_2 resurfacing is still a viable alternative for patients with significant lines and botulinum toxin A will enhance and prolong the efficacy of this procedure. During the consultation, it is important to explain that BoNT-A will soften, but not completely prevent or obliterate vertical lip lines. It should also be clearly explained and stated on consent forms that injecting lip lines may decrease the ability to purse lips. This action is used for kissing or putting on lipstick, whistling, drinking from a straw, and creating a seal around a spoon. Knowing this, one should avoid treating patients who play a wind instrument or plan on scuba diving or snorkeling in the next few months. In addition, such pursing of the lips is required to some extent for enunciating words with 'p,' 'b,' and sometimes 'j and g.' You can illustrate this for patients by having them say 'peanut butter and jelly.' Patients in professions that require perfect phonation may not be good candidates for this treatment area.

The effect of treatment usually lasts several weeks less than in other regions, averaging about 7–10 weeks duration of treatment in our experience[17]. In addition, because the dosages used are so small, these patients are followed up 2 weeks after treatment to evaluate efficacy by comparing current photos to pre-treatment photos, and touching-up if occasionally necessary. Treatment should involve the upper and lower lip. In our experience, some of the patients who just wanted upper lip treatment vaguely expressed that it 'felt funny' until the lower lip was treated as well.

Injection technique for lips

Treatment of the lips usually hurts more than other sites. Thus, these patients should ice the perioral area prior to the injection. Our usual $1\,cm^3$ dilution for other sites is diluted by a factor of 5:1 for the lips. The dose for this area being only 6–9 units and we use the dilution to obtain a more even relaxation.

In the upper lip, two injection points are used. They are along the vermillion border on each side of the upper lip spaced about 1.5 cm apart, as well as another more superior injection site between them 1 cm above the vermillion border. Maintenance of symmetry is very important to ensure preservation of the philtrum midline. For the lower lip, we inject only along the vermillion border – using two sites on each side of the lip, also spaced about 1.5 cm apart. Like the forehead, we press down on the injection sites for a few seconds after the treatment to facilitate some mild diffusion.

15.6.3 'Gummy smile'

The 'gummy smile' refers to excessive showing of the gums above their maxillary teeth (probably responsible for the expression of 'being long in the tooth'). This can be treated by targeting the levator labii superioris aleque nasi muscle. This muscle may be identified by asking the patient to move the tip of his or her nose[18]. Injection of between 1–3 units of BOTOX® at each superior medial nasolabial fold will relax this muscle. Without the elevation provided by this muscle the upper lip will be lowered enough to cover the upper portion of the teeth while the patient is smiling. Improvement of this area may be enhanced with a filler substance used adjunctively to diminish prominent superior nasolabial folds. This treatment is best for younger patients with significant upper gum show when smiling, sometimes called the 'extreme canine smile.' Caution should be exercised when treating older patients as treatment can cause an accentuation of mid-face flattening and cutaneous upper lip vertical elongation, which normally occurs with aging, and may be undesirable in those patients. Treatment of the levator labii superioris aleque nasi should be reserved for those physicians with a great deal of experience injecting botulinum toxin A in the lower aspect of the face. Complications seen in this area may include asymmetry of the lips and depression of the corners of the mouth.

15.6.4 'Downturned smile'

The 'downturned smile' can misrepresent emotions, imparting a sad or concerned appearance. This may be corrected with botulinum toxin injections of the depressor anguli oris (DAO) muscle. This muscle can be identified for injection by palpating along the jawline as the patient frowns or pulls down the corners of the mouth. The average doses of BOTOX® is between 3–5 units per side. Injections are made into the posterior-aspect of DAO. This permits the zygomaticus muscle to act unopposed and elevate the corners of the mouth to a horizontal, more aesthetically pleasing position. Great care should be exercised in treating this area as a medial injection can diffuse to the depressor labii inferioris causing slurred speech. This area should be avoided in patients who play wind instruments, sing or are broadcast journalists or scuba divers.

Perhaps more than any other, this area is typically treated in conjunction with a filler such as Restylane®.

15.6.5   Mentalis-'golf ball chin'

Excessive wrinkling of the chin is produced by the mentalis muscle, which originates on the canine fossa and inserts into the dermis of the chin. This pebbly appearance is made more prominent when speaking or chewing. Injections of this area with BoNT-A will alleviate these rhytids and impart a more youthful appearance to the lower face. The mentalis muscle may be triggered by asking the patient to push his or her lower lip downwards. Injections of the area may be made with 4–8 units BOTOX® injected at the bony part of the chin (either as a single midline injection or as two injections approximately 1 cm apart) (Figure 15.6). This treatment can also be used to soften mental crease. Be cautious however, as too lateral an injection can diffuse to depressor labii inferioris, resulting in slurred speech. Just above this area of musculature lies the mental crease. Treatment of a prominent mental crease can be enhanced with fillers.

15.6.6   'Vertical neck bands' and 'horizontal necklace lines'

After weight loss, chin/neck liposuction or general ageing changes, some patients complain of prominent vertical bands in their neck. These hyperfunctional platysmal bands differ from horizontal lines, which are believed to be from prominent SMAS. The platysmal bands can be relaxed by experienced botulinum toxin A injectors. The specific injection sites are determined at rest, and

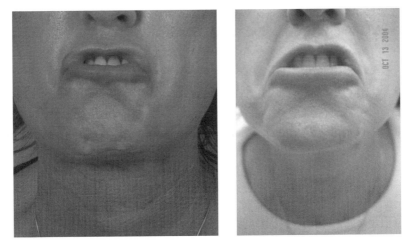

Figure 15.6   A 52-year-old woman who complained of dimpling in her chin when speaking and chewing gum. She was treated with two three-unit injections of BOTOX® into the mentalis (in addition, her horizontal neck bands were treated the same day with a total of 10 U BOTOX®). Photos: Joel L. Cohen, MD.

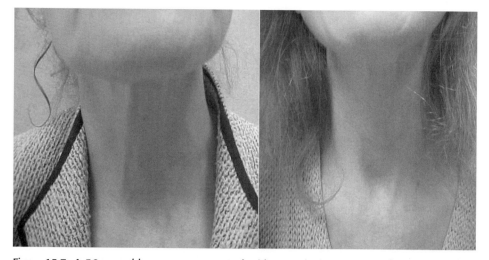

Figure 15.7 A 56-year-old woman was treated with a total of 18 U BOTOX® for vertical neck bands present at rest. The right band was treated with 12 U and the left band 6 U. Photos: Joel L. Cohen, MD.

without animation. Typically 20—35 units total are used, with re-treatment 2—3 weeks later for undercorrection. Injections of between 1—3 units are spaced approximately 1.5 cm apart along the band or horizontal line (Figure 15.7). Grasp the band between thumb and forefinger and ensure that each injection is superficially placed. Deeper or larger injections may possibly relax the platysma enough to allow the elevators of the lower face to more effectively lift the neck and jowls. However, one report of severe dysphagia occurred following injection with 60 units[17]. This patient required a nasogastric tube feeding for 6 weeks and caution should be exercised when treating the neck. If a patient complains of swallowing difficulties following a procedure they should be evaluated immediately. Treatment should consist of soft foods, metoclopramide to stimulate upper GI motility and ENT evaluation. This procedure is best for our young patients with good skin tone, post-submental liposuction, or post-face/necklift.

15.6.7 Newer indications for treatment with botulinum toxins

Radish calf

Hypertrophic gastrocnemius muscles are the cause of psychological stress for women affected by enlarged muscles of the calf area. BoNT-A has been used to reduce the girth and improve the contour of the calves of oriental women. One study treated so called 'radish calves' with botulinum toxin type A. (Ref. PRS OCT. 2003) Doses ranging from 32, 48 and 72 units were injected into the medial head of the gastrocnemius muscle. The results from this study demonstrated an improvement of leg contour with a 'slight' decrease in girth.

There was no apparent detriment to any functional component of the muscle group and the improvement lasted for about 6 months. Not surprisingly, the authors noted that there was a low patient satisfaction with this procedure as there was apparently little change rendered by the treatment. Injections of radish calves will most likely be limited to very select patients who are greatly distressed by the contour and size of their calves.

15.6.8   Adjunctive uses of botulinum toxins

One of the most interesting aspects of botulinum toxins is their use in conjunction with other minimally invasive procedures such as injection of soft tissue augmentation products and with lasers and other light sources. Combinations of these procedures is virtually unlimited.

The use of toxins with fillers

The combination of fillers with botulinum toxins makes sense, as many patients desiring treatment of dynamic rhytids also need volume replacement. From a mechanistic perspective, the use of toxins makes eminent sense, as they will tend to reduce the ability of muscles to pump fillers out of their sites of injections. Among the fillers that are used with botulinum toxins include collagen, calcium hydroxylapatite (Radiesse®), hyaluronic acids and poly-L-lactic acid (Sculptra®). Permanent fillers that may be used with toxins include silicone and Artefill®.

Many of the dynamic rhytids treated with botulinum toxins will have some static component at the time of treatment. Despite adequate inhibition of muscle activity, these resting wrinkles persist. Fillers offer an additional opportunity to correct the static rhytid. Areas amenable to correction with non-permanent fillers and toxins include the glabella, periorbital area, mentalis, perioral area and in limited cases, the nasolabial creases.

Materials used in conjunction with BoNT in the glabella include collagens and hyaluronic acids. Although calcium hydroxylapatite may be used, caution should be exercised when injected near the trochlear plexus of vessels. Collagens that may be used for glabella treatment include those that are non-crosslinked (e.g. Zyderm® I and II and Cosmoderm® I and II). Isolagen® will most likely also be an acceptable filler for this area. The crosslinked collagens are not recommended for this area.

Useful hyaluronic acid products in this area in concentrations between $5.5\,\mathrm{mg\,ml^{-1}}$ and $20\,\mathrm{mg\,ml^{-1}}$ include those that are animal derived as well as those that are non-animal derived. Large particle size is best avoided for a filler for the glabella.

More durable fillers such as Radiesse® may be used in the glabella in conjunction with botulinum injections. Paralysis afforded by the toxin will allow the scaffolding of the calcium hydroxyapatite to remain relatively immobile and may help to improve the ingrowth of fibroblasts and collagen. The major caveat with using this product in this area is that injection of thick products has resulted in intravascular injection of material with resulting necrosis of the skin. In addition, the vascular plexus for the eye may be the unintended recipient of filler via retrograde flow.

The same caution exercised when injecting the glabella when not using toxins must also be used when providing combination therapy. Fillers such as silicone and Artefill® should be used only by experienced injectors. Poly-L-lactic acid should also be used by experienced injectors in this area.

When treating the glabella with a filler and botulinum toxin, it is recommended that the filler be injected prior to the injection of the toxin. This will reduce the risk of untoward migration and unintended paralysis of levator muscles.

The periorbital area may also benefit from use of toxins with fillers. As with the glabellar area, fillers will help to alleviate the static component of the rhytid while the BOTOX® will prolong the duration of the soft tissue correction by decreasing the muscular pumping action.

Collagens have long been used to fill the periorbital areas. The thin skin of the area mandates that one of the thinner collagens is used (such as Cosmoderm® or Zyderm®). Using one of the crosslinked products is not recommended for this area. Hyalouronic acids are also helpful for adjunctive treatment of this area and products intended for superficial or mid-dermal placement (but not deep dermal or sub-cutaneous placement) are tolerated well in these areas. As with any periorbital injection, care should be taken to avoid intravascular injection.

Rhytids of the upper lip are one of the best places to use combinations of fillers and toxins. Patients that have static and dynamic perioral rhytids will greatly benefit from the synergistic effect of the two treatments. Fillers that are effective when used with botulinum toxins include collagens (the type depends on the thickness of the wrinkle and of the skin) and the hyaluronic acids (particularly ones with small particle size). Care should be exercised when using Sculptra® in this area as it may result in subcutaneous papule formation. Silicone may be useful as long as a micro-droplet technique is used and enough toxin is given to minimize the risk of silicone migration during the encapsulation process. There is not enough data to know whether Radiesse® may be used for this area, but, if one uses toxin and allows the product to remain immobile, it might be an acceptable long-term alternative.

Injection of the depressor anguli oris in conjunction with volume replacement of the marionette lines is another combination that is synergistic. The toxin not only helps to reduce the depressor function (allowing for less filler to restore proper positioning of the corner of the mouth) but will also decrease the muscular pumping that tends to move fillers out of their intended locations.

Fillers used for the marionette lines include collagens, hyaluronic acids, poly-L-lactic acid, silicone and calcium hydroxylapatite. As with other locations, each has its relative risks and benefits for this location.

Mentalis creases are also ideally treated with combinations of fillers and toxins. The use of typical amounts of toxin in this area will relax most of the dynamic rhytids associated with muscle actions here. Depending on the degree of static rhytids, fillers can often make the difference between a patient that is not satisfied and one that is thrilled. As with the marionette lines, the choice of filler for this area depends on the experience and preference of the physician and patient.

Adjunctive use of fillers for neck treatment is an area that will most likely receive attention in the future. One filler that seems to enhance the performance of the botulinum toxins is poly-L-lactic acid, which adds volume to this area. Hyaluronic acids, collagens, calcium hydroxyapatite and silicone are helpful for treating this area but require large volumes.

15.7 Conclusions

Botulinum toxins are frequently used for cosmetic indications. Areas once thought not to be amenable to treatment are now routinely treated. Newer uses of these drugs in conjunction with other cosmetic procedures have enhanced the utility not only of the toxins, but also of these adjunctive treatments. What an exciting time to be in cosmetic dermatology!

REFERENCES

1. Carruthers, J. D. and Carruthers, J. A. (1992). Treatment of glabellar frown lines with *Clostridium botulinum*-A exotoxin. *Journal of Dermatologic Surgery and Oncology,* **18**(1), 17–21.
2. Hsu, T. S., Dover, J. S. and Arndt, K. A. (2004). Effect of volume and concentration on the diffusion of botulinum exotoxin A. *Archives of Dermatology,* **140**(11), 1351–4.
3. Dover, J. S. and Arndt, K. A. (2002). Pain associated with injection of botulinum A exotoxin reconstituted using isotonic sodium chloride with and without preservative: a double-blind, randomized controlled trial. *Arch. Dermatol.,* **138**(4), 510–14.
4. Lewis, C. (2002). Botox cosmetic: a look at looking good. *FDA Consumer,* **36**(4), 11–13.
5. Goodman, G. (2003). Diffusion and short-term efficacy of botulinum toxin A after the addition of hyaluronidase and its possible application for the treatment of axillary hyperhidrosis dermatologic surgery. *Dermatologic Surgery,* **29**(5), 533–8.

6. Finn, C., Cox, S. E. and Earl, F. (2003). Social implications of hyperfunctional facial lines. *Dermatol. Surg.*, **29**, 450–5.

7. Carruthers, A., Carruthers, J. and Said, S. (2005). Dose-ranging study of botulinum toxin type A in the treatment of glabellar rhytids in females. *Dermatologic Surgery*, **31**(04), 414–22.

8. Carruthers, A. and Carruthers, J. (2005). Prospective, double-blind, randomized, parallel-group, dose-ranging study of botulinum toxin type A in men with glabellar rhytids. *Dermatologic Surgery*, **31**(10), 1297–303.

9. Carruthers, J. A., Lowe, N. J., Menter, M. A., Gibson, J., Nordquist, M., Mordaunt, J., Walker, P. and Eadie, N. (2002). A multicenter, double-blind, randomized, placebo-controlled study of the efficacy and safety of botulinum toxin type A in the treatment of glabellar lines. *Journal of American Academy of Dermatology*, **46**, 840–9.

10. Carruthers, A., Carruthers, J. and Cohen, J. (2003). A prospective, double-blind, randomized, parallel group, dose-ranging study of BOTOX® in female subjects with horizontal forehead rhytids. *Dermatologic Surgery*, **29**, 462–7.

11. Kane, M. A. (2003). Classification of crow's feet patterns among caucasian women: the key to individualizing treatment. *Plastic and Reconstructive Surgery*, **112**(Suppl. 5), S33–S39.

12. Goldman, M. (2003). Festoon formation after infraorbital botulinum-A toxin: a case report. *Dermatologic Surgery*, **29**(5), 560.

13. Lowe, N. *et al.* (2005). Double-blind, randomized, placebo-controlled, dose-response study of the safety and efficacy of botulinum toxin type A in subjects with crow's feet. *Dermatologic Surgery*, **31**(3), 257–62.

14. Cohen, J. and Dayan, S. (2005). Botulinum toxin type A in the treatment of dermatochalasis: a prospective study evaluating temporal brow elevation. *American Academy of Dermatology*, **52**(Suppl. 3), 86.

15. Flynn, T., Carruthers, J. A., Carruthers, A. and Clark, R. (2003). Botulinum A toxin (BOTOX®) in the lower eyelid: dose-finding study. *Dermatol. Surg.*, **29**(9), 943–50.

16. Tamura, B., Odo, M., Chang, B., Cuce, L. and Flynn, T. (2005). Treatment of nasal wrinkles with botulinum toxin. *Dermatologic Surgery*, **31**(03), 271–5.

17. Carruthers, J. and Carruthers, A. (1999). Practical cosmetic Botox® techniques. *Journal of Cutaneous Medicine and Surgery*, **3**(Suppl. 4), S49–52.

18. Pessa, J. E. (1992). Improving the acute nasolabial angle and medial nasolabial fold by levator alae muscle resection. *Annals of Plastic Surgery*, **29**(1), 23–30.

Other clinical neurological uses of botulinum toxin

Michael P. Barnes

Walkergate Park, International Centre for Neurorehabilitation and Neuropsychiatry, Newcastle upon Tyne, UK

16.1 Introduction

This chapter will highlight some of the less common but nevertheless helpful uses of botulinum toxin for a variety of neurological conditions. The list of potential uses of botulinum toxin is growing each year and this chapter does not attempt to offer a completely comprehensive guide to every case report in every potential neurological condition. This chapter discusses the reasonably established use in the following conditions:

- Tics
- Myoclonus
- Stiff person syndrome
- Parkinson's disease
- Tremor
- Limb dystonia including occupational cramps

Each section will give a brief overview of the condition itself and then give some thoughts with regard to the place of botulinum toxin in the treatment of the condition. None of these conditions yet constitute a licensed indication for botulinum toxin type A or type B. Indeed the conditions and indications are so rare that it is unlikely that definitive trials will be undertaken in order to satisfy the licensing regulations. However, the lack of a license indication can still mean that botulinum toxin may be a useful addition to our therapeutic armoury in these conditions, which are often difficult to ameliorate.

16.2 Tics

16.2.1 Background

A tic is a sudden rapid recurrent non-rhythmic stereotyped motor movement or vocalization[1]. Tourette's syndrome is characterized by both multiple motor

Clinical Uses of Botulinum Toxins, eds. Anthony B. Ward and Michael P. Barnes. Published by Cambridge University Press. © Cambridge University Press 2007.

and vocal tics. Tics are extremely common in childhood and some studies indicate a prevalence of up to a quarter of all children being affected at some point during their childhood[2].

Tics can range from simple to complex. Simple motor tics can just consist of a brief movement such as blinking, grimacing or shrugging of shoulders. More complex motor tics can involve elaborate stereotyped actions of whole limbs or the whole body. The tics are involuntary but, in contrast to many other movement disorders, can be temporarily suppressed but only at the expense of an increasingly irresistible urge to perform the tic.

The cause of tics is unknown although almost certainly involves abnormal basal ganglia function. An autoimmune cause for Tourette's syndrome has been suggested but has not been confirmed. A genetic predisposition to some forms of tic is also likely and indeed the familial transmission of Tourette's syndrome is well established. However, no clear genetic cause has yet been determined. In a very small number of cases the tic disorder is secondary to another underlying disease. As in all movement disorders a drug cause should be excluded, particularly neuroleptic medication.

16.2.2 Natural history

In the great majority of cases simple motor tics occurring in childhood will fade during adolescence and not reoccur during adult life. However, as a generalization, the more complex the tic then the more likely it is to extend into adulthood. The prognosis is somewhat worse in boys than girls. It is also worse if the tic is also associated with other problems such as obsessive compulsive disorder, self mutilation and attention deficit hyperactivity disorder (ADHD) − all of which can occur in association with a tic. Rarely tics can occur in adult life when they are usually secondary to another underlying cause, such as Huntington's disease or neuroacanthocytosis but in general movement disorders appearing for the first time in adult life are unlikely to be tics.

16.2.3 Management

Children with mild tics probably need no treatment. Explanation, reassurance and information are usually adequate. Indeed focusing too much on the condition can cause additional stress and anxiety that can worsen the problem. The benign nature of the condition and the high likelihood of remission should be emphasized. Tics should only be treated if they are severe enough to cause significant disability. If treatment is necessary then clearly any medication needs to be combined with appropriate counselling, explanation and information.

Treatment is usually focused on oral medication. Neuroleptics and α-2 adrenergic agonists are the mainstay of treatment, despite the fact that neuroleptic medication can also cause tics in a few individuals. Many centres would now use risperidone or clonidine. Both agents have recently been studied in comparison with placebo and shown to be equally effective[3,4]. Obviously adverse events are of concern in children and such side effects include sedation, tremor and depression – in those taking risperidone. Tricyclic antidepressants, particularly desipramine can also be tried, as can methylphenidate[1]. The latter is useful in children with Tourette's syndrome in combination with ADHD. Improvement in tics have also been reported with tetrabenazine, low dose dopamine agonists, clonazepam and calcium channel blockers. However, robust studies are lacking with many of these medications.

16.2.4 The role of botulinum toxin

Botulinum toxin has a small role to play in the management of tics. The obvious difficulty is that tics are intermittent by definition whereas botulinum toxin lasts for the entire duration of the treatment period of usually 10–12 weeks. This can mean that although botulinum toxin can be useful for the tic itself that there is a risk of unnecessary muscle weakness in between the tics. This can, of course, be as disabling as or more disabling than the tic itself. However, if the tic is reasonably localized to one or a few muscle groups then botulinum toxin can be considered. This is particularly the case if individuals cannot be suitably treated with oral medication, or develop unacceptable side effects with such medication. Simple motor tics will tend to be better treated than more complex stereotyped tics which often involve many muscle groups. Clearly there is a limit to how many muscle groups can be effectively injected with botulinum toxin.

Many of the studies have been small scale and not controlled. However, the efficacy has been confirmed. The largest study involved 35 patients (30 male and 5 female) treated with botulinum toxin type A for the most problematic tics[5]. The response to botulinum toxin was based on a 0–4 clinical rating scale and the scale was supplemented by questionnaires to evaluate the patient's subjective impressions. The tics were well established with a mean duration of 15 years. The sites of injection differed considerably but most were in the cervical or upper thoracic area (17 people), upper face (14 people) and lower face (7 people). The response to the botulinum toxin was as expected in terms of the duration of action, latency to onset and side-effect profile. The mean dose used was around 100 BOTOX® units for each visit. A total of 21 people (84%) of the 25 people with premonitory sensation derived marked relief of these symptoms with a mean of 70.6 per cent benefit. The authors concluded that botulinum was an effective and more tolerated treatment for motor tics particularly for providing relief of premonitory sensations.

Similar positive results were found by Marras and colleagues[6]. In this study 18 patients with simple motor tics were randomized to receive either botulinum toxin or placebo in a double-blind cross-over design. The primary outcome measure was the number of treated tics per minute on a video tape recording. Other outcome measures included a numerical assessment of the urge to perform the treated tic as well as record the premonitory sensation and global impression of change. The reduction in treated tics per minute with botulinum toxin was 39 per cent versus a 5.8 per cent increase in the placebo phase. The average change in urge scores was −0.46 in the treatment phase and +0.49 in the placebo phase. The other secondary outcome measures were not significantly different between the two groups. The authors found that botulinum was useful not only in reducing tic frequency but also the urge associated with the tic. Other authors have found similar positive benefits in small series[7,8].

Some authors have also confirmed the benefit for vocal tics in the context of Tourette's syndrome. Porta and colleagues[9] assessed the effect of botulinum toxin on phonic tics in a total of 30 patients with Tourette's syndrome. Each received 2.5 BOTOX® units into both vocal cords. In these patients vocal tics improved after treatment in 93 per cent of cases and 50 per cent were tic free. Premonitory sensation dropped from 53 per cent to 20 per cent. Quality of life measures improved. Hypophonia was the only side-effect of note which occurred in 80 per cent of patients. This was a very encouraging result confirming the efficacy and safety of botulinum in these circumstances. This larger scale study had built on previous successful case reports[10,11].

Thus, although a number of studies have confirmed the efficacy of botulinum toxin, particularly for simple motor tics and vocal tics, there are no clear criteria for patient selection. Sensible criteria would seem to be individuals with persistent and disabling simple motor tics or vocal tics, unresponsive or poorly responsive to oral medication or in those in whom medication produces undesirable side effects. It could be argued that in those with disabling tics localized to just one or a few muscle groups then botulinum toxin may be used as a first line treatment, given its safety and excellent side-effect profile in contrast to the complex and troublesome side-effect profiles of the oral medications.

16.3   Myoclonus

16.3.1   Background

Myoclonus involves sudden shock-like muscle jerks. The jerks are involuntary and not associated with loss of consciousness. There are a number of different classifications of myoclonus, some based on clinical features (e.g. generalized, multifocal, segmental or focal myoclonus) and others based on the proposed pathophysiological mechanism (e.g. cortical myoclonus, reticular reflex myoclonus, subcortical myoclonus, spinal myoclonus and peripheral myoclonus). Finally there is a classification based on aetiology (see Table 16.1).

It is not the purpose of the section to provide a definitive review of myoclonus. It is simply important to emphasize that there are a variety of different causes of myoclonus, some of which clearly require specific treatments

Full investigation is important and should almost certainly include electro-encephalogram (EEG) and magnetic resonance imaging (MRI) scans, particularly for the assessment of brainstem and spinal segmental myoclonus.

16.3.2   Other treatments

Obviously some forms of myoclonus require a specific treatment, such as tumours or arteriovenous malformations (AVMs), or attention may be needed to the various metabolic causes such as liver and renal failure. Cortical myoclonus can

Table 16.1. Aetiology of myoclonus

Essential myoclonus	
Myoclonic epilepsy syndromes	
Acquired metabolic disorders	Liver failure
	Renal failure
	Hyponatraemia
Post hypoxic myoclonus	
Focal lesions of the brain	Tumour
	Trauma
	Demyelination
	Encephalitis
	AVM
	Ischaemia
	etc.
Progressive cerebral disorders	Alzheimer's disease
	Creutzfeldt–Jacob disease
	Huntington's disease
	Corticobasal degeneration
	Diffuse Lewy body disease
	Spinocerebellar degeneration
	Mitochondrial diseases and neuronal storage diseases
	Other rarer progressive cerebral disorders

respond very well to clonazepam, sodium valproate or other conventional anti-epileptics. Piracetam has also shown to be effective in both cortical and subcortical myoclonus[12]. Myoclonus with a neurophysiological origin below the cortex tends to respond less well to antimyoclonic medication. However reticular reflex myoclonus can sometimes respond to clonazepam or fluoxetine and spinal myoclonus can also respond to clonazepam[13]. Palatal myoclonus is a specific entity characterized by myoclonic jerking movements of the palate sometimes with synchronous movements of the tongue, face, neck or arms. One form is associated with lesions in the Guillain–Mollaret triangle (dentate–red nucleus–inferior olivary circuit). It is sometimes associated with specific brainstem lesions such as demyelination or cerebral ischaemic disease. It can respond to clonazepam, anticholinergic or antidepressant medication.

More recently there has been some evidence of efficacy of levetiracetam which is a novel anti-epileptic agent for various myoclonic disorders. Gamma-hydroxybutyric acid (GHB) has also been shown to be efficacious in alcohol sensitive myoclonic dystonia[14]. Alcohol can also suppress myoclonus in some patients, particularly those with essential myoclonus. Zonisamide has been particularly effective in progressive myoclonic epilepsy[15]. A recent review by Agarwal and Frucht gives a good and up-to-date review of medication in the treatment of myoclonus[16].

Severe focal cortical myoclonus can sometimes respond to surgical resection of the cortical lesion.

16.3.3   The role of botulinum toxin

There have been no controlled studies of the use of botulinum toxin for the treatment of myoclonus. Most of the literature involves single case reports. Botulinum toxin is likely to be most useful when there is persistent focal myoclonus in just one or a few localized muscle groups that has been resistant to oral medication. For example Polo and Jabbari[17] describe a 16-year-old girl with a pulmonary vascular anomaly who suffered from an acute spinal cord infarct at the age of 11. In addition to paralysis of the right leg and bladder problems she also developed involuntary myoclonic movements of the left thigh confirmed by electromyography. Treatment with botulinum toxin led to complete cessation of the pain associated with these movements and a marked reduction in the amplitude of the movements, both clinically and electromyographically. Lagueny and colleagues[18] report similar improvement after botulinum toxin injection of the left trapezius for a patient with stimulus sensitive spinal segmental myoclonus. Awaad and colleagues[19] describe the use of botulinum toxin in nine children with myoclonus of various aetiologies. The patient details are sketchy but they report a 'dramatic' reduction of painful myoclonus with improvement of functional skills. Indeed one patient who was a non-ambulatory prior to treatment was able to walk afterwards. There have also been a few case reports of the efficacy of botulinum toxin for palatal myoclonus. Bryce and Morrison[20] report two patients injected with botulinum toxin into the tensor veli palitini muscle which resulted in the relief of tinnitus and cessation of the palatal contractions. Two other authors have demonstrated benefit for palatal myoclonus after injection into the tensor veli palitini muscle and the levator veli palitini muscle at small doses of BOTOX® (2.5 units in one case). These cases were associated with side effects of nasal regurgitation and swallowing difficulties[21,22]. Obviously such injections require considerable expertise and involvement of an injector with intimate knowledge of the local anatomy.

In summary there are just a few case studies of the use of botulinum toxin for myoclonus. Most forms of myoclonus respond quite well to oral medication and botulinum toxin is likely to only be used in a few resistant cases with focal and limited muscle spasm. The same problem applies to myoclonus as previously described in tics. The myoclonus will tend to be intermittent and botulinum toxin obviously has a longer term duration which can result in troublesome muscle weakness in between the myoclonic jerks. Thus there needs to be a clinical decision regarding the balance between potential benefits of muscle relaxation against potential drawbacks.

16.4 Stiff person syndrome

16.4.1 Background

Stiff person syndrome is a rare progressive rigidity of the trunk and proximal limbs often associated with stimulus sensitive spasms. It was first described by Moersch and Woltman in 1956[23]. The original case was a 49-year-old man with episodic tightness of the neck muscles slowly spreading to involve muscles at the shoulder and back and upper part of the legs over 4 years. The rigidity was produced by continuous muscle contraction which obviously made voluntary movements slow and awkward. Prolonged and painful muscle spasms were superimposed on the background rigidity. Cases classically arise in mid-life and commonly involve the trunk. There is often a hyperlordotic posture with severe rigidity of the lumbar and abdominal muscles. Painful muscle spasms are often superimposed upon the fixed rigidity. A variety of other associated features can occur including autonomic dysfunction, ataxia and seizures.

The disorder is thought to be autoimmune in origin[24]. Antibodies to glutamic acid decarboxylase (GAD) are found in many, but not all, cases. These antibodies cross react with pancreatic islet cells and gastric parietal cells. There is an association with diabetes in about a third of cases. Other autoimmune disorders can also co-exist. In some individuals the problem is paraneoplastic and associated with different auto antibodies[25].

The condition is sometimes subdivided into the stiff trunk syndrome and stiff limb syndrome which simply describes the predominant areas of muscle stiffness. A third variant is progressive encephalomyelitis with rigidity which is often associated with more severe muscle rigidity and spasms and is characterized by rapid progression but with clinical evidence of active encephalomyelitis. The onset in such cases is sub-acute over weeks or months and obviously may be associated with other neurological problems such as sensory disturbance and muscle weakness due to the active encephalomyelitic process affecting the brainstem and spinal cord[26]. There is an excellent review of stiff people by Thompson[27]. The review is now a little out of date but nevertheless it is the most comprehensive review of the subject.

16.4.2 Treatments

Standard medication for stiff person syndrome consists of the usual anti-spastic medication. Oral and intrathecal baclofen have been used successfully as have diazepam, tizanidine and clonazepam. However, reports tend to be based on individual cases or small uncontrolled studies and there is no sound evidence base. There are some reports of improvements with steroids and plasma exchange and also from intravenous immunoglobulin therapy[28]. Most anti-spastic treatment is sedative and given the severe spasticity high doses often have to be employed. Side-effects, particularly sedation, are common.

The role of botulinum toxin

It is not surprising that botulinum toxin has been tried for the stiff person syndrome. However, as the muscle stiffness is extensive in this syndrome it is also not surprising that the effects of botulinum toxin have not been dramatic. Botulinum can only be used in a few muscle groups and cannot be injected throughout the entire trunk and limbs. However, botulinum can be used to alleviate some specific symptoms, particularly if a few muscle groups seem to be more troublesome than other areas. There is very limited published literature. Davis and Jebbari produced the first description in 1993[29]. This is a case study of a single individual. Botulinum (BOTOX®) was injected into five sites in the lumbar paraspinal region with around 20 units per site. There were no reported side effects and there was some symptomatic relief in the injected areas. Ligouri and colleagues reported a similar response in two patients[30]. A variety of muscles were injected in these two individuals over a 2-year period. There was a significant cumulative dose of Dysport toxin (4200−5200) units. Relief of symptoms was reported in the injected muscles with only minimal side effects.

However, it is not realistic to expect the botulinum will be a treatment in isolation for the diffuse muscle spasm in stiff person syndrome. It is only likely to relieve localized muscles and other treatments are likely to be needed in addition. However, such localized pain relief and relief of muscle spasm may produce worthwhile benefit in troublesome and severe cases. Botulinum toxin is worthwhile in stiff person syndrome and in other disorders characterized by muscle rigidity and cramps.

16.5 Parkinson's disease

16.5.1 Background

Obviously botulinum toxin is not a treatment for Parkinson's disease per se. The mainstay treatment clearly still remains the use of dopamine replacement therapy. However there are some troublesome symptoms in Parkinson's disease that may be alleviated by the judicious use of botulinum toxin. A brief résumé is as follows.

16.5.2 Sialorrhoea (dribbling)

Dribbling is regrettably a common problem in Parkinson's disease, particularly in the latter stages. It is a major social embarrassment and often in itself a reason for social isolation. The treatment of sialorrhoea is covered in Chapter 10 by Alberto Albanese.

16.5.3 Dystonia

Dystonia can be a significant part of Parkinson's disease either in isolation or as part of the spectrum of dopamine-associated complications. If a dystonia coexists then botulinum toxin should be the treatment of choice. The response for the localized dystonia should be no different from other forms of dystonia but obviously the dystonia will only be one part of the whole symptom complex of Parkinson's disease and as such the alleviation of those symptoms may be less dramatic than in isolated dystonia. The various forms of dystonia are described in other chapters in this book and limb dystonia is described later in this chapter[31].

16.5.4 Blepharospasm/apraxia of lid opening

Blepharospasm can also be associated with Parkinson's disease. Occasionally the problem can be so severe that functional blindness can result. Obviously some alleviation can be gained by manipulation of dopaminergic agents but, particularly in later stages, it can be extremely difficult to achieve a balance between dyskinesias, including blepharospasm, and rigidity. If the problem is not remediable by dopaminergic manipulation then botulinum toxin can be used for localized improvement of the problem. The treatment in the context of Parkinson's disease is the same as idiopathic blepharospasm or isolated apraxia of lid opening and the treatment technique and dosages are described in Chapter 13.

16.5.5 Isolated muscle spasm

Sometimes people with Parkinson's disease have a troublesome muscle spasm in isolated muscle groups. Clenched fist, for example, is not uncommon as is the so-called striatal toe. In the latter condition the great toe is persistently and painfully dorsiflexed. This can cause problems with footwear as well as worsening balance and gait. The treatment of clenched fist is the same as treatment of upper limb spasticity in the context of stroke or multiple sclerosis and is covered in Chapter 8. The treatment of striatal toe consists of an injection of botulinum toxin into the extensor digitorum hallucis longus. The muscle can usually be palpated when it is in isolated spasm and clinical injection without electromyographic (EMG) control is usually quite straightforward. However, EMG can also be used for localization of the injection into the muscle belly. There are no controlled studies but a dose of 100−200 Dysport units of botulinum toxin is probably sufficient to alleviate the problem for the usual duration of 2−3 months.

16.5.6 Gastrointestinal problems

Constipation is extremely common in Parkinson's disease. Chapter 14 outlines the use of botulinum toxin for anismus. It can be a complication of Parkinson's disease and thus a cause of stubborn constipation. Obviously it is not the only cause of constipation in the context of Parkinson's disease but nevertheless for this specific entity botulinum toxin may be useful[32].

16.5.7 Freezing

Freezing is a common symptom of Parkinson's disease and usually consists of a sudden cessation of gait where both feet appear to be 'glued' to the floor. It can occur at any time although it commonly occurs during initiation of gait or a change of direction. Although freezing of gait is the commonest problem, it can also occur in terms of speech or hand function, such as during writing or other daily living involving hand function. Sometimes the freezing is irritating but only transient and at other times it can be very functionally disabling and last for several minutes. It probably occurs more commonly in other forms of parkinsonism than in Parkinson's disease and can be a particular problem in progressive supranuclear palsy and multiple system atrophy. The phenomenon is sometimes related to dopaminergic dose variations, often occurring towards the end of dose but often there is no clear pattern. It can sometimes be alleviated by dosage manipulations but in many people can still remain troublesome even when there is best possible balance between dopaminergic drugs over the course of the day.

The condition can often be helped by various cueing techniques. A simple and useful technique is for the individual to imagine that they need to step over an object. There are a number of other visual cue techniques including the use of simple walking aids.

In 2001 Giladi and colleagues published a study demonstrating the efficacy of botulinum toxin on gait freezing[33]. In this open study botulinum toxin was injected into the calf muscles of 10 parkinsonian patients who demonstrated gait freezing as a predominant symptom. Their response was assessed subjectively on a four-point scale. Seven of the patients reported improvement in 15/17 therapeutic sessions. Four patients were markedly improved and the mean duration of improvement was 6 weeks. The patients demonstrated definite deterioration after the injections had worn off. One patient responded in an additional single blind study with botulinum toxin injections but not to saline injections. This was an encouraging early report and the authors suggested that before any firm conclusions could be drawn further studies, particularly double-blind placebo-controlled trials, would be required. In this case BOTOX® was used with a dose of 300 units. The injection was mainly into the gastrocnemius/soleus/tibialis posterior and extensor hallucis longus muscles.

16.5.8 Rigidity

Rigidity in Parkinson's disease refers to a constant increase in muscle tone which can be felt throughout the full range of passive movement. It is often described as lead pipe rigidity when the resistance is uniform in all directions. Occasionally there is superimposed tremor which gives rise to the term cogwheel rigidity. Rigidity is well known as one of the key features of parkinsonism although it is not pathognomic of the disorder. The most efficacious treatment of rigidity is manipulation of dopamine replacement therapy. In the latter stages it can be very difficult to get the most helpful balance between rigidity and dyskinesia and indeed sometimes a good balance is not achievable. The rigidity is usually widespread and botulinum toxin only has a limited role to play. However, if the rigidity is more localized in one or a few muscle groups then botulinum toxin might be helpful. There is only a very limited literature on the subject. Polo and Jebbari described the use of botulinum toxin and rigidity in just two people with progressive supranuclear palsy and noted marked improvement in both individuals[34]. The same authors produced a further report the following year describing a total of eight people with progressive supranuclear palsy as well as Parkinson's disease and corticobasal degeneration. In this series they reported improvement in 7/8 patients with regard to rigidity for 3–4 months. A variety of muscles were injected, particularly in the arms[35].

Finally, Vanek and Jankovic[36] injected botulinum toxin into painful dystonic areas in six people with corticobasal degeneration. Two reported marked improvement of both dystonia and pain while the other four had less marked improvement. There were no complications. Clearly further studies are required but nevertheless for certain selected patients with marked and resistant rigidity in localized muscle groups botulinum toxin may have a role to play.

16.5.9 Tremor

One of the major characteristics of parkinsonism is tremor. Dopamine replacement therapy is the treatment of choice for parkinsonian tremor but occasionally the tremor can be disabling and not responsive to drugs. Surgery can be very useful but for such resistant disabling tremor botulinum toxin could be considered. The treatment of tremor for a variety of conditions including Parkinson's disease is outlined in the section below.

16.6 Tremor

16.6.1 Background

Tremor can be defined as a rhythmic oscillatory movement of a body part. There are various classifications and the commonest is a description of the tremor according to the circumstances in which a tremor mainly occurs – rest tremor, action tremor, postural tremor, intention tremor and task specific tremor. Other classifications depend on the frequency of the tremor. Low frequency tremors (around 2.5–3.5 Hz) include tremors in association with cerebellar, brainstem disease or dystonic tremor. Faster tremors (around 8 Hz and above) include physiological tremors, drug intoxication and primary orthostatic tremor. There are a host of conditions which can cause tremor. The commonest cause of rest tremor is Parkinson's disease and the commonest cause of postural and kinetic tremor is essential tremor. Less common causes include multiple sclerosis, drug-induced tremors, cerebellar disease and alcohol-induced tremor, post-traumatic tremor and task-specific tremors such as primary-writing tremor. It is not the role of this brief article to discuss the differential diagnosis and investigation of tremor but, as with myoclonus, it is worth emphasizing that the symptom of tremor needs full neurological investigation. Some causes of tremor will have a specific treatment but unfortunately most causes of tremor do not have a specific treatment and symptomatic treatment is all that can be offered.

16.6.2 Other treatments

Many mild tremors including enhanced physiological tremor do not need treatment. Accurate diagnosis is still essential but if the symptoms are mild then reassurance and explanation are all that may be required. Many people will be concerned that they have Parkinson's disease. Treatment of tremor usually focuses on oral medication. Enhanced physiological tremor and essential tremor can respond to beta-blockers. Sometimes these tremors are also very sensitive to alcohol. Regrettably some of the tremors can be so sensitive to alcohol that there is a serious risk of alcoholism. Primidone can also be a useful treatment for essential tremor. However, side effects can be troublesome. Recent studies have confirmed the efficacy of topiramate for essential tremor in doses of around 400 mg per day. Adverse events included appetite suppression with weight loss and parathesiae[37]. Gabapentin has also shown recent promise, particularly for tremor in multiple sclerosis and orthostatic tremor, although many of the studies have been small and larger scale studies are required[38]. Atypical neuroleptics can also be tried for essential and other tremors. Olanzapine showed some efficacy in a study of 37 patients[39]. Tremor of Parkinson's disease will often respond to dopaminergic agents, anticholinergic drugs or amantadine. If such therapy fails it is probably safe to use beta-blocker therapy although a recent Cochrane review of beta-blockers in parkinsonian tremor produced inconclusive results[40]. Other specific modalities are the use of isoniazid for multiple sclerosis tremor and D-penicillamine in Wilson's disease[41].

If tremors are drug resistant then stereotatic surgery can be used. Unilateral thalamotomy can be efficacious but a number of studies have now shown the usefulness of bilateral thalamic deep brain stimulation[42]. The technique has also been used specifically in Parkinson's disease with electrodes planted into ventral intermedial nucleus of the thalamus[43].

Overall the drug management of tremor is often disappointing and associated with a number of side effects. It is often a matter of simply trying one medication after another until the best balance between benefit and side effects is found. Thus, the use of oral medication, whilst sometimes efficacious, can often be a long and frustrating progress with eventually unsatisfactory results.

16.6.3 The role of botulinum toxin

A simple rationale for using botulinum toxin is to dampen the agonist and antagonist muscles in an attempt to reduce the severity of the oscillations. It may also be a valid principle to deliberately unbalance the agonists and antagonists by injecting more botulinum toxin into one group than the other which can have the effect of disrupting the tremor oscillations. The disadvantage of botulinum toxin is clearly that muscle weakness may ensue, producing functional disability which may or may not be worse than the original tremor. However, for a functionally disabling tremor that has proved to be drug-resistant treatment with botulinum toxin is certainly worthwhile. Indeed, given the unsatisfactory nature of oral medication, a severe localized disabling tremor might be treated primarily with botulinum toxin given the safety and reversibility of the injection.

There are no clear published protocols of when botulinum toxin should be used in the context of tremor and at the moment such decisions need to be based on clinical judgement. The first description of botulinum toxin treatment for tremor was published by Jankovic and Schwartz in 1991[44]. This was a report of an open trial of botulinum toxin (BOTOX® variety) in the treatment of 51 people with disabling tremors including dystonic tremor, essential tremor, parkinsonian tremor and tremor secondary to brain tumour. The average age of the patients was around 56 years with a long duration of symptoms of around 14 years. Thirty-five patients (67%) reported improvement with a latency of 6.8 days and an average duration of improvement of around 10.5 weeks. The expected range of side effects was noted including dysphagia, when injected for head tremor, as well as transient neck weakness and local pain. Six patients (60%) of those with hand tremor noted transient focal hand weakness. However, the results of this pilot study certainly indicated that the botulinum toxin injections could be used to control tremor when other forms of therapy had failed. Other more specific and better controlled studies followed.

Pahwa and colleagues published the results of a double-blind placebo-controlled study on the effects of botulinum toxin in patients with essential head tremor[45]. Each subject received two treatments, one with botulinum toxin and one with normal saline into the stylomastoid and splenius capitis muscles for essential head tremor. There was marked to moderate improvement in clinical ratings in five subjects after botulinum toxin and just one subject after placebo. There was marked to moderate subjective improvement also in five patients with botulinum toxin and three with placebo. The side effects were mild and transient. Although the results were not dramatic the authors concluded that botulinum toxin could be useful for those with essential head tremor who have failed to benefit from oral medication.

Slightly more promising results were produced by Jankovic and colleagues in 1996 in the context of essential hand tremor[46]. In this study 25 people with hand tremor, of moderate to severe severity, were randomized to receive either 50 units of BOTOX® or placebo injected into the wrist flexors and extensors of the dominant limb. Rest, postural and kinetic tremors were evaluated at 2–4 week intervals over a 16-week study period. A significant improvement in the tremor severity rating scale at 4 weeks was noted after the injection in people treated with

BOTOX® compared to the placebo and it was maintained for the duration of the study. In total 75 per cent of the botulinum-treated patients improved compared to 47 per cent in the placebo group. There were reports of finger weakness but there were no severe or unexpected problems.

Further larger scale studies followed and one of the largest published so far is by Brin and colleagues[47]. In this study 133 patients with essential hand tremor were randomized to low dose (50 BOTOX® units) or high dose (100 BOTOX® units) or placebo treatment. Injections were into the wrist flexors and extensors. Both doses of botulinum toxin significantly reduced postural tremor on the clinical rating scales after 4 weeks although measures of motor function were not consistently improved with the botulinum treatment. Grip strength was reduced compared to placebo group. Other measures confirmed the efficacy of botulinum toxin type A for essential hand tremor in terms of significant improvement of postural tremor but not kinetic tremor, with only limited results in terms of function and efficacy. However, it is fair to point out that there are few valid reliable hand function scales that are capable of showing change in the context of tremor. In the absence of such robust objective measures of functional disability then patients subjective opinion needs to carry significant weight. In this context Pacchetti attempted to demonstrate improvement of activities of daily living self-questionnaire scores and severity tremor scales in an open study of 20 patients with disabling essential tremor. After botulinum toxin treatment there was a significant reduction in both severity and functional rating scale scores and tremor amplitude as measured by accelerometry and EMG. The authors used accelerometry and surface electromyography to identify the arm muscles with tremorogenic activity. Adverse events were again limited to a slight degree of finger extension weakness[48].

The use of EMG recordings for determining muscles to be injected is not uniformly accepted in the literature. Some authors use clinical landmarks for palpable tremor oscillation whilst others use EMG recordings. Some use a combination of both techniques. Wissel and colleagues used both clinical muscle palpation and standardized simultaneous electromyographical recordings to determine where to inject in 43 patients with significant head tremor[49]. There were 29 patients classified as either suffering from tremor or cervical dystonia and 14 with head tremor without dystonia. They received a mean dose of 400 Dysport units of botulinum toxin (range 160–560) distributed between the two splenius capitis muscles. A mean of three muscles were injected for more complicated problems with tremorless cervical dystonia. The condition of all patients with head tremor and 26/29 patients with tremorless cervical dystonia improved subjectively. The total on the Tsui scale as well as pain scales also decreased significantly following treatment.

There is no clear basis in the literature for determining the muscles to be injected and in the present state of our knowledge we must depend on clinical judgement. However, in general terms a 'no–no' head tremor will probably benefit from a bilateral injection to the splenius capitis and/or the sternomastoid. The 'yes–yes' head tremor may benefit from the same muscle injections in addition to bilateral semi spinalis. Hand tremor would usually involve injections into flexor carpi radialis and flexor carpi ulnaris as well as extensor carpi radialis and extensor carpi ulnaris. The technique for muscle selection and identification of the muscles is obviously the same in tremor as it would be for arm spasticity or cervical dystonia – as described in other relevant chapters in this book.

Finally, some other specific tremors have been reported to improve following botulinum injection. Hertegard and colleagues reported an improvement in essential voice tremor[50]. Fifteen patients with a diagnosis of essential voice tremor were treated with botulinum toxin injection into the thyrohyoid muscles and in some cases the cricothyroid and thyrarytenoid muscles. Evaluations were based on subjective judgement by the patients as well as perceptual and acoustic analysis of voice recordings. Subjective evaluations showed benefit in 67 per cent of the patients. Perceptual evaluation shows significant decrease in voice tremor during speech. Acoustic analysis showed a significant decrease in fundamental frequency during sustained vowel phonation. The authors concluded that the treatment was successful in around 50–65 per cent of the patients depending on the method of evaluation. Improvements in central palatal tremor have also been reported in case studies in a similar fashion to the related condition of palatal myoclonus (see above). The rare condition of hereditary trembling chin has also been reported to improve with the use of botulinum toxin injections. This is an autosomal dominant condition characterized by recurrent bouts of tremor involving the chin and there was a report of one such family being treated successfully with botulinum injections into the mentalis muscle[51].

There are limited reports on the efficacy of botulinum toxin injections for disabling stuttering[52]. Brin and colleagues also treated 14 adults with persistent glottal block who previously failed standard speech therapy. A total of 125 BOTOX® units were injected into the thyroarytenoid (vocalis) muscle. Improvement in fluency was documented by a number of rating instruments.

Overall there is sufficient literature on the treatment of tremor with botulinum toxin to merit a trial of this therapy, after failure of medication. There are no clear protocols for the muscles that should be injected and at which dose and, at the present state of our knowledge, treatment still has to rely on experience and a certain amount of trial and error.

16.7 Limb dystonias and occupational cramps

16.7.1 Background

The commoner forms of dystonia have been described in Chapters 6 and 7. However dystonia can affect any group of voluntary muscles. The commoner forms that have not been described in preceding chapters are the focal limb dystonias, especially of the lower limb and commonly involving the foot and the ankle. The other important group of dystonias are those that are secondary to a particular task, mainly involving the arm and hand. The limb is relatively normal at other times. The commonest of these task specific dystonias is writers cramp but there are other types. This section will briefly look at the efficacy of botulinum toxin for focal limb dystonias and task specific dystonias.

16.7.2 Focal limb dystonias

Any voluntary muscle can be affected by dystonia. Whilst the potential range of limb dystonias is wide and varied, the commoner dystonias involve the ankle, usually with inversion and plantar flexion. Other dystonias include dorsiflexion of the great toe (striatal toe – see Section 16.5) and dystonia in the arm, particularly involving finger and elbow flexion or extension and sometimes proximal dystonias involving the shoulder. As with all dystonias the conditions need full evaluation. In those with hemi-dystonia an MRI scan may be worthwhile to detect contra-lateral cerebral pathologies such as tumour or AVM. However, in common with other forms of adult onset focal dystonia, there is often no specifically treatable condition found. Primary treatment of choice in such cases is probably botulinum toxin even though there are no large placebo-controlled studies confirming efficacy in these rare conditions. However it is not unreasonable to assume similar efficacy and safety as in other dystonic conditions.

Often the goal of treatment will focus on improvement of function but another goal can be alleviation of pain. It is preferable to have some form of objective assessment but this is often difficult. Range of movement could be recorded or other simple functional measures made such as a timed 10 metre walking test for those with focal foot dystonia. A simple visual analogue scale can be used to monitor an effect on pain. Patients' subjective impression of improvement should not be forgotten as a valid measure of efficacy.

Obviously botulinum toxin should be injected into the muscles most involved in the dystonic process. There is no clear evidence that EMG guided control provides better efficacy than clinical identification and palpation of the muscles by known surface landmarks. In the absence of evidence it is probably valid to use clinical identification in the larger muscles with clear cut surface landmarks but use stimulation or EMG guided techniques for smaller muscles which are more difficult to locate or in those in whom the anatomy is distorted. The dose of botulinum toxin injected will depend on the size and number of the muscles involved and the number of necessary injection sites. A typical dose may range from 100 Dysport units (around 25–30 BOTOX® units) for forearm flexor or extensor muscles up to 200–250 Dysport units (around 75 BOTOX® units) for larger calf muscles, such as the gastrocnemius. Lower doses clearly need to be used for the small muscles of the hand or feet and larger doses for the larger muscles, such as quadriceps and hamstrings. In general, the recommendations outlined in the spasticity chapter will apply to dystonic muscles in the limbs. There are really no studies of large numbers of individuals to determine the efficacy but improvement in pain and function would be expected in the majority of patients. The onset of duration of action and side effects will be as expected with the commoner forms of injection. The only likely functional problems following injection in the limbs would be the induction of unacceptable limb weakness and a balance needs to be determined between benefits of muscle relaxation compared to the drawbacks of such relaxation. However, the safety and efficacy of botulinum toxin would usually result in a relatively low threshold of trying the effect of botulinum toxin for focal limb dystonias.

16.7.3   Occupational task specific dystonia

Task specific dystonias are a fascinating group of conditions characterized by focal action dystonia, usually of the arm. It is usually restricted to a particular task, often occupational or recreational in origin. There are many examples cited in the literature. The commonest and best known is writer's cramp but there are many others often involving musicians (pianists, violinists, drummers, saxophonists, cellists and others). Other varieties are found in sportsmen such as golfers (yips), snooker and dart players and specific professions such as typists, painters, letter sorters, shoemakers, stonemasons, watchmakers and many others. The onset of automation is probably responsible for reducing the incidence of such conditions. The great majority of publications have been related to writer's cramp and this brief section will review the use of botulinum toxin in this condition. However, the same principles apply to other conditions and it is likely that other conditions will share the same efficacy as well as the same problems that are associated with the treatment of writer's cramp.

Although writer's cramp is described in the nineteenth century, the first large scale descriptive study was produced by Sheehy and Marsden in 1982[53]. The condition is uncommon with an estimated prevalence of around 1/37 000 individuals. Our own epidemiological survey in dystonia in the town of

Darlington in North East England showed this prevalence with an average age of onset of 37 years and time to diagnosis of just over 6 years[54].

In most individuals the dystonia occurs just during the act of writing and all other tasks are normal. However, in some people other hand tasks are also involved from the beginning, albeit to a lesser degree. In some individuals the condition is somewhat more progressive and begins as a task specific problem but becomes non-task specific and a more permanent dystonic feature over time. It is slightly commoner in men than women and there is occasionally a family history. The condition usually begins gradually and often there is no obvious precipitating cause. However, some do report some minor trauma to the limb that appears to have started the condition.

The condition is characterized by difficulty writing. The muscles of the forearm and hand will tend to tighten as soon as a pen or pencil is grasped. The muscle spasm can spread to involve the whole arm, even the proximal muscles. The condition is not usually painful but nevertheless is uncomfortable. The hand and arm can adopt most abnormal postures whilst the individual tries to write. The muscle spasms then characteristically cease as soon as the pen is released. In many people the writing eventually becomes slow, painful and often illegible. In common with cervical dystonia some individuals find a sensory trick that can alleviate the problem such as gently touching part of the hand. Many people experiment with altering the grip, changing hands or writing with thicker pens or adopting a different writing style. Sometimes these measures produce longer term success but often only result in temporary alleviation. Although many individuals can now perform writing tasks through the computer keyboard there are still a number of occupations in which writing is essential. In any case even if the occupational changes can be made then social tasks, such as writing a cheque, can become disabling for many people.

Unfortunately the chance of remission is poor. Although few actually give up writing completely, a significant number have long-term problems and major social difficulties. Remission is most unusual. In some individuals the problem is compounded by a primary writing tremor.

The diagnosis is usually made from the history and simply watching the patient write. Occasionally focal neurology can confuse the diagnosis such as peripheral nerve entrapment, radiculopathy or other overuse disorders such as tenosynovitis. Other investigations are rarely needed but might include nerve conduction studies and EMG to aid with a differential diagnosis.

16.7.4   Other treatments

In milder cases the best treatment is probably further experimentation with different hand postures and writing styles. Oral medication is associated with a very poor response rate and often with unacceptable side effects. Overall only around 20 per cent of individuals can eventually find some oral medication that is of benefit to them without unacceptable side effects[53]. A wide variety of drugs can be used. Probably the more efficacious are anticholinergic agents. Other possibilities include anti-spastic drugs such as baclofen, tizanidine and dantrium as well as gabapentin and clonazepam. There have been individual case reports of treatment with other physical modalities such as biofeedback and relaxation techniques. However, regrettably no oral medication or other physical treatments have been subject to any robust trials. No clear preference of one modality above another can be recommended from the literature.

16.7.5 The role of botulinum toxin

Botulinum toxin may be helpful for task specific dystonias by selectively reducing muscle overactivity. Obviously the drawback of this treatment is the muscle weakness that may be induced. This is particularly a problem for the intermittent task specific dystonias where the dystonic problem only occurs during a particular task and obviously the patient does not wish to have a relaxed and weaker muscle during other activity. This is the main effect that limits both the efficacy and the dosage that can be employed. The other main difficulty of botulinum toxin treatment is identifying the correct muscles to be injected. It is anatomically difficult to identify the muscle but more particularly it is difficult to know which muscles are primarily involved in the dystonic process and which may be secondarily involved in terms of antagonizing the action of the primary muscles. The crude overall efficacy of dystonia for writer's cramp is in the order of 50 per cent as an 'average' of the existing literature. That is half the individuals injected will have sufficient benefit to wish for a repeat injection whereas the other half will have only limited benefit, no benefit or even find that their overall functional abilities are worse. However, this response rate is much superior to other treatment modalities. Probably botulinum toxin would be the first choice for the treatment of writer's cramp and other task specific dystonias – when the problems are sufficiently disabling to warrant any treatment at all.

Early open label studies showed good results. One of the earliest by Poungvarin[55] described treatment of 25 patients with writer's cramp. The mean age was nearly 37 years and the mean duration of the problem was nearly 6 years with a range of 1–30 years. The majority had simple writer's cramp (72%) and the remainder had dystonic writer's cramp. Twenty-one patients were eventually injected with 2–4 divided doses into the overactive forearm muscles observed during writing but without EMG guidance. Two-thirds of the subjects showed definite improvement in handwriting whilst the rest only improved minimally or not at all. Arm pain in patients who had such a symptom was abolished.

About a third had transient finger, hand and arm weakness. In the same year Rivest and colleagues[56] showed subjective improvement in 92 per cent of 12 patients and such improvement was significant in the majority. Other open label studies showed similar levels of improvement.

There have been very few placebo-controlled blinded trials. Results have been somewhat mixed and a study by Tsui and colleagues[57] showed only 6/20 patients reporting improvement although 12 demonstrated improvement in a computerized test of pen control. This demonstrates the subjective nature of the problem and emphasizes the need to listen to the patient rather than rely on objective testing. A somewhat more positive result was reported by Cole and colleagues[58]. This was a study of just 10 patients and objective benefit was confirmed in eight patients. In another study 7/9 patients improved[59]. Some individuals would be quite happy with modest improvement which is enough to enable them to write their signature, for example. Others require a high degree of skill and precision as part of their job. This particularly applies to professional musicians affected by task specific dystonia. Many depend on a very high degree of hand and arm co-ordination in order to play at a professional level. Obviously these individuals are far more critical of the response than those with lesser occupational needs. The author recalls a professional accordion player who had had to stop playing all together because of his dystonia. Botulinum toxin injection improved the condition sufficiently for him to take up the accordion again but he never achieved the same level of professional expertise and was forced to retire from professional playing. Many would have considered his treatment a success but obviously in terms of his own high standards and professional abilities this was not the case.

The injection technique in writer's cramp is frankly fraught with problems. The best idea of the muscle to be injected can be gained from prolonged observation of the individual during a number of different writing and drawing tasks. Probably the commonest pattern is flexion of one or more of the fingers at the same time as extension of the wrist. However, a number of flexor and extensor patterns are possible. However, many postures are simply compensatory for the dystonia and analysis of the muscles primarily involved can be very complicated and often is no more than inspired guesswork.

The author's own experience and the review of the literature indicates that most benefit probably ensues from injection of the forearm flexors and extensors rather than attempts to inject the smaller muscles of the hand. It is probably reasonable to suggest that EMG is difficult to use to choose the muscles for injection but EMG may be useful for guiding the injection into the required target muscles which have been identified by clinical observation. The value of EMG for selecting muscles in comparison to pure clinical observation has not been robustly studied.

There is certainly no substitute for a working knowledge of the normal actions of the muscles of the hand and their surface anatomy. It is, of course, quite possible that precise localization is not essential as the toxin in any case will spread at least a few centimetres from the site of the injection. There is no clear consensus on the dose to be used. A reasonable starting dose for the extensor and flexor muscles of the forearm would be in the order of 50 Dysport units (10–15 BOTOX® units) with perhaps 1–2 injections per muscle. Many individuals would inject with a needle that could also record EMG or can help localize the muscle by electrical stimulation. Others would use simple clinical palpation and surface markers. The injected volumes are likely to be small and dilutions of one vial of Dysport (500 units) or BOTOX® (100 units) with 2 ml of normal saline are probably acceptable. However, there is no study that has compared different dilutions in terms of overall efficacy.

Overall, the treatment of task specific dystonia is not entirely satisfactory. However, botulinum toxin clearly has advantages over other treatment modalities in terms of overall response rate. There are no clear protocols for the technique and injectors must rely on a considerable amount of clinical experience mixed with a little inspired guess work. However, the technique is safe and associated with few side effects and certainly worth trying in these disabling disorders.

REFERENCES

1. Pringsheim, T., Davenport, W. J. and Lang, A. (2003). Tics. *Curr. Opin. Neurol.*, **16**(4), 523–7.
2. Snider, L. A., Seligman, L. D., Ketchen, B. R. *et al.* (2002). Tics and problem behaviors in schoolchildren: prevalence, characterization, and associations. *Paediatrics*, **110**, 331–8.
3. Dion, Y., Annable, L., Sandor, P. and Chouinard, G. (2000). Risperidone in the treatment of Tourette syndrome: a double-blind, placebo-controlled trial. *J. Clin. Psychopharmacol.*, **22**, 31–9.
4. Gaffney, G. R., Perry, P. J., Lund, B. C. *et al.* (2002). Risperidone versus clonidine in the treatment of children and adolescents with Tourette's syndrome. *J. Am. Acad. Child. Adolesc. Psychiatry*, **41**, 330–6.
5. Kwak, C. H., Hanna, P. A. and Jankovic, J. (2000). Botulinum toxin in the treatment of tics. *Arch. Neurol.*, **57**, 1190–3.
6. Marras, C., Andrews, D., Sime, E. and Lang, A. E. (2001). Botulinum toxin for simple motor tics: a randomized, double-blind, controlled clinical trial. *Neurology*, **56**, 605–10.
7. Jankovic, J. (1994). Botulinum toxin in the treatment of dystonic tics. *Movement Disorders*, **9**, 347–9.
8. Awaad, Y. (1999). Tics in Tourette syndrome: new treatment options. *J. Child. Neurol.*, **14**, 316–19.

9. Porta, M., Maggioni, G., Ottaviani, F. and Schindler, A. (2004). Treatment of phonic tics in patients with Tourette's syndrome using botulinum toxin type A. *Neurol. Sci.*, **24**(6), 420–3.

10. Scott, B. L., Jankovic, J. and Donovan, D. T. (1996). Botulinum toxin injection into vocal cord in the treatment of malignant coprolalia associated with Tourette's syndrome. *Movement Disorders*, **11**(4), 431–3.

11. Trimble, M. R., Whurr, R., Brookes, G. and Robertson, M. M. (1998). Vocal tics in Gilles de la Tourette syndrome treated with botulinum toxin injections. *Movement Disorders*, **13**(3), 617–19.

12. Brown, P., Steiger, M. J., Thompson, P. D. *et al.* (1993). Effectiveness of piracetam in cortical myoclonus. *Movement Disorders*, **8**, 63–8.

13. Obeso, J. A. (1995–96). Therapy of myoclonus. *Clin. Neurosci.*, **3**, 253–7.

14. Priori, A., Bertolasi, L., Pesenti, A. *et al.* (2000). Gamma-hydroxybutyric acid for alcohol-sensitive myoclonus with dystonia. *Neurology*, **54**(8), 1706.

15. Leppik, I. E. (1999). Zonisamide. *Epilepsia*, **40**(Suppl.), S23–9.

16. Agarwal, P. and Frucht, S. J. (2003). Myoclonus. *Curr. Opin. Neurol.*, **16**(4), 515–21.

17. Polo, K. B. and Jabbari, B. (1994). Effectiveness of botulinum toxin type A against painful limb myoclonus of spinal cord origin. *Movement Disorders*, **9**(2), 233–5.

18. Lagueny, A., Tison, F., Burbaud, P. *et al.* (1999). Stimulus-sensitive spinal segmental myoclonus improved with injections of botulinum toxin type A. *Movement Disorders*, **14**, 182–5.

19. Awaad, Y., Tayem, H., Elgamal, A. and Coyne, M. F. (1999). Treatment of childhood myoclonus with botulinum toxin type A. *J. Child. Neurol.*, **14**, 781–6.

20. Bryce, G. E. and Morrison, M. D. (1998). Botulinum toxin treatment of essential palatal myoclonus tinnitus. *J. Otolaryngol.*, **27**, 213–16.

21. Saeed, S. R. and Brookes, G. B. (1993). The use of *Clostridium botulinum* toxin in palatal myoclonus. A preliminary report. *J. Laryngol. Otol.*, **107**(3), 208–10.

22. Varney, S. M., Demetroulakos, J. L., Fletcher, M. H. *et al.* (1996). Palatal myoclonus: treatment with *Clostridium botulinum* toxin injection. *Otolaryngol. Head Neck Surg.*, **114**(2), 317–20.

23. Moersch, F. P. and Woltman, H. W. (1956). Progressive fluctuating muscular rigidity and spasm ('stiff man' syndrome): report of a case and some observations in 13 other cases. *Mayo Clin. Proc.*, **31**(15), 421–7.

24. Blum, P. and Jankovic, J. (1991). Stiff-person syndrome: an autoimmune disease. *Movement Disorders*, **6**, 12–20.

25. Levin, K. H. (1997). Paraneoplastic neuromuscular syndromes. *Neurol. Clin.*, **15**, 597–614.

26. Barker, R. A., Revesz, T., Thom, M. *et al.* (1998). Review of 23 patients affected by the stiff man syndrome: clinical subdivision into stiff trunk (man) syndrome, stiff limb syndrome, and progressive encephalomyelitis with rigidity. *J. Neurol. Neurosurg. Psychiatry*, **65**, 633–40.

27. Thompson, P. D. (1994). Stiff people. In C. D. Marsden and S. Fahn, eds., *Movement disorders 3*. Oxford: Butterworth Heinemann, pp. 373–405.

28. Barker, R. A. and Marsden, C. D. (1997). Successful treatment of stiff man syndrome with intravenous immunoglobin. *J. Neurol. Neurosurg. Psychiatry*, **62**, 426−7.

29. Davis, D. and Jabbari, B. (1993). Significant improvement of stiff-person syndrome after paraspinal injection of botulinum toxin A. *Movement Disorders*, **8**, 371−3.

30. Liguori, R., Cordivari, C., Lugaresi, E. and Montagna, P. (1997). Botulinum toxin A improves muscle spasms and rigidity in stiff-person syndrome. *Movement Disorders*, **12**, 1060−3.

31. Jankovic, J. and Tintner, R. (2001). Dystonia and parkinsonism. *Parkinsonism Relat. Disord.*, **8**, 109−21.

32. Albanese, A., Maria, G., Bentivoglio, A. R. *et al.* (1997). Severe constipation in Parkinson's disease relieved by botulinum toxin. *Movement Disorders*, **12**, 764−6.

33. Giladi, N., Gurevich, T., Shabtai, H. *et al.* (2001). The effect of botulinum toxin injections to the calf muscles on freezing of gait in parkinsonism: a pilot study. *J. Neurol.*, **248**, 572−6.

34. Polo, K. B. and Jabbari, B. (1994). Botulinum toxin-A improves the rigidity of progressive supranuclear palsy. *Ann. Neurol.*, **35**(2), 237−9.

35. Grazko, M. A., Polo, K. B. and Jabbari, B. (1995). Botulinum toxin A for spasticity, muscle spasms, and rigidity. *Neurology*, **45**, 712−17.

36. Vanek, Z. and Jankovic, J. (2001). Dystonia in corticobasal degeneration. *Movement Disorders*, **16**(2), 252−7.

37. Connor, G. S. (2002). A double-blind placebo-controlled trial of topiramate treatment for essential tremor. *Neurology*, **59**, 132−4.

38. Faulkner, M. A., Bertoni, J. M. and Lenz, T. L. (2003). Gabapentin for the treatment of tremor. *Ann. Pharmacother.*, **37**, 282−6.

39. Yetimalar, Y., Irtman, G., Gurgor, N. and Basoglu, M. (2003). Olanzapine efficacy in the treatment of essential tremor. *Eur. J. Neurol.*, **10**(1), 79−82.

40. Crosby, N. J., Deane, K. H. and Clarke, C. E. (2003). Beta-blocker therapy for tremor in Parkinson's disease. *Cochrane Database of Systematic Reviews*, (1): CD003361.

41. Hallett, M., Lindsey, J. W., Adelstein, B. D. and Riley, P. O. (1985). Controlled trial of isoniazid therapy for severe postural cerebellar tremor in multiple sclerosis. *Neurology*, **35**, 1374−7.

42. Berk, C. and Honey, C. R. (2002). Bilateral thalamic deep brain stimulation for the treatment of head tremor: Report of two cases. *J. Neurosurg.*, **96**, 615−18.

43. Benabid, A. L., Pollak, P., Gao, D. *et al.* (1996). Chronic electrical stimulation of the ventralis intermedius nucleus of the thalamus as a treatment of movement disorders. *J. Neurosurg.*, **84**, 203−14.

44. Jankovic, J. and Schwartz, K. (1991). Botulinum toxin treatment of tremors. *Neurology*, **41**, 1185−8.

45. Pahwa, R., Busenbark, K., Swanson-Hyland, E. F. *et al.* (1995). Botulinum toxin treatment of essential head tremor. *Neurology*, **45**(4), 822−4.

46. Jankovic, J., Schwartz, K., Clemence, W. *et al.* (1996). A randomized, double-blind, placebo-controlled study to evaluate botulinum toxin type A in essential hand tremor. *Movement Disorders*, **11**, 250−6.

47. Brin, M. F., Lyons, K. E., Doucette, J. et al. (2001). A randomized, double masked, controlled trial of botulinum toxin type A in essential hand tremor. *Neurology*, **56**, 1523–8.

48. Pacchetti, C., Mancini, F., Bulgheroni, M. et al. (2000). Botulinum toxin treatment for functional disability induced by essential tremor. *Neurol. Sci.*, **21**, 349–53.

49. Wissel, J., Masuhr, F., Schelosky, L. et al. (1997). Quantitative assessment of botulinum toxin treatment in 43 patients with head tremor. *Movement Disorders*, **12**(5), 722–6.

50. Hertegard, S., Granqvist, S. and Lindestad, P. A. (2000). Botulinum toxin injections for essential voice tremor. *Ann. Otol. Rhinol. Laryngol.*, **109**, 204–9.

51. Gordon, K., Cadera, W. and Hinton, G. (1993). Successful treatment of hereditary trembling chin with botulinum toxin. *J. Child. Neurol.*, **8**, 154–6.

52. Brin, M. F., Stewart, C., Blitzer, A. and Diamond, B. (1994). Laryngeal botulinum toxin injections for disabling stuttering in adults. *Neurology*, **44**, 2262–6.

53. Sheehy, M. P. and Marsden, C. D. (1982). Writer's cramp – a focal dystonia. *Brain*, **105**(Pt. 3), 461–80.

54. Butler, A. G., Duffey, P. O., Hawthorne, M. R. and Barnes, M. P. (2004). An epidemiologic survey of dystonia within the entire population of northeast England over the past nine years. *Advances in Neurology*, **94**, 95–9.

55. Poungvarin, N. (1991). Writer's cramp: the experience with botulinum toxin injections in 25 patients. *J. Med. Assoc. Thai.*, **74**(5), 239–47.

56. Rivest, J., Lees, A. J. and Marsden, C. D. (1991). Writer's cramp: treatment with botulinum toxin injections. *Movement Disorders*, **6**(1), 55–9.

57. Tsui, J. K., Bhatt, M., Calne, S. and Calne, D. B. (1993). Botulinum toxin in the treatment of writer's cramp: a double-blind study. *Neurology*, **43**(1), 183–5.

58. Cole, R., Hallett, M. and Cohen, L. G. (1995). Double-blind trial of botulinum toxin for treatment of focal hand dystonia. *Movement Disorders*, **4**, 466–71.

59. Yoshimura, D. M., Aminoff, M. J. and Olney, R. K. (1992). Botulinum toxin therapy for limb dystonias. *Neurology*, **42**, 627–30.

Index

acetylcholine 2, 3, 9, 10, 12, 15–17, 21, 45, 66, 114,
    175, 176, 180, 182, 202, 211, 231, 250, 297,
    301, 302. *See also* botulinum toxin:
    mechanism of action
achalasia 64, 283, 318
Action Research Arm Test 152
acupuncture 87
acyclovir 177
adenosine triphosphate (ATP) 301
adenovirus 40
adipocytes, effect of botulinum toxin on 38
adrenergic agonists and antagonists
    α- 294, 297, 334, 350
    β- 230, 361. *See also* specific drug
adrenoreceptors 303
AIDS 85
akinesia 204
alcoholism 317
alfusozin 295
Allergan, Inc. 4, 28, 29, 33, 59, 252, 256, 288,
    309, 313
allergies, treatment with botulinum toxin 39
alpha-bungarotoxin 262, 263
amantadine 361
amblyopia 265
American Urological Association (AUA)
    symptom index 293, 295, 297
amino acid disorders 85
aminoglycoside antibiotics 75, 255
aminoquinoline antimalarial compounds 74
ammonium chloride 15
amyotrophic lateral sclerosis (ALS) 204, 220
anal
    disorders and their treatment 298–311
    fissure 64, 283, 303–11
    haemorrhoidectomy 316
    pain 315
    sphincter. *See* sphincter: external anal (EAS);
        sphincter: internal anal (IAS)
    tone 299
analgesics 5, 6, 177, 230, 231, 246, 247,
    250. *See also* codeine; morphine; opioids;
    paracetamol; pain: anaesthesia for
anhidrosis 181. *See also* euhydrosis; hyperhidrosis

anismus 65
antibodies for botulinum
    toxin. *See* immunoresistance to
    botulinum toxin
anti-cholinergic drugs 80, 87, 88, 180, 207, 361
anticoagulants 264
anticonvulsants 230, 247
antidepressants 177, 230, 247, 351
apraclonidine hydrochloride (IOPIDINE®) 334
apraxia of eye opening 6, 275–6
    as cause of abnormal neck posture 87
    definition of 275
    non-response to botulinum toxin 275
Artefill® 345, 346
Ashworth Scale 73, 138, 145, 148, 149, 151–4
assays for botulinum toxin. *See* botulinum
    toxin: assay
atrial natriuretic peptide 175
atropine 11, 180, 208
attention deficit hyperactivity disorder (ADHD)
    350, 351

baclofen 80, 88, 128, 134, 135, 138, 141,
    368. *See also* gamma-aminobutyric acid
    (GABA)
back pain
    activity modification for 246
    analgesics for 246
    anaesthetics for 249
    bed rest for 245
    botulinum toxin for 28, 245, 250–1, 253–5
    diagnosis and assessment 245, 255
    economic costs of 1, 244
    from acute muscle spasms 66
    management of 244
    muscle relaxants for 247
    percutaneous radiofrequency neurotomy for 249
    physical therapy for 248–9
    prevalence of 243
    steroids for 249
    surgery for 249
    trigger points in 253–6. *See also* neck: pain
basal ganglia, in cervical dystonia 80
Bean strain of botulinum toxin 33